An Osteopathic Approach
to Diagnosis and Treatment

Andrew T. Still

An Osteopathic Approach to Diagnosis and Treatment

EDITED BY

Eileen L. DiGiovanna, D.O., F.A.A.O.

Assistant Dean of Student Affairs
Professor and Chairperson
J. C. Griswold Department
of Osteopathic Principles and Practice
New York College of Osteopathic Medicine
New York Institute of Technology
Old Westbury, New York
Fellow of the American Academy
of Osteopathy

Stanley Schiowitz, D.O., F.A.A.O.

Academic Dean
Professor and Former Chairperson
J. C. Griswold Department
of Osteopathic Principles and Practice
New York College of Osteopathic Medicine
New York Institute of Technology
Old Westbury, New York
Fellow of the American Academy
of Osteopathy

With 23 Contributors

J.B. Lippincott Company
PHILADELPHIA   NEW YORK
HAGERSTOWN   LONDON

We dedicate this book

To our grandchildren who were born as this book was written:

Diona Marie Amen and Justine Esta Ellis.

To osteopathic students and physicians who share our belief that our hands are channels of healing.

To our patients who have taught us so much.

Acquisitions Editor: Charles McCormick, Jr.
Assistant Production Manager: Lori J. Bainbridge
Production: Editorial Services of New England, Inc.
Compositor: Compset, Inc.
Printer/Binder: Arcata Graphics/Halliday

6 5 4

Library of Congress Cataloging-in-Publication Data

An osteopathic approach to diagnosis and treatment / edited by Eileen
    L. DiGiovanna, Stanley Schiowitz : with 23 contributors.
        p.   cm.
    Includes bibliographical references and index.
    ISBN 0-397-51001-2
    1. Osteopathy.   I. DiGiovanna, Eileen L.   II. Schiowitz, Stanley.
    [DNLM: 1. Osteopathic Medicine.   WB 940 084]
    RZ302.078   1991
    615.5'33—dc20
    DNLM/DLC
    for Library of Congress   90-13685
                                                           CIP

The authors and publisher have exerted every effort to ensure that drug selection and dosage set forth in this text are in accord with current recommendations and practice at the time of publication. However, in view of ongoing research, changes in governmental regulations, and the constant flow of information relating to drug therapy and drug reactions, the reader is urged to check the package insert for each drug for any change in indications and dosage and for added warnings and precautions. This is particularly important when the recommended agent is a new or infrequently employed drug.

Any procedure or practice described in this book should be applied in accordance with professional standards of care used with regard to the unique circumstances that apply in each practice situation. Care has been taken to confirm the accuracy of information presented and to describe generally accepted practices. However, the authors, editors, and publisher cannot accept any responsibility for errors or omissions or for consequences from application of the information in this book and make no warranty, expressed or implied, with respect to the contents of the book.

Contributors

NANCY BROUS, D.O.
Family Practice Resident
Stony Brook University Hospital
Stony Brook, New York

DENNIS CARDONE, D.O.
Intern
J. C. Griswold Department
of Osteopathic Principles and Practice
New York College of Osteopathic Medicine
New York Institute of Technology
Old Westbury, New York

LISA R. CHUN, D.O.
J. C. Griswold Department
of Osteopathic Principles and Practice
New York College of Osteopathic Medicine
New York Institute of Technology
Old Westbury, New York

ALBERT J. DeRUBERTIS, D.O.
Resident
Physical Medicine and Rehabilitation
University of Illinois Hospital
Chicago, Illinois

EILEEN L. DiGIOVANNA, D.O., F.A.A.O.
Assistant Dean of Student Affairs
Professor and Chairperson
J. C. Griswold Department
of Osteopathic Principles and Practice
New York College of Osteopathic Medicine

New York Institute of Technology
Old Westbury, New York
Fellow of the American Academy
of Osteopathy

JOSEPH A. DiGIOVANNA, D.O.
Attending Physician
Massapequa General Hospital
Seaford, New York
Attending Physician
Central General Hospital
Plainview, New York

MICHAEL J. DiGIOVANNA, JR., D.O.
Attending Physician
Massapequa General Hospital
Seaford, New York
Attending Physician
Central General Hospital
Planview, New York

DENNIS J. DOWLING, D.O.
Assistant Professor
J. C. Griswold Department
of Osteopathic Principles and Practice
New York College of Osteopathic Medicine
New York Institute of Technology
Old Westbury, New York

BARRY S. ERNER, D.O.
Private Practice
Ryebrook, New York

HUGH ETTLINGER, D.O.
Clinical Associate
J. C. Griswold Department
of Osteopathic Principles and Practice
New York College of Osteopathic Medicine
New York Institute of Technology
Old Westbury, New York
Osteopathic Consultant
St. Barnabus Hospital
Bronx, New York

JONATHAN F. FENTON, D.O.
Resident
Department of Physical Medicine–Rehabilitation
St. Vincents Hospital
New York, New York

BONNIE RITT GINTIS, D.O.
Adjunct Professor
J. C. Griswold Department
of Osteopathic Principles and Practice
New York College of Osteopathic Medicine
New York Institute of Technology
Old Westbury, New York

RAYMOND B. GOLDSTEIN, D.O.
Retired Director of Emergency Room Services
Baptist Medical Center
Brooklyn, New York

DONALD V. HANKINSON, D.O.
Attending Physician
Osteopathic Hospital of Maine
Portland, Maine

MARY E. HITCHCOCK, D.O., F.A.A.O.
Associate Professor
J. C. Griswold Department
of Osteopathic Principles and Practice
New York College of Osteopathic Medicine
New York Institute of Technology
Old Westbury, New York

DAVID J. MARTINKE, D.O.
Private Practice
Brownstown, Pennsylvania

TONI MURPHY, D.O.
Internal Medicine Resident
Delaware Valley Medical Center
Langhorne, Pennsylvania

DONALD E. PHYKITT, D.O.
Family Practice Resident
Warren Hospital
Phillipsburg, New Jersey

BARBARA POLSTEIN, D.O.
Intern
J. C. Griswold Department
of Osteopathic Principles and Practice
New York College of Osteopathic Medicine
New York Institute of Technology
Old Westbury, New York

PAULA D. SCARIATI, D.O.
Intern
J. C. Griswold Department
of Osteopathic Principles and Practice
New York College of Osteopathic Medicine
New York Institute of Technology
Old Westbury, New York

STANLEY SCHIOWITZ,, D.O., F.A.A.O.
Academic Dean
Professor and Former Chairperson
J. C. Griswold Department
of Osteopathic Principles and Practice
New York College of Osteopathic Medicine
New York Institute of Technology
Old Westbury, New York
Fellow of the American Academy
of Osteopathy

LILLIAN SOMNER, D.O.
Intern
Massapequa General Hospital
Seaford, New York

SANDRA D. YALE, D.O.
Family Practice Resident
Buffalo General Hospital
Deaconess Hospital
Buffalo, New York

Preface

The instruction of students in the concepts and principles of osteopathic medicine, as well as in the skills of manipulative medicine, began in a tiny frame building in Kirksville, Missouri, almost 100 years ago today. Andrew Taylor Still was the founder and professor of that school. He wrote down many of his thoughts and ideas, which were later collected into the first books of this profession.

Since that time, only a few books have been published on osteopathy, with most of the educational process relying on personal instruction and demonstration. To add to this, much of the information is scattered in obscure journals not available to everyone. Those texts which are available are generally limited to one or a few types of techniques.

Our goal here has been to prepare a text that organizes currently taught concepts and techniques into one comprehensive volume which might then serve as a reference for osteopathic medical students, as well as practicing physicians. The result is a book which presents an integrated method for both the diagnosis and treatment of somatic and visceral problems manifesting in the soma. We have also added an extensive section on practical applications to serve as a demonstration of examples of osteopathic concepts integrated into the management of some commonly encountered conditions.

The osteopathic approach to diagnosis and treatment is unique. We hope this text will make it more readily available to all osteopathic medical students.

E.L.D.
S.S.

Acknowledgments

We wish to acknowledge the able assistance given us in preparing this book by a group of dedicated fellows of osteopathic principles and practice from our department. We also wish to express our gratitude to Anna Moon and Adele Gordon for their help in preparing and handling the manuscript and correspondence. A special thanks goes to the New York College of Osteopathic Medicine of the New York Institute of Technology for allowing us the time to complete this work, as well as to Charles McCormick of J. B. Lippincott Company for encouraging us to do it. And of course, thanks to our spouses, Joseph DiGiovanna, D. O., and Lillian Schiowitz for being there.

Contents

1

Introduction to Osteopathic Medicine

WHAT IS OSTEOPATHIC MEDICINE?
Eileen L. DiGiovanna

Osteopathic medicine represents one of two distinct schools of medicine in the United States. Osteopathic medical institutions issue D.O. degrees, while allopathic medical institutions issue M.D. degrees. The educational process is similar in both kinds of institutions. Most applicants to osteopathic medical schools have an undergraduate degree, exceeding the requirement of three years of an undergraduate education; and many have earned a master's or other postgraduate degree. The four years in osteopathic medical school are spent in the study of basic and clinical sciences, much as in allopathic medical schools, with added focus on osteopathic concepts and manipulation. After graduation the D.O. assumes a rotating internship for one year and may then specialize in any branch of medicine. The D.O. is qualified to write prescriptions, perform surgery, deliver babies, and undertake other medical services as needed for promoting good patient health. As of April 1985, D.O.'s were certified in all specialties, including general practice.

The uniqueness of osteopathic medicine lies in the application of osteopathic concepts. Allopathic (Gr. *allos*, other; Gr. *pathos*, disease) medicine denotes a therapeutic system in which the treatment delivered is designed to be antagonistic to, or incompatible with, the ongoing existence of

the condition under treatment. Osteopathic (Gr. *osteon*, bone; Gr. *pathos*, disease) medicine, while in a limited sense denoting the treatment of bone disease, in a broader sense refers to a therapeutic system based on the belief that the body, in normal structural relationship and with adequate nutrition, is capable of mounting its own defenses against most pathologic conditions. Osteopathic medical practitioners therefore follow accepted methods of physical and surgical diagnosis and treatment, but are primarily interested in the achievement of normal body mechanics as central to good health.

Osteopathic medicine thus recognizes the neuromusculoskeletal system as salient to the full expression of life. The viscera subserve the neuromusculoskeletal system by providing nourishment to it and removing its wastes. Disease processes frequently manifest in the musculoskeletal system, so that findings here are of diagnostic utility to the physician. As George Northup noted in *Osteopathic Medicine, An American Reformation*, "The musculoskeletal system is intimately connected with all other systems of the body through both the voluntary and the involuntary nervous systems. . . . Thus, indications are that the musculoskeletal system is a mirror of both health and disease, responding as it does to inflammation and pain from disorder in other body systems." Therefore, the osteopathic physician considers the body as an integrated unit, comprising multiple complex functions and interrelated structures, when assessing a patient.

In addition to the central role assigned to the neuromusculoskeletal system, another important principle in osteopathic medicine is that structure governs function. An abnormality in the structure of any body part can lead to abnormal function, whether expressed locally or distantly from the deranged structure. To correct the mechanical disorders of the body, the osteopathic physician undertakes therapeutic manipulations. Osteopathic manipulation is gentle and controlled; it may be directed toward joint motion or directed toward the muscles or fascia. It is utilized to affect circulation, lymphatic drainage, and nervous impulses.

The heart of osteopathy is the recognition of the body's ability to cure itself, with some external help, of many pathologic conditions. This tenet echoes the belief enunciated by Hippocrates more than 2,000 years ago: "Our natures are the physicians for our diseases."

Osteopathic medicine continues to grow even as it remains in a minority position in the health care system in the United States. The five schools in 1962 increased to 15 in the 1980s. Norman Gevitz in *The D.O.s* reported 1,004 new D.O.'s graduating in 1979 and projected a figure of 1,844 new graduates in 1989, or an increase of 84%. In January 1990 the American Osteopathic Association estimated that 1,673 students would graduate in 1990. Based on government estimates, Gevitz suggested that in 1982, when his findings were published, D.O. physicians and surgeons provided health care services for more than 20 million Americans, or in excess of 10% of the population. Most osteopathic physicians were in primary care practice, often in underserved areas.

The osteopathic profession has changed even as it has grown. It has achieved recognition as a significant part of the American health care system. It is now carefully defining its special contribution to medicine, and is undertaking various kinds of research to prove the effectiveness of its manipulative techniques. With these and similar steps toward full realization of the potential of osteopathic medicine, the profession is securing its position in the modern medical climate.

HISTORY OF OSTEOPATHY
Eileen L. DiGiovanna

Andrew Taylor Still, the founder of osteopathy, was born in 1828 in Lee County, Virginia. He was of Scottish-Irish descent. His father was a circuit-riding minister in the Methodist Church, a physician, a farmer, and a millwright.

As a young boy, Still suffered severe headaches. One day, during such a headache, he went to sit in a rope swing his father had hung for him from a tree branch. Feeling ill, he removed the board from the swing and lay on the ground with the back of his neck resting against the rope. The pain eased, and he fell asleep. When he awoke the headache was gone. This observation later led to the development of osteopathic manipulation.

Still's formal education was in small schoolhouses, and his medical education was primarily by preceptorship, a common practice in America at that time. Still constantly pursued an interest in anatomy. As a hunter, he studied the muscles and bones of his game. He was issued an M.D. degree by the state of Missouri.

Even as a youth, Still held strong opinions on controversial subjects. One of the first concerned abolition. He, like his father, was strongly against slavery. Missouri was a border state with pro-slavery sentiments. Eventually the Stills had to move from Missouri to Kansas. In Kansas, Andrew Taylor Still continued his fight against slavery and was elected to the Kansas legislature. He was instrumental in Kansas's achieving statehood.

When the Civil War broke out, the young physician joined the Union Army as a captain in the Kansas militia. He saw active duty and rose to the rank of major.

The times in which Still practiced medicine were significant in guiding his career. In the 1850s and 1860s, American medical practitioners were frequently poorly trained and had little understanding of the causes of disease. Treatments were unsophisticated to the point of being dangerous. Some common remedies used in those years included laxatives, purgatives, blood-letting (sometimes to the point of unconsciousness), calomel (a mercury compound), narcotics, and drugs in alcohol bases. Drug addiction, alcoholism, and mercury poisoning were among the results. Often the treatments were more dangerous than the illness.

An epidemic of meningitis took the lives of three of Still's children; orthodox medicine was unable to save them. In his autobiography, Still reflected on this episode: "In sickness, had God left man in a world of guessing? Guess what is the matter? What to give and guess the result?" Pushing away confusion and despair, Still sought a systematic method of treating illness that would eliminate guesswork and bring some order to the hodgepodge of therapy. He worked largely with the musculoskeletal system and recognized the importance of the vascular system, particularly arteries. He believed in natural immunity, and that the body had its own "pharmacy" for healing itself. He developed a form of manipulation to help keep the body fit with unobstructed circulation and innervation.

Still broke with allopathy, as he called orthodox medicine, on June 22, 1874, when he "flung the banner of osteopathy to the breeze." He eventually moved back to Missouri to establish his practice in the town of Kirksville. As his fame grew, huge crowds would gather for his new treatment. However, Still wanted to teach his beliefs to others, so he attempted to have osteopathy included in the curriculum at Baker University in Baldwin, Kansas, an institution to which he and his brothers had contributed substantial financial support. He was not successful; osteopathy was regarded as quackery.

In 1892 Still opened the American School of Osteopathy in Kirksville, Missouri. The first graduating class, in 1893, included five women, opening the door to the practice of osteopathy to women before they were well accepted into other medical schools.

Still died in 1917 at the age of 89. He left a strong but struggling profession. Ahead were battles for acceptance into the American health care system. Although many schools offering the D.O. degree sprang up, only a few survived. By 1960 there were six colleges, located in Kirksville, Kansas City, Chicago, Philadelphia, Des Moines, and Los Angeles.

In 1961 the profession suffered a major setback. The American Medical Association changed its policy of fighting osteopathy, and offered an alliance to D.O.'s in California. The AMA urged osteopathic physicians to join the California Medical Society. They turned the California school into an M.D. degree-granting institution and offered the M.D. degree to all California D.O.'s (and for a small fee to D.O.'s all over the country). To the amazement of the AMA, most D.O.'s rejected this offer, and, although the profession lost the California school and many California D.O.'s, it survived and its numbers continued to grow. A new California Osteopathic Medical Society and a new college in Pomona have regained much of the lost ground.

As of 1990 there are 15 schools of osteopathic medicine. D.O.'s are licensed in all 50 states— Vermont was the first and Mississippi the last to license them. Osteopathic physicians are recognized by all major insurance carriers and are commissioned in the military.

THE PHILOSOPHY OF OSTEOPATHIC MEDICINE
David J. Martinke

The precepts discussed in this section are ideals. Realistically, few physicians consistently hold to these ideals. However, those who do incorporate them into their practice will have a more realistic view of health and disease. Therefore, osteopathic physicians maintain that, as Still stated, "if we cannot swallow all, we can taste."

Osteopathic medicine is not merely a combination of allopathic medicine and osteopathic manipulations. Rather, the principles and philosophy of osteopathic medicine apply not only to manipulative therapy but also to surgery, obstetrics, emergency medicine, internal medicine, geriatrics, and many other areas of care traditionally subsumed by allopathic medicine. Osteopathic principles and philosophy in fact permeate all aspects of health maintenance and disease prevention and treatment.

It is appropriate at this point to review the difference between a philosophy and a principle. The *American Heritage Dictionary* defines a philosophy as an "inquiry into the nature of things based on logical reasoning rather than empirical methods." In philosophy, logical reasoning, not experimental design, is the guide. Philosophical knowledge is gained by the pursuit of wisdom by intellectual means, not by laboratory analysis. By contrast, a principle is defined as a "rule or law concerning the functioning of natural phenomena or mechanical process." Examples are Fryette's law of vertebral motion, or Einthoven's law concerning the primary unipolar leads of the electrocardiogram. Unlike philosophies, these rules or laws can be proved by experimental design or laboratory analysis. With these definitions in mind, it will be clear that the precepts outlined below are properly termed philosophies, not principles, since for the most part they are based on logical reasoning rather than on experimental design.

The first four of the following precepts were developed in 1953 by the osteopathic faculty committee at Kirksville College of Osteopathic Medicine, Kirksville, Missouri. The rest, which were added by common usage, were enunciated by Sarah Sprafka, Robert C. Ward, and David Neff, in the Journal of AOA, September 1981.

1. "The body is a unit."

The human body does not function as a collection of separate parts but as an integral unit. Obviously the body does consist of parts—the heart, the lungs, the musculoskeletal system, and so forth—all working to benefit the organism in totality. However, the osteopathic physician refrains from exalting any part above the whole. The kidneys, of interest to a nephrologist, or the heart, of interest to a cardiologist, are regarded by the osteopathic physician as components subserving the greater interest of the body. Uniting the body's parts is the fascia, a deep fibrous tissue investing the muscles and organs and acting as a ground substance to support the arteries, veins, lymphatics, and nerves. The tubular collagen fibrils unite the whole body in a fluid matrix from head to foot. Thus the fascia is a fluid mechanism of profound functional significance. Still regarded the fascia almost as the dwelling place of "the soul of man with all the streams of pure living water." Osteopathic medicine, a bit less imagistically, understands the body as a unit whose component parts, linked by fasciae, work to benefit the whole organism.

2. "Structure and function are reciprocally interrelated."

Any body part carries out a function dictated by its structure. As an example, lung structure dictates that gases, carried by the red blood cells and dissolved in the blood, pass through the pulmonary arteries to the small capillaries in close approximation to the alveoli, where gas exchange takes place. As structure governs function, similarly, abnormal structure governs dysfunction. In the case of abnormal lung structure, as in pulmonary fibrosis or interstitial pneumonia, the gradient between the alveolar gases and blood gases is increased, resulting in decreased gas exchange.

3. "The body possesses self-regulatory mechanisms."

Many examples of this precept can be considered. First, neuronal reflex mechanisms are constantly monitoring body functions. For example, the carotid sinus and baroreceptors monitor blood pressure and adjust the heart rate and cardiac contractility in response to changes in blood pressure. Second, hormonal pathways are involved in self-regulation. The releasing hormones of the hypothalamus cause the release of the stimulating hormones from the pituitary, which causes release of end-organ products (such as hormones or steroids); these products in turn provide feedback and regulate the activity of the hypothalamic-pituitary axis. These hormonal pathways are part of the complex endocrine system that is involved in the self-regulation of the body. Third, many organs such as the heart and kidneys are able to regulate blood flow. This vascular autoregulation allows the organ to maintain the appropriate blood flow in the setting of a changing vascular status. These examples represent only a few of the many ways in which the body can regulate its functions.

4. The body has the inherent capacity to defend itself and repair itself.

The first lines of defense commonly recognized are the skin and mucous membranes. Once these are violated, neutrophils, macrophages, and lymphocytes—elements of the cellular immune system—are called on to protect the body from present and future invaders. Defense mechanisms are constantly working to protect the body as it contacts thousands of microorganisms daily.

The body's ability to repair itself is easily substantiated by observing the healing of a laceration or a fracture. It is the laying down of granulation tissue and the regenerative properties of certain tissues that allow healing to take place. The physician may provide the environment for the healing to take place, but the inherent capacity of the body to repair itself brings about the actual healing. The physician's contribution is to remove obstacles to the body's performance.

5. When normal adaptability is disrupted, or when environmental changes overcome the body's capacity for self-maintenance, disease may ensue.

Disease is caused by adverse environmental factors that overwhelm the body's defenses, or by the body's inability to adapt to a situation. Thus a cause-and-effect relationship is established. The cause may be the body's inability to adapt, as in the case of an abnormal structure (e.g., the abnormal hemoglobin structure of sickle cell anemia), which yields an abnormal function, or the effect (e.g., sickling of the red blood cell). This cause-and-effect relationship is fundamental to the practice of osteopathic medicine. The physician is presented with a symptom, dysfunction, or disease—the effect—and then embarks on a search for the cause. A physician who treats a disease is merely treating an effect and will have no great impact on the cause. The osteopathic physician corrects the cause by restoring proper structure (at either the organ, tissue, or cellular level) so that proper function or adaptability may ensue. Once the cause is corrected, the body will heal itself through its inherent capacity for repair.

6. Movement of body fluids is essential to the maintenance of health.

The arteries and other tubular structures play a crucial role in carrying nutritive elements to their destination and carrying away waste materials to be expelled. Disturbances in the circulation will produce pathology, such as acute or chronic inflammation, atrophy, irritation, or trauma. If the blood vessels to these areas are compromised by intrinsic or extrinsic damage, blood flow will be inadequate, potentially leading to increasing hypoxia and relative acidosis of the tissues involved. Such an environment could delay or even stop the healing process. For example, if the compromised artery is a coronary artery, angina or myocardial infarction might ensue.

The osteopathic physician focuses on areas of structural dysfunction that influence the circulation to an area involved by a pathologic process. If such dysfunction is corrected, oxygen delivery by the arteries might increase, the venous congestion be dispelled, and the healing process initiated. This process frees the body to make the repairs necessary for return of health.

7. The nerves play a crucial part in controlling the fluids of the body.

Since the nervous system is a major factor controlling blood flow, dysfunction of the nervous system can cause a disturbance of blood flow and compromise health. Impaired autonomic nervous control of the upper thoracic spinal cord traveling to the cervical sympathetic ganglia can produce a vast array of vascular changes in the somatic dermatomes supplied by these nerves. The somatic changes possible when such a dysfunction occurs include increased temperature locally, moisture, tenderness, and edema. These signs, recognizable on palpation, are normal vascular responses to an abnormal autonomic nervous supply.

Once the dysfunction has been corrected, a more normal autonomic tone should ensue, the vascular changes should resolve, and a higher level of health should result. Therefore, thinking osteopathically requires a knowledge of vascular and autonomic nervous system anatomy and the ability to reason from the region of pathologic manifestation to the site of autonomic control, not ignoring any of the tissues enroute that may contribute to their dysfunction.

8. There are somatic components to disease that are not only manifestations of disease but also are factors that contribute to maintenance of the diseased state.

The somatic component of the disease process may be caused by a direct bodily injury (such as a blow to the skeletal structures) or it may represent the response of viscera to pathology. One need not explain how a broken arm manifests a major somatic component; however, with visceral disease the somatic component is a bit more elusive, though still generally recognized by clinicians of all schools of practice.

For example, in abdominal visceral pathology, such as acute appendicitis or peritonitis, one may observe spasm or guarding of the abdominal musculature. Other musculoskeletal effects may develop at a segmentally related spinal region, creating osteopathic somatic dysfunctions. These somatic components of the visceral disease are major diagnostic clues. The mechanism of this somatic response is probably the segmentally integrated viscerosomatic reflex. The nervous system is the most important system connecting and integrating the visceral and skeletal organs.

One can now understand that in many instances, illness is a disparity between the neuromuscular system and the visceral systems. This disparity must be mitigated before the body can heal itself.

Osteopathic manipulative treatment was not mentioned in the eight precepts of osteopathic philosophy. When Still first announced his philosophy in 1874, he did not mention manipulation, and it was about five years later that he began using manipulation as a tool for diagnosis and treatment. Manipulation is not the only aspect of osteopathic philosophy, nor is it the most important. However, with recognition of the importance of the somatic component of disease, the value of manipulation will be correspondingly better appreciated.

What is so "osteopathic" about the eight precepts? Still's purpose was not to violate or rewrite the basic scientific principles of his time, but rather to elucidate them and position them centrally on a system of therapeutics that deemphasized interventions in favor of promoting the body's ability to regulate itself toward health, given an appropriate environment and adequate nutrition. Osteopathic medicine is generally applicable to all disease states; the osteopathic physician does not address one organ system or structure at the expense of another but considers the body as an integral unit.

SOMATIC DYSFUNCTION
Eileen L. DiGiovanna

The term *somatic dysfunction* has been adopted by the osteopathic profession as a substitute for the older designation, *osteopathic lesion.* Somatic dysfunction refers to a condition of the musculoskeletal system that is recognized solely by the osteopathic profession and was first defined by Ira Rumney. The accepted definition in the *Glossary of Osteopathic Terminology* is as follows:

Somatic Dysfunction is an impaired or altered function of related components of the somatic (body framework) system: skeletal, arthrodial and myofascial structures, and related vascular, lymphatic, and neural elements.

It is apparent that the term can be applied to a wide variety of problems and therefore is a little too general in scope.

Not all somatic lesions are somatic dysfunctions. Fractures, degenerative processes, and inflammatory processes are not somatic dysfunctions. A useful observation has been given by Fred Mitchell, Sr.: "Implicit in the term 'somatic dysfunction' is the notion that manipulation is appropriate, effective, and sufficient treatment for it."

A somatic dysfunction is a change in the normal functioning of a joint and is diagnosed by using specific criteria. These criteria may be re-membered as the A-R-T of diagnosis.

1. A denotes asymmetry. The position of the ver-tebra or other bone is asymmetrical.
2. R denotes restriction of motion within the bounds of physiologic motion. The involved joint does not have a full, free range of motion. The restriction involves one or more planes; it most frequently involves the minor motions of any given joint. This restriction is found by mo-tion testing the joint in all planes.
3. T denotes tissue texture changes. The soft tis-sues around a joint in somatic dysfunction undergo palpable changes. These changes oc-cur in the skin, fascia, or muscle.

Asymmetry

On palpation of a joint involved in somatic dys-function, the bone involved will be found to lie in an asymmetric position with respect to its nor-mal position and to the position of bones contig-uous to it. For example, the spinous process of a vertebra involved by somatic dysfunction may lie to one side of the line formed by the spinous pro-cesses of other vertebrae (which should lie in the midline), or one transverse process may lie more posterior than the contralateral one. There may be an approximation of one transverse process to the vertebra below while the opposite transverse process is separated from the one below it.

Barriers to Motion

A joint involved by somatic dysfunction has a re-stricted range of motion. It is said to meet an ab-normal "barrier" to motion. In the normally

Figure 1-1. Barriers to motion.

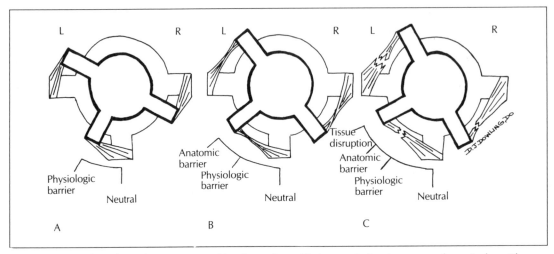

Figure 1-2. (**A**) Physiologic barrier engaged by the patient. (**B**) Anatomic barrier engaged passively, with ligaments stretched. (**C**) Anatomic barrier has been passed, causing tissue disruption.

functioning joint there are two barriers to motion (Fig. 1-1):

1. The *physiologic barrier* is that point to which the patient may actively move any given joint; it represents a functional limit within the anatomic range of motion. Passive motion is still possible (Fig. 1-2A).
2. The *anatomic barrier* is that point to which the joint may be passively moved beyond the physiologic barrier (Fig. 1-2B). Restriction at this point occurs due to bone, ligament, or tendons. To pass the anatomic barrier, a disruption of tissue would have to occur (Fig. 1-2C).

A pathologic barrier may occur as the result of disease or trauma. An example is joint fusion due to spondylitis or osteophytes in an arthritic joint. Inflammation or joint effusion will restrict normal motion. The osteopathic pathologic barrier is one that lies within the physiologic range of motion and prevents a joint from moving symmetrically within the physiologic range of motion (Fig. 1-3).

In somatic dysfunction, a joint is restricted, or meets a barrier, in one or more planes of motion. Motion in the opposite direction is normal or free. For example, a vertebra may move freely into flexion but not be able to move all the way to the physiologic motion barrier of extension.

Tissue Texture Changes

Tissue texture changes are a significant diagnostic tool. They occur in response to a variety of factors, including the following:

A. Neurologic factors
  1. Somatic manifestations
    a. Hyperresponsiveness of segmentally related functions
      i. Hypertonic muscles
      ii. Muscle spindle overactivity
    b. Sudomotor activity either increased or decreased
    c. Vasomotor activity, either constriction or dilation of vessels
  2. Reflex manifestations
    a. Tenderness to palpation
    b. Rigidity of tissues at reflex site
    c. Sudomotor activity may increase or decrease
    d. Changes in pulse rate (increase or decrease)
    e. Changes in skin temperature
B. Circulatory factors
  1. Macroscopic changes
    a. Temperature changes
    b. Erythema
    c. Swelling
    d. Changes in pulse and cardiac rate

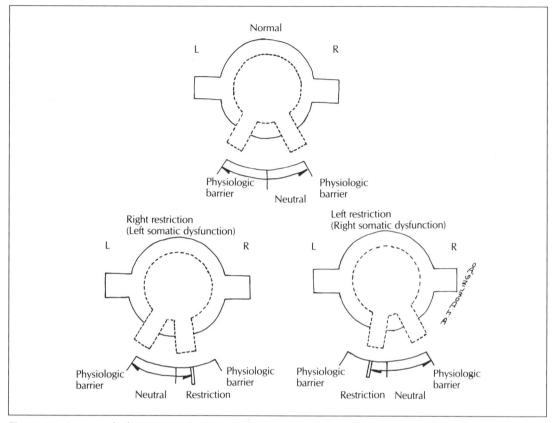

Figure 1-3. Somatic dysfunction, with illustration of rotational restrictions.

2. Microscopic changes
   a. Hyperemia of soft tissues
   b. Congestion and dilation
   c. Edema of subcutaneous tissues
   d. Minute hemorrhages
   e. Fibrosis
   f. Local ischemia
   g. Atrophy

Criteria for Evaluation of Soft Tissues

Tissue texture changes vary somewhat between acute and chronic somatic dysfunctions. In the spinal area the changes tend to occur at the articulations of the vertebrae, over the transverse processes, and over the spinous process. The following is a chart of findings in acute and chronic somatic dysfunctions:

	Acute	Chronic
Temperature	Increased	Slight increase or decrease (coolness)
Texture	Boggy, more rough	Thin, smooth
Moisture	Increased	Dry
Tension	Increased, rigid, boardlike	Slight increase, ropy, stringy
Tenderness	Greatest	Present but less
Edema	Yes	No
Erythema test	Redness lasts	Redness fades quickly or blanching occurs

Definitions of some of these terms from the *Glossary of Osteopathic Terminology* are as follows:

Bogginess. A tissue texture abnormality characterized by a palpable sense of sponginess in the tissue, interpreted as resulting from congestion due to increased fluid content.

Ropiness. A tissue texture change characterized by a cord or stringlike feeling.

Stringiness. A palpable tissue texture abnormality characterized by fine or stringlike myofascial structures.

Diagnosing Viscerosomatic Somatic Dysfunctions

A tenet of osteopathic medicine is that visceral reflexes to the soma are an important cause of somatic dysfunction and are of major diagnostic significance. Dysfunctions caused by these reflexes may be either acute or chronic. Acute viscerosomatic reflex dysfunctions are probably indistinguishable from any other acute somatic dysfunction. Chronic viscerosomatic dysfunctions have a few characteristics which may aid in differentiating them from somatic dysfunctions of other causes.

1. The skin tends to be more atrophic over the involved area.
2. The tissues display a firm, dry sponginess, as opposed to the bogginess of an acute dysfunction. The texture is very firm.
3. Joint motion is more restricted and seems more fixed than the usual dysfunction. Attempts to elicit motion in the involved joint produce a sluggish, rigid movement. When such dysfunction is corrected, it will return to a dysfunctional state within 24 hours.

It is important to know the location of sympathetic innervation in relation to the thoracic vertebrae so that viscerosomatic reflex dysfunctions may be utilized for diagnostic purposes.

Naming Somatic Dysfunctions

A standard terminology has been devised for the purpose of recording somatic dysfunctions. In the case of vertebrae, it is traditional to refer to a functional vertebral unit, consisting of two vertebrae and the intervening disc, with the upper of the vertebrae being the one with restricted motion. The somatic dysfunction is always named for its freedom of motion, i.e., the directions in which the vertebra can move most easily. For example, if the C3 veretbra is restricted in the motions of extension, side bending to the right, and rotation to the right, C3 is said to be flexed, side-bent to the left, and rotated to the left on C4. This is denoted as C3 FSl Rl. The terminology reflects the fact that the vertebra assumes the position of its freedom of motion. T7 ESr Rr indicates that the seventh thoracic vertebra is extended, side-bent to the right, and rotated right on T8. In this case the seventh thoracic vertebra is restricted in the motions of flexion, side bending left, and rotation to the left.

Somatic dysfunctions are classified as Type I or Type II dysfunctions. Type I dysfunctions follow Fryette's first principle of physiologic motion (see Chap. 4, Physiologic Motion of the Spine) and are group curves involving more than one vertebra. If rotation and side bending are involved, the rotation is opposite to the side bending. Although Type I dysfunctions are group curves, they are distinct from idiopathic scoliosis.

Type II dysfunctions follow Fryette's second principle of physiologic motion. Rotation and side bending are in the same direction. These are single dysfunctions and are often traumatic in origin.

Predisposing Factors

Certain factors that predispose to the development of a somatic dysfunction are as follows:

1. Posture
   a. Habitual
   b. Occupational
2. Gravity
3. Anomalies
   a. Abnormal size or shape of vertebra
   b. Abnormal facets
   c. Fusion or lack of fusion
      i. Lumbarization
      ii. Sacralization
4. Transitional areas (These areas are especially prone to the development of somatic dysfunction.)
   a. Occipito-atlantal
   b. C7–T1
   c. T12–L1
   d. L5–S1

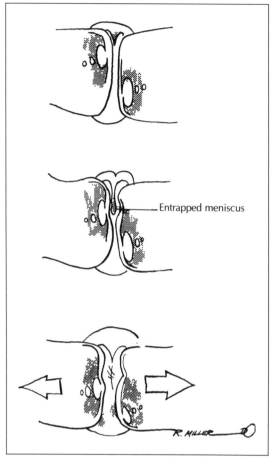

Figure 1-4. Meniscus entrapment theory. With joint motion the meniscus is trapped between the joint surfaces. Traction is required to free the meniscus.

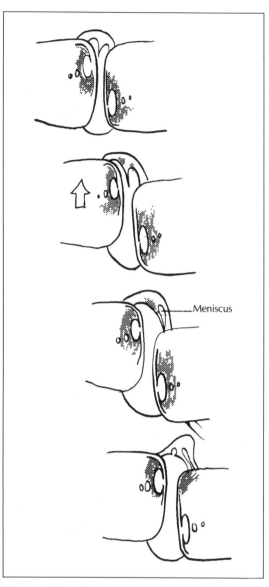

Figure 1-5. Meniscus extrapment theory. As the joint is flexed. The meniscus moves above the articular surface and occasionally is trapped there as the joint begins to extend. With further extension the meniscus bends, causing pain.

5. Muscle hyperirritability
   a. Stress
   b. Infection
   c. Reflex from another somatic or visceral area
6. Physiologic locking of a joint, "close pack position"
7. Adaptation to stressors—spontaneously reversible
8. Compensation for other structural deficits—stable.

Etiology

The exact cause of somatic dysfunction is often debated. Some feel there is a true facet locking.

Some theories postulated in support of this include the following:

1. Meniscoid entrapment
2. Meniscoid extrapment
3. Capsular compression

The meniscoid theory was proposed by Kos and Wolf (Bogdvk and Jull) as a mechanism of "acute locked back" and was elaborated by Bogdvk and Jull. This theory is based on the premise that there are wedge-shaped menisci in the lumbar zygapophysial joints. It is speculated that the apex of the wedge may become trapped between the articular surfaces or, on flexion, outside the joint cavity (Figs. 1-4, 1-5). Most osteopathic physicians today believe that abnormal neural impulses to muscles are the most significant factor in causing joint restriction and pain. Trauma is probably the major factor triggering an abnormal neural impulse.

Type I somatic dysfunctions may be due to any of the following:

1. Muscle imbalance
2. Short leg
3. Occupation
4. Trauma
5. Visceral reflexes
6. Disease/infection

The ability to diagnose somatic dysfunction is of utmost importance to the osteopathic physician, who then assumes the responsibility of correcting all such dysfunctions that he or she finds.

NEUROPHYSIOLOGIC MECHANISMS RELATED TO OSTEOPATHIC DIAGNOSIS AND TREATMENT
Dennis J. Dowling

The body is artificially divided into groups of structures identified as organs, glands, ligaments, muscles, neural tissue, vessels, bone, and skin. This differentiation is anatomically correct but functionally misleading. The somatic and visceral components act synergistically to fulfill the body's needs and functions. However, this interaction is often visualized as a strictly mechanistic process in which one part of the body causes the action to be initiated, either automatically or volitionally, and the rest of the body simply carries out orders. By contrast, osteopathic medicine holds that each part of the body is in some manner responsible for and responsive to every other part.

The spinal cord is the organizer of information, which is processed from the brain to other regions. Feedback from these areas to the brain helps maintain normal function. A difficult concept to grasp is that parts of the body may communicate directly with one another without the brain's intervention. In these communications, the neurologic system is less like a two-way intercom system in a large apartment house than like a fully interactive telephone system with the brain acting as the operator. A common example is the knee-jerk reflex, which occurs automatically in response to appropriate stimuli without direct intervention from the brain.

The Autonomic Nervous System
The autonomic nervous system can be thought of as an involuntary manager. It is divided into sympathetic and parasympathetic nervous systems. The autonomic nervous system controls the moment-by-moment activity of the viscera. Its components, often described as antagonistic, are more realistically understood as cooperative or complementary.

The somatic component is often discussed as a totally independent, voluntary system responsible for the musculoskeletal system. It is not customarily thought of as interacting with the autonomic nervous system. However, the somatic component has undeniable effects on the autonomic nervous system, and vice versa.

The Sympathetic Nervous System
The sympathetic chains of ganglia are bilaterally oriented in a cephalad-caudad direction at the levels of the first thoracic segment to the second or third lumbar segment. The fibers exit the cord

along with the somatic motor axons as the ventral roots via the intervertebral foramina. These preganglionic fibers exit the root along the white ramus and into the ganglia. They synapse with postganglionic nerves at various levels of the chain. The postganglionic axons return to the spinal nerve via the gray ramus. For much of their course, the sympathetic nerves travel intimately with the somatic axons.

Another important anatomic feature of the sympathetic chain is its relationship to the ribs. The ganglia lie inferior to the junction between the head and neck of the ribs but posterior to the pleura. The range of influence is further extended superiorly as far as the sympathetic plexuses to the head by the cervical ganglion and to the lower extremities by the lumbar splanchnic nerves.

The sympathetic nervous system assists the body in managing the stresses and requirements of the external environment. It is responsible for the "flight or fight" response. Reactions are constantly moderated and adjusted in response to information received by higher centers. Visceral function is fine tuned. Circulation, metabolism, smooth muscle tone, intestinal motility, cardiac function, and pulmonary response are regulated (Fig. 1-6).

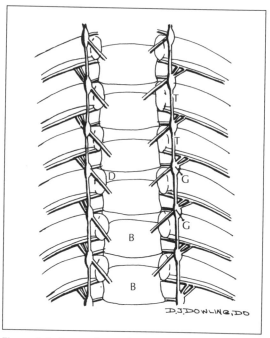

Figure 1-6. Sympathetic chain. *B,* vertebral body; *G,* sympathetic trunk ganglion; *T,* sympathetic trunk; *D,* intervertebral disk.

The Parasympathetic System

The parasympathetic system is also known as the craniosacral portion of the autonomic nervous system, owing to the sites of origin of the preganglionic fibers. The cranial portion has ganglia associated with the third, seventh, ninth, and tenth cranial nerves. Spinal cord segments S2, S3, and S4 make up the sacral portion.

The parasympathetic ganglia are located close to the innervated organ. Fibers from the oculomotor, facial, and glossopharyngeal nerves supply ganglia for organs found in the head, while the remainder of the visceral organs receive their innervation from the vagus and the sacral axis. The vagus alone supplies the heart, lungs, trachea, liver, gallbladder, esophagus, stomach, pancreas, spleen, kidneys, small intestine, and the ascending and transverse colons. The nervi erigentes, constituting the pelvic nerve, send fibers to sex organs, external genitalia, and the bladder and its sphincters.

The visceral organs are under dual control of the sympathetic and parasympathetic nervous systems. The process is a synergistic rather than a competitive one, with activation usually occurring reciprocally. The primary function of the parasympathetic system is internal maintenance, including digestion and excretion. Among other functions, the cranial axis causes constriction of the pupil and decreases in heart rate. The parasympathetic division operates most effectively during times of recovery and rest.

Skeletal Muscle System

The skeletal or somatic nervous system is under voluntary control, although some processes can be performed automatically. The typical spinal nerve is formed by a joining of the ventral and dorsal roots inside the vertebral canal. Sensory fibers have their cell bodies in the dorsal root ganglion and then synapse in the dorsal horn. The ventral root contains the motor neurons. The rami of the 31 pairs of spinal nerves split into a dorsal and ventral ramus. These in turn are subdivided into other branches. The structure is fairly consis-

Figure 1-7. Sympathetic pathways. *D*, dorsal root; *V*, ventral root; *DRG*, dorsal root ganglion; *S*, splanchnic; *R*, recurrent meningeal; *g*, gray rami communicantes; *W*, white rami communicante·; *G*, sympathetic trunk ganglion; *T*, sympathetic trunk.

tent but is best represented by the thoracic nerves. All of the skeletal muscle nerves arise or terminate in common origins in the spinal cord and exit via the vertebral foramina. The sympathetic pathways are shown in Figure 1-7.

Segmentalization

Dermatome mapping of the cutaneous innervation is an established method of localizing a disease process to a particular segment. Although variations might exist in a given individual, the overall pattern is fairly consistent (Fig. 1-8). A different type of segmentalization is not as well known: the sympathetic system also shows segmental preference in regard to the visceral organs. According to *Gray's Anatomy*, the afferent fibers that accompany the preganglionic and postganglionic fibers of the sympathetic system occur in a segmental arrangement. Painful stimuli to the viscera are carried back to the cord via the sympathetics (Fig. 1-9). When all clues are combined,

knowledge of this segmentalization can assist in the diagnosis of visceral disorder. For example, pain fibers from the heart pass to the first five thoracic spinal cord segments mainly through the middle and inferior cardiac nerves. Ischemia of the heart muscle often produces pain substernally with radiation to the chest, shoulder, neck, jaw, and abdomen.

Pain secondary to appendicitis is generally noted to be periumbilical. Anatomically the appendix is not within this region of the abdomen. However, the innervation for the appendiceal region is derived from the tenth thoracic segment as is the area around the umbilicus. This segmental relationship demonstrates the intertwining of different regions anatomically.

Viscerosomatic Reflexes

A viscerosomatic reflex is one in which disruption, irritation, or disease of an internal organ or tissue results in reflex dysfunction of a segmen-

Figure 1-8. Dermatome map of cutaneous innervation.

tally related musculoskeletal region. In 1907, Louisa Burns attempted, through experiments on animals, to demonstrate the physiologic processes occurring in viscerosomatic and somatovisceral reflexes. By stimulating various visceral organs, she elicited contractions of segmentally related muscles. Irritation of the visceral pericardium and the heart muscle initiated contractions in the second through sixth intercostal and spinal muscles. Stimulation of abdominal organs similarly yielded results predictable from segmental distributions. More recent investigators (Beal, 1983; Cox et al., 1983) have experimentally ex-

amined both cardiac patients and normal subjects for the extent of distribution of thoracic somatic dysfunction, with results similar to those obtained by Burns.

Musculoskeletal pain related to visceral dysfunction may be the sole presenting symptom of a viscerosomatic reflex. As a diagnostic aid, the viscerosomatic reflex has played an important role in medicine, whether or not the physician understood the mechanism. A common dictum in physical diagnosis is that 90% of the information needed is derived from the history and physical examination. Hematologic, radiologic, physiochemical, pathologic, and other tests are properly used for confirmation of a suspected disease.

Somatovisceral Reflexes

The term *somatovisceral* refers to neuromusculoskeletal disturbances, also known as somatic dysfunctions, that disrupt the function of visceral organs. The somatic nerves from one segmental region are intimately involved with the sympathetic nerves originating at that segment.

Thomas Brown in 1828 discussed the nature of "spinal irritation" of visceral organs resulting from a disturbed vertebra. In 1863 John Hilton, an anatomist and surgeon, described "sympathies" that correlated segmentally related tender spots with visceral pain (Gevitz).

Disturbances in the tissue and structure of the surrounding neural tissue are usually discussed in macroscopic terms: subluxations, "pinched nerves," herniated disks, fractures. However, some alteration in function can be induced by small impingments of the neural and vascular tissue. Within the intervertebral foramina are nerves and roots covered by their sheaths, connective tissue, periosteum, blood vessels, and fat. Normally, with movement, the nerve should glide within its sheath. Irritative forces induced by adhesion, traction, inflammation, compression, torsion, or spasm can induce disturbances of conductivity and excitability. Such disruptions frequently are not radiologically apparent. Also, much of the course of the spinal nerves is through skeletal muscle. Localized contraction resulting from strain may further compress an already agitated nerve. The blood vessels in the region may narrow and produce ischemic changes.

Burns' examination of the somatovisceral reflex in the early 20th century entailed visual observation of visceral organs of animals during stimu-

Figure 1-9. Segmentalization of the sympathetic nervous system.

lation of the deep paravertebral tissues. She noted a decrease in vascular supply, as shown by a lightening of the color. Cessation of the irritation resulted in a subsequent return to normal color. Later studies on animals with transected spinal cords produced contraction of ipsilateral visceral organs after stimulation of segmentally related paravertebral muscles.

Somatic dysfunctions, especially in the thoracic region, cause disruption of underlying tissues. At times, this stimulation reaches proportions sufficient to cause symptoms. The sympathetic nerves in the region may be under constant stimulation, which for the different organs may constitute either stimulation or inhibition. The gastrointestinal system becomes less motile. The cardiovascular system may demonstrate tachycardia, elevated blood pressure, vasoconstriction, or other changes. Medicinal intervention may temporarily reduce the symptoms. However, the cause will most probably remain. Treatment of the cause—neuromusculoskeletal in these examples—is the only logical course.

Axonal Transport and the Trophic Function of Nerves

Maintenance of the distal portions of a neuron depends on the delivery of fresh cytoplasm. The axon and its branches act as the delivery system for the manufactured substances, including neurotransmitters. Flow proceeds at a rate of 1 to 11 mm/d and may occur in wavelike fashion. These nutritive substances are not limited to the neural tissue but have been found in innervated muscle tissue (Korr, 1966; Korr, Wilkinson, and Chornock, 1966, 1967; Korr, Chornock, Cole, and Wilkinson, 1967; Korr and Appeltauer, 1970). The importance of these findings has yet to be determined, but it is readily apparent that disruption

by compression would limit or eliminate any benefits obtained from this nutrition. With complete separation of the axon, Wallerian degeneration occurs and innervated fibers are lost.

Facilitation

Facilitation indicates that an area of impairment or restriction develops a lower threshold for irritation and dysfunction when other structures are stimulated. It may be activated by reflexes of either the somatosomatic or viscerosomatic type. These low-threshold segments showed reflex hyperexcitability in response to pressure placed on the corresponding spinous processes, in response to pressure placed on the spinous processes of distant, high-threshold segments, and in response to impulses from proprioceptors associated with positioning, from remote areas of skin, and from higher centers (Denslow et al., 1947) (Fig. 1-10). Facilitated segments are chronically hyperirritable and hyperresponsive. Muscles in the region are maintained in a hypertonic state, which constricts the available spinal motion. All of the sup-

Figure 1-10. Facilitated vertebral segment. (**A**) Facilitated segment (*shaded region*) shows increased activity. (**B**) Force or stress applied some distance away from the facilitated segment produces hyperreactivity. (**C**) Both the stressed segment and the facilitated segment exhibit hyperreactivity.

portive structures and their innervations may become afferent sources of facilitation.

Reasonably, the neural controls would be expected to accommodate to the high level of activity, and this does occur in some cases. According to one theory, the muscle spindles, which monitor muscle length through gamma neuron control, are improperly set and therefore react inappropriately to stimuli. In comparison with messages sent from normally reactive neighboring neural tissue, messages sent from inappropriately reactive tissues are presented to the spinal cord and higher centers as confused. In other theories the spinal cord itself is considered able to adapt to the higher activity level and to channeling impulses to the affected region as if it were a "neurologic lens" (Korr, 1986).

Manipulation

The goal of manipulation is to restore the whole body to a state of homeostasis. This is not some standardized posture to be rigidly applied in all cases but is individually tailored to the patient. The discovery of somatic dysfunctions describes the regions to be treated. In the case of facilitated segments, whether one imagines resetting the gamma gain or reestablishing a coherent neural communication, the end effect is to bring about normal, comfortable motion.

Somatovisceral reflexes produce unmeasured changes on the internal organs. Sympathetic stimulation may promote or maintain a disease process. Relief of this source, if performed early enough, should alleviate the symptoms and the disease process. The viscerosomatic reflex is less amenable to cure. Manipulating the affected soma should have a beneficial effect in reducing symptoms, but the overall effect on the visceral component is indeterminable at this time. If we postulate a "tape loop" that promotes the whole process, then anything that breaks the cycle is of importance.

References

American Heritage Dictionary. 1969. W. Morris, Ed. Boston: Houghton Mifflin.

Beal MC 1983. Palpatory testing for somatic dysfunction in patients with cardiovascular disease. J Am Osteopath Assoc 82(11):822–831.

Bogdvk N, Jull G. 1985. The theoretical pathology of acute locked back: A basis for manipulative therapy. Manual Medicine 1:78–82.

Booth ER. 1905. History of Osteopathy and Twentieth-Century Medical Practice. Cincinnati: Press of Jennings and Graham.

Burns L. 1907. Viscero-somatic and somato-visceral spinal reflexes. J Am Osteopath Assoc 7:51–60.

Chaitow L. 1974. Osteopathy: Head to Toe Health Through Manipulation. Wellingborough, Northamptonshire: Thorsons Publishers Limited.

Chusid JG. 1976. Corrective Neuroanatomy & Functional Neurology. 16th Ed. Los Angeles: Lange.

Cox JM, Gorbis S, Dick LM, Rogers JC, Rogers FJ. 1983. Palpable musculoskeletal findings in coronary artery disease: Results of double-blind study, J Am Osteopath Assoc 82(11):832–836.

Denslow JS, Korr IM, Krems AD. 1949. Quantitative studies of chronic facilitation in human motoneuron pools. Am J Physiol 150:229–238.

Educational Council on Osteopathic Principles. 1982. Glossary of Osteopathic Terminology. Chicago: American Osteopathic Association.

Fryette HH. 1954. Principles of Osteopathic Technic. Kirksville, Missouri: Journal Printing Co. 9.

Frymann VM. 1976. The philosophy of osteopathy. Osteopath Ann 4:102–112.

Gevitz N. 1982. The D.O.'s: Osteopathic Medicine in America. Baltimore: Johns Hopkins University Press.

Haycock W. 1959. The osteopathic lesion and body unity in relation to diagnosis, prophylaxis, and therapeutics. In: Yearbook of the American Academy of Osteopathy. American Academy of Osteopathy.

Hix EL. 1976. Reflex viscerosomatic reference phenomena. Osteopath Ann 4(12):496–503.

Hoag JM. 1970. Theoretical analysis of osteopathic lesions. In: Yearbook of the American Academy of Osteopathy. Colorado Springs: American Academy of Osteopathy.

Jones BE. 1978. The difference a D.O. makes. Oklahoma City: Times-Journal Publishing Co.

Kimberly PE. 1980. Formulating a prescription for osteopathic manipulative treatment. J Am Osteopath Assoc 43–50.

Korr IM. 1947. The neural basis of the osteopathic lesion. J Am Osteopath Assoc 47:191–193.

———. 1967. The nature and basis of the trophic function of nerves: Outline of a research program. J Am Osteopath Assoc 66:74–78.

———. 1986. Somatic dysfunction, osteopathic manipulative treatment and the nervous system: A few facts, some theories, many questions. J Am Osteopath Assoc 86(2):109–114.

———, Appeltauer, GSL. 1970. Continued studies on

axonal transport of nerve proteins to muscle. J Am Osteopath Assoc 69:76–78.

————, Chornock FW, Cole WV, Wilkinson PN. 1967. Studies in trophic mechanisms: Does changing its nerve change a muscle? J Am Osteopath Assoc 66:79–80.

————, Wilkinson PN, Chornock FW. 1966. Studies in neurotrophic mechanisms (abstr). J Am Osteopath Assoc 65:990–991.

————, Wilkinson PN, Chornock FW. 1967. Axonal delivery of neuroplasmic components to muscle cells. J Am Osteopath Assoc 66:1057–1061.

————, Wright HM, Thomas PE. 1962. Effects of experimental myofascial insults on cutaneous patterns of sympathetic activity in man. J Neural Transm 23:22, 330–355.

Laughlin GM. 1924. The scope of osteopathy. J Osteopathy 31.

Magoun HI. 1948. Osteopathic diagnosis and therapy for the general practitioner. J Am Osteopath Assoc 48(4):169–172.

Mitchell F, Jr. 1979. Towards a definition of "somatic dysfunction." Osteopath Ann 7:12–25.

Nicholas AS. 1978. Palpation in osteopathic medicine. Osteopath Ann 6:304–310.

Northup GW. 1969. Orientation. In: Osteopathic Medicine. New York: McGraw-Hill.

Northup GW. 1979. Osteopathic Medicine, An American Reformation. Chicago: American Osteopathic Association.

Pansky B, Delmas JA. 1980. Review of Neuroscience. New York: Macmillan.

Postgraduate Institute of Osteopathic Medicine and Surgery. 1970. The Physiological Basis of Osteopathic Medicine. New York: The Postgraduate Institute of Osteopathic Medicine and Surgery.

Rumney I. 1976. The relevance of somatic dysfunction. In: Yearbook of the American Academy of Osteopathy. Colorado Springs: American Academy of Osteopathy.

Schmidt RF. 1978. Fundamentals of Neurophysiology. New York: Springer.

Siehl D. 1984. Andrew Taylor Still memorial lecture: The osteopathic difference—Is it only manipulation? J Am Osteopath Assoc 83:348–352.

Still AT. 1908. Autobiography. Kirksville, Missouri: Andrew T. Still.

Still AT. 1899. Philosophy of Osteopathy. Kirksville, Missouri: Published by the author.

Still AT. 1920. The Philosophy and Mechanical Principles of Osteopathy. Kansas City, Missouri: Hudson-Kimberly.

Special Committee on Osteopathic Principles and Osteopathic Techinic, Kirksville College of Osteopathy and Surgery. 1953. An interpretation of the osteopathic concept: Tentative formulation of a teaching guide for faculty, hospital staff and student body. J Osteopathy 60:8–10.

Sprafka S, Ward RC, Neff D. 1981. What characterizes an osteopathic principle? Selected responses to an open question. J Am Osteopath Assoc 81:81–85.

Stoddard A. 1959. The osteopathic spinal lesion. In: Yearbook of the Academy of Osteopathy. Carmel, California: American Academy of Osteopathy.

Truhlar RE. 1950. Doctor A.T. Still in the living. Cleveland, Ohio: R.E. Truhlar.

Walton WJ. 1971. The osteopathic lesion (somatic spinal complex). In: Yearbook of the American Academy of Osteopathy. Colorado Springs: American Academy of Osteopathy.

Warwick R, Williams PL, eds. 1973. Gray's Anatomy, 35th British Edition. Philadelphia: W.B. Saunders.

2

Soft Tissues

THE SKIN
Eileen L. DiGiovanna

The skin is the largest organ in the body. It is in constant contact with the environment, and many of its important functions have to do with protecting the body from environmental insults or with regulating the internal milieu as the external environment changes. The skin safeguards the internal structures from chemical and mechanical irritants and seals in bodily fluids to maintain a fluid internal environment. Salt and waste products are excreted through the skin. Dilation and constriction of blood vessels in the skin and evaporation of sweat from the surface of the skin aid in regulating body temperature. Finally, the skin acts as a sensory organ, relaying information about the environment to the central nervous system.

Skin Structures
The skin consists of three layers. From exterior to interior, there are the epidermis, the dermis, and the fascia. The outer, epidermal layer is made up of dead and dying cornified cells. It has no vasculature and very few nerve endings. The middle and most important dermal layer is the least dense, consisting of about five layers of cells. It contains capillaries, small vessels, and most nerve endings. Hair and nails, specialized protec-

tive structures of the skin, are derived from dermal tissue. The deep, fascial layer of skin connects to the subcutaneous tissues. More vessels and nerve endings lie in this layer.

The circulatory elements of the skin have two functions: to conduct heat and to carry nutrition to the skin. Heat conduction, perhaps the more important of these functions, is performed by venous plexi and arteriovenous anastomoses. Nutritive components are carried by the arteries and capillaries. Other structures in the skin include two types of glands, *sudiferous*, or sweat-producing glands, and *sebaceous*, or oil-producing glands.

Innervation and Sensation
The skin is innervated by the autonomic (sympathetic) nervous system and the peripheral (sensory) nervous system. Sympathetic innervation affects the blood vessels, the muscles of the hair follicles, and the glands in the skin. Sympathetic innervation of the blood vessels in the skin contributes to vasoconstriction and vasodilation. The ends of the vasoconstrictor fibers apparently secrete norepinephrine, and it is believed vasodilation results from the secretion of acetylcholine at

some of the endings. Vasodilation raises the temperature of the skin, which then becomes red, in pale-complexioned persons, or darkens, in dark-complexioned persons. Vasoconstriction results in cooling of the skin and a bluish color due to the increase in deoxygenated blood. With severe or prolonged vasoconstriction the skin hue pales as blood is squeezed out of the vessels. Sympathetic stimulation also causes sweating. These effects of sympathetic stimulation contribute to osteopathic diagnosis. Increased or decreased temperature, sweating, and changes in skin texture are associated with somatic dysfunctions in the involved area.

The skin is responsive to four types of sensation—touch (pressure), heat, cold, and pain. These sensations are detected by mechanoreceptors that are expanded nerve endings in the skin. Also present are some unmyelinated, or free, nerve endings. All four sensations are elicited in skin where only free nerve endings exist; thus, the free nerve endings apparently respond to all types of stimuli. The mechanoreceptors or expanded nerve endings (Merkel's disks and Ruffini endings) and encapsulated endings (Pacini corpuscles, Meissner's corpuscles, and Krause's end bulbs) (Fig. 2-1) appear to be sensation specific. Merkel's disks are sensitive to touch (two-point discrimination). Meissner's corpuscles are sensitive to touch, and Pacini corpuscles to deep pressure. It has been postulated that Ruffini endings are sensitive to heat and Krause's end bulbs to cold, but this is open to debate.

The Physician's Skin

Mechanoreceptors and other neural elements in the skin of the palpating physician's hand convey information about the patient. Because the dorsum of the hand is thinner skinned than the palm, temperature is best palpated with the dorsum. Merkel's disks are most numerous in the palm and especially in the finger pads, which makes the finger pads most sensitive to touch. Thickening of the skin, as in calluses, decreases sensitivity. Because the receptors fatigue, the physician may find it necessary to rest or change fingers during palpation to ensure maximum sensitivity.

Figure 2-1. Mechanoreceptors in the skin.

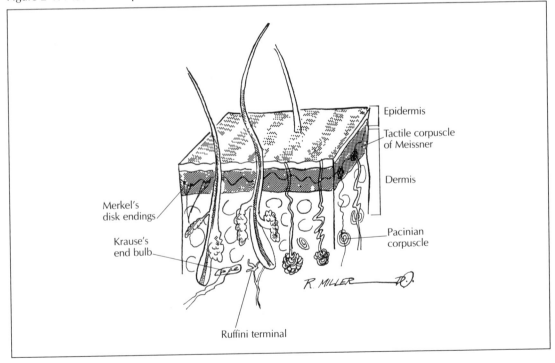

FASCIA
Nancy Brous

Anatomists define fascia as a dissectable mass of fibroelastic connective tissue. The osteopathic physician defines fascia as all the connective tissue of the body that has a supportive function, including ligaments, tendons, dural membranes, and the linings of body cavities.

Fascia is very extensive. If all other tissues and organs were removed from the body, with the fascia kept intact, one would still have a replica of human anatomy. Fascia surrounds every muscle and compartmentalizes muscle masses. It surrounds and compartmentalizes organs in the face, neck, and mediastinum. Fascia forms sheaths around nerves and vessels. It envelops the thoracic and abdominopelvic organs. It forms the pleura, pericardium, and peritoneum. Fascia connects bone to bone, muscle to bone, and forms tendinous bands and pulleys.

Fascia is continuous throughout the body. The majority of the fascial planes are arranged in a longitudinal direction. Areas of hypertonicity or muscular imbalance can impose functional restriction on the natural longitudinal glide of the body's fascial sheets. Therefore, one area of restriction can influence adjacent and distal areas.

Several functional transverse diaphragms exist in the body. Restrictions of these diaphragms can cause major alterations in the function of surrounding structures. The respiratory diaphragm permits passage of the aorta, vena cava, azygous veins, thoracic duct, vagus, and phrenic nerves. The urogenital diaphragm supports the pelvic viscera, allows sacrococcygeal mobility, and transmits the anal canal, urethra, vagina, lymphatics, and neurovascular bundles. The cranial base and dura transmit the jugular veins and cranial nerves IX, X, and XI through the jugular foramen. Any restrictions in these major transverse diaphragms will inhibit longitudinal fascial motion above and below and thus affect function of those structures it encompasses.

The fascia has varied functions. It acts to stabilize and maintain upright posture through the lumbodorsal fascia, the iliotibial band, the gluteal fascia, and the cervical fascia. Fascia also protects and supports organs, muscles, neurovascular bundles, and lymphatic channels. It restrains and binds, enclosing muscle groups while defining their motion. This delimiting function channels muscle energy into specific action, while simultaneously preventing muscles from rupturing and tearing. Therefore, fascia coordinates the action of muscle and muscle groups for a smoother, coordinated motion.

Fascia aids the circulation of body fluids. It keeps veins open and widens them as it is tensed during muscle contraction. Fascia is inherently contractile and elastic. As it contracts along the muscle, it compresses the veins within it, increasing venous return. The elasticity of the fascia pulls the veins open after they have been squeezed by contractility, resulting in a milking action. Any contraction, tension, or imbalance in the fascia can impede or inhibit this dynamic contractile-elastic activity and result in decreased venous return and congestion.

The distribution of arterial blood to any part of the body requires adequate blood pressure and unobstructed arterial channels. The heart must be able to contract freely in the thorax without fascial or bony restrictions. Innervation to the heart must be free from mechanical irritation along its distribution. Adequate venous return is needed. Again, any restrictions in fascial sheaths housing the neurovascular bundles or even in neighboring fascial planes can decrease blood flow to an area.

The lymphatic vessels are arranged in a superficial and a deep set. Both pierce the fascia and accompany the veins. Therefore, lymphatic drainage can also be affected by restrictions in the fascial planes.

As the immediate external environment of every living cell, fascia directly or indirectly influences the metabolism of these cells. Abnormal pressure or tension will alter the diffusion of nutrients and the elimination of wastes, resulting in alterations in cell function. A cell needs proper maintenance of osmotic pressure and tissue tension of the surrounding interstitial fluid and ground substance for proper metabolism.

The most abundant cellular component of fascia is the fibroblast. The fibroblast is under control of the endocrine system. Fibroblasts are responsible for the production of collagen and ground substance, and their response to physico-chemical changes is important. Under pressure, fibroblasts produce collagen organized along the same stress lines as the direction of force. There-fore, fascia can adapt to external stresses by cross-linking of collagen. This increase in strength can also decrease fascial flexibility and can cause re-strictions and potential compression of vessels and nerves.

Fascia directly or indirectly influences the health of the body through coordination with the musculoskeletal system, cooperation in circulat-ing body fluids, and by allowing generous passageway for nerves. Derangement in the fascial planes can result in venous congestion, abnormal reflexes, and a decreased range of motion. Thus, myofascial techniques are crucial in eliminating fascial restrictions and allowing the body to re-turn to a healthier state.

NEUROPHYSIOLOGY RELEVANT TO OSTEOPATHIC MANIPULATION
Paula D. Scariati

Neurophysiology is a complex subject; many dif-ferent types of neurons and synaptic pathways must be understood. Nevertheless, such knowl-edge is essential to understanding the mecha-nisms employed in osteopathic manipulation.

Some definitions follow:

Afferent nerve. A nerve carrying impulses to-ward the central nervous system (CNS).
Efferent nerve. A nerve carrying impulses from the CNS.
Ventral horn. The anterior portion of the gray matter in the spinal cord where efferent motor neurons leave the spinal cord.
Dorsal horn. The posterior portion of the gray matter of the spinal cord where afferent sensory nerves enter the spinal cord.
Contraction. Physiologic shortening of muscle length from its usual resting length.
Contracture. Abnormal, fixed shortening of muscle length.
Agonist. Muscle or muscle groups primarily re-sponsible for performing some motion (i.e., flexion).
Antagonist. Muscle or muscle groups that op-pose the motion of the agonist and produce an opposite motion (i.e., extension).

Neuroanatomy and Neurophysiology
Sensory nerves carry impulses from sense organs to the spinal cord or brain. In either case they en-ter the spinal cord via the dorsal horn. Those des-tined to terminate locally end in the gray matter of the spinal cord, where they produce local seg-mental responses such as excitation, facilitation, and reflex actions. Those with distant termina-tions travel to integrative areas higher in the spi-nal cord, the brain stem, or the cerebral cortex.

The changes created by osteopathic manipula-tive treatment are mediated at a local level but have the potential to be far-reaching and interac-tive. Proper control of muscle function depends on local excitation in conjunction with continu-ous feedback from the brain about muscle status.

Ventral motor neurons give rise to two types of nerves that exit the anterior horn to innervate skeletal muscle, alpha motor neurons and gamma motor neurons. Alpha motor neurons transmit impulses via Ar nerve fibers to innervate large skeletal muscle fibers. A single alpha motor neu-ron excites a few to several hundred skeletal mus-cle fibers known as the *motor unit.* Gamma motor neurons transmit impulses via Ar nerve fibers to innervate small skeletal muscle fibers called in-trafusal fibers. These fibers compose the muscle spindle (Fig. 2-2).

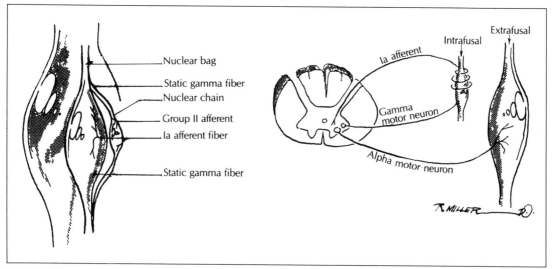

Figure 2-2. Innervation of the intrafusal muscle fiber.

Interneurons, as the name implies, are bipolar neurons that connect two other neurons. They are located in all areas of the spinal cord, not just the anterior horn. Interneurons are small, highly excitable, and often spontaneously active. They can fire as rapidly as 1,500 times per second.

Certain interneurons located in the anterior horn in close association with the motor neurons constitute the Renshaw inhibitory system, which causes inhibition of neurons surrounding the motor neuron carrying a given excitatory impulse. This phenomenon is known as *recurrent inhibition*. The function of the Renshaw inhibitory system is to sharpen the signal of the motor unit. It prevents the signal from diffusing into adjacent nerve fibers, which would weaken the signal.

Neuromuscular Reflexes

Every muscle has two separate reflex patterns, each with a different function. The muscle spindle reflex sends information to the nervous system about muscle length or the rate of change in muscle length. The Golgi tendon reflex sends information to the nervous system about muscle tension or the rate of change in tension. Both reflexes function at a subconscious level.

MUSCLE SPINDLE REFLEX

Muscle spindles are mechanoreceptors that are widely distributed between skeletal muscle fibers in the belly of the muscle. They occur in parallel with the skeletal muscle fibers, and the connective tissue around the muscle spindles is continuous with the connective tissue around the other muscle fibers. In conjunction with feedback contraction of the skeletal muscle fibers (mediated through the Golgi tendon organs), the muscle spindles mediate a response to a load placed on the muscle; this is known as the *load reflex*. Muscle spindles have a dampening function as well: they prevent some types of oscillation and jerkiness in body movement. Finally, in addition to serving at a subconscious level, the muscle spindle reflex is invoked in voluntary motor activity.

Muscle spindles are composed of *intrafusal muscle fibers*, which come in two types: nuclear bag fibers, so called because their nuclei appear to be bunched in the center of the cell, as in a bag, and nuclear chain fibers, so called because their nuclei are lined up in single file in the center of the fiber. There are two to five nuclear bag fibers and six to ten nuclear chain fibers in a typical muscle spindle. The components of an intrafusal muscle spindle are diagrammed in Figure 2-3.

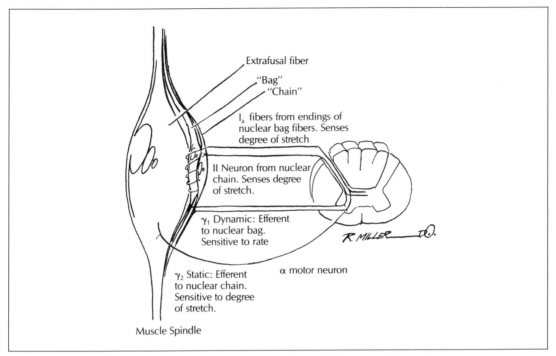

Figure 2-3. Components and innervation of the intrafusal muscle fiber (muscle spindle).

The sensory afferents of the muscle spindle comprise group Ia fibers (primary endings), which send branches to every intrafusal fiber in the muscle spindle, and group II fibers (secondary endings), which innervate the nuclear chain endings only. The larger primary endings (Ia) surround the center of the muscle spindle, while the smaller secondary endings (II) terminate on either side of the primary endings.

Motor efferents of the muscle spindle consist of static and dynamic gamma fibers, which make different contributions to the stretch reflex mediated by the muscle spindle. Static gamma fibers primarily innervate nuclear chain fibers, producing tonic activity in Ia afferent fibers. Dynamic gamma fibers primarily innervate nuclear bag fibers, generating phasic activity in Ia afferent fibers. Overall, the gamma motor neurons serve two functions. (1) They cause the intrafusal fibers to contract, thereby stretching the muscle spindle and causing it to fire. This is the mechanism for maintaining postural tone. (2) They cause the intrafusal fibers to contract sufficiently to stretch the muscle spindle toward threshold, thereby in-

creasing the sensitivity of the muscle spindle apparatus.

Stretch reflex. Stimulation of the muscle spindle occurs either with lengthening of the whole muscle, which stretches the midpoint and excites the receptor, or with contraction of the end points of the intrafusal fibers, which also stretches the midpoint and excites the fiber. Stretching the muscle spindle increases the rate of firing, while shortening the muscle spindle decreases the rate of firing. Thus, the musculoskeletal system can send a positive or negative signal to the spinal cord to indicate the status of the muscle.

Slow stretch of the length of the receptor portion of the muscle spindle produces the *static stretch reflex.* The number of impulses transmitted from both the primary and secondary endings increases in proportion to the amount of stretch, and signals are transmitted as long as the muscle is stretched. The static stretch reflex is thought to be mediated primarily by nuclear chain fibers, since these are the only fiber type innervated by both primary and secondary endings. The static gamma fibers, which mainly excite the nuclear

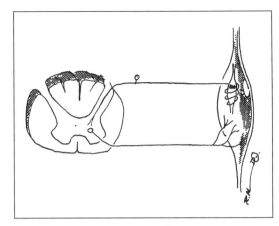

Figure 2-4. Dynamic stretch reflex.

chain fibers, enhance the static reflex but contribute little to the dynamic reflex.

Sudden lengthening of the muscle spindle receptor produces the *dynamic stretch reflex* (Fig. 2-4). The dynamic reflex, more powerful than the static reflex, is mediated by primary (Ia) endings only; and because only Ia endings innervate the nuclear bag fibers, it is assumed that nuclear bag fibers are responsible for the dynamic response. The dynamic gamma motor fibers enhance the muscle spindle's dynamic stretch reflex but have little effect on the static reflex.

Neuronal circuitry of muscle spindle reflexes. The monosynaptic pathway, in which sensory input fibers synapse directly with motor output fibers, governs the primary endings (Ia) that mediate the dynamic stretch reflex. The type II fibers may occasionally terminate monosynaptically, but most terminate on multiple interneurons in the gray matter of the spinal cord. Type II fibers transmit more delayed signals to the anterior motor horn.

GOLGI TENDON REFLEX

Golgi tendon organs, sometimes called tendon spindles, are encapsulated sensory mechanoreceptors located in mammalian tendons between the muscle and the tendon insertions. There is one tendon organ for every three to 25 muscle fibers. Golgi tendon organs detect the degree of skeletal muscle tension and convey this information to the CNS; similarly, they aid in maintaining the degree of muscle tension dictated by the CNS. The Golgi tendon organs are in series with the extrafusal fibers and are stretched whenever the muscle contracts.

Neural pathway. Afferent neurons from the Golgi tendon mechanoreceptors are larger, myelinated neurons of the Ib group. Upon entering the gray matter of the spinal cord, the afferent Ib neuron synapses with inhibitory interneurons. It also synapses with other interneurons that ascend to higher CNS levels. The inhibitory interneurons synapse with the large alpha motor neurons located in the anterior gray horn of the spinal cord. The alpha motor neurons that are inhibited are the ones to the same muscle in which the Ib afferents originate (Fig. 2-5).

Basic reflex. Like the muscle spindle, the Golgi tendon organ has a dynamic and a static response.

Figure 2-5. Golgi tendon reflex.

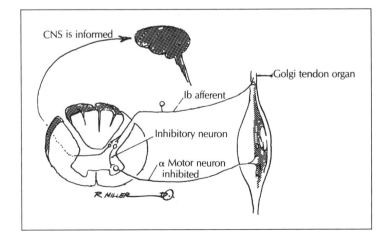

Increased tension in a skeletal muscle distorts the Golgi tendon organ, producing a generator potential that initiates an action potential; the action potential travels over the Ib neurons to the spinal cord. Afferent action potentials activate the interneurons, which inhibit the alpha motor neurons back to the skeletal muscle. The increased muscle tension that initiates the reflex can result from contraction of the skeletal muscle or from marked passive stretch of the muscle.

Since the basic Golgi tendon reflex results in inhibition of the muscle—the opposite effect of the stretch reflex produced by the muscle spindle—this reflex is called the *inverse stretch reflex*, or *autogenic inhibition*, more commonly known as the lengthening reaction or the clasp-knife reflex.

Flexor Reflexes
CROSSED EXTENSOR REFLEX
The crossed extensor reflex is the response elicited, by stimulation of a given muscle (e.g., the biceps of the right arm, causing flexion), on the muscle of opposite function on the opposite side of the body (e.g., contraction of the triceps in the left arm, creating extension). The crossed extensor reflex is mediated via many sensory and motor interneurons in the spinal cord. It usually occurs in response to prolonged stimulation (200–500 msec) after a pain stimulus and continues long after the provoking stimulus has been withdrawn (Fig. 2-6).

RECIPROCAL INNERVATION
Reciprocal innervation is the stretching of a given muscle, stimulating the contraction of that muscle as well as the inhibition of the antagonist muscle.

Causes of Muscle Pain
Muscle spasms of diverse origin can cause pain. Prolonged muscle contractions irritate the splinting muscle and the associated ligaments and ten-

Figure 2-6. Flexor reflex. Shown is the crossed extensor reflex with reciprocal inhibition.

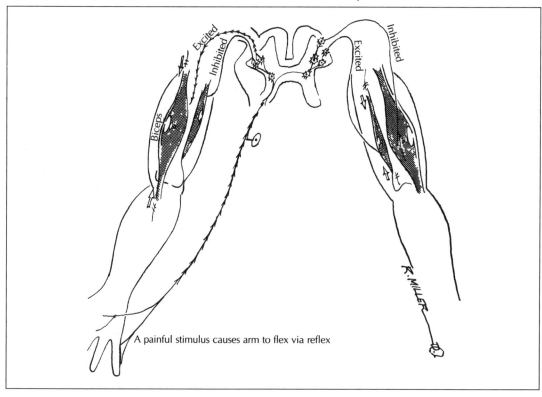

A painful stimulus causes arm to flex via reflex

dons, producing further spasm and initiating a pain cycle. The severity of the pain reflects the duration of a sustained contraction.

Ischemia, or localized anemia due to obstruction of blood at a specific site, is a well-known cause of muscle pain, occipital tension headaches, and intermittent claudication. Retention of irritating metabolites also causes muscle pain. Blood flow to the area must be increased in order to remove these substances.

Pain due to trauma or irritation (e.g., by an osteophyte) can be alleviated with the use of therapies that decrease muscle tension and improve local tissue circulation, affording subjective and objective relief from pain and spasm.

Failure of calcium to accumulate in the sarcoplasmic reticulum, abnormal interaction between the muscle fibril's actin and myosin, and anxiety may all cause muscle pain.

Practical Applications of Neurophysiology in Osteopathic Manipulative Treatment

MYOFASCIAL/MUSCLE TECHNIQUES

1. **Stretch reflex:** Quick stretch of a muscle excites the muscle spindle, causing reflex contraction. To prevent this reflex, myofascial therapy is done slowly for correction of contracted or contractured muscles. A quick stretch can be employed if the goal of therapy is to stimulate muscle tone.
2. **Moist heat** applied to muscle usually increases its elastic response to stretch. It also aids in increasing circulation.
3. Connective tissue placed under prolonged **mild tension** shows plastic elongation.
4. **Servo-assist function of the muscle spindle reflex:** Should the extrafusal fibers contract less than the intrafusal fibers, the muscle spindles will maintain a stretch reflex to further excite the extrafusal fibers. This technique is used in active resistive myofascial therapy.
5. **Golgi tendon organ reflex:** When tension on the tendon becomes extreme, the inhibitory effect from the tendon organ can become so great that it causes a sudden relaxation of the entire muscle. This technique is used in active resistive myofascial therapy.
6. **Reciprocal innervation:** When a stretch reflex excites one muscle, it simultaneously inhibits the antagonist muscle. Reciprocal innervation

is of use in active myofascial therapy, with or without resistance.
7. **Crossed extensor reflex:** When a stretch reflex excites one muscle, it simultaneously excites the contralateral antagonist muscle; the motion created crosses from one side of the spine to the other side in an X pattern. The crossed extensor reflex is helpful in active myofascial therapy, usually with resistance.

COUNTERSTRAIN TREATMENT

The theories of counterstrain treatment are discussed in Chapter 5; here we will consider only the neurophysiologic underpinnings of the theories.

Prolonged shortening of a muscle allows shortening of both the intrafusal (muscle spindle) and extrafusal fibers. The gamma motor neurons then increase their firing rate to maintain tone in the muscle, resulting in hypersensitive muscle spindle fibers in the shortened muscle. If the shortened, hypersensitive muscle is now lengthened rapidly (the muscle spindle responds to both length and rate of change of length), a reflex overstimulation of the alpha motor neurons will occur and muscle spasm will ensue. The sensory signals also travel to the higher centers of the CNS, which are not capable of interpreting them properly and thus respond with excessive gamma motor stimulation, which maintains the spasm.

Reshortening the muscle allows the muscle spindle to shorten and resume normal firing. The CNS is now able to interpret the signals properly so it resets its gamma motor neurons. This takes about 90 seconds to accomplish.

MUSCLE ENERGY TECHNIQUES

Muscle energy treatment combines elements of the Golgi tendon reflex, reciprocal innervation, and elastic stretch. Muscle energy techniques that use the Golgi tendon reflex are much like active myofascial techniques in that extreme tension is used to create an inhibitory effect that will produce a sudden relaxation.

In reciprocal innervation when a stretch excites one muscle, it simultaneously inhibits its antagonist.

Direct muscle pull causes an elastic stretch, such as occurs during periods of relaxation between active contractions and also at the passive stretch administered at the end of muscle energy treatment.

PALPATION
Eileen L. DiGiovanna

Palpation is a particularly important means of uncovering information. Palpation can disclose subtle changes in the texture of the soft tissues of the body—the skin, fascia, muscles, ligaments, and tendons. Tissue changes that occur in response to the effects of sympathetic innervation may be manifested by an increase or decrease in skin temperature or moisture. Edema of the underlying soft tissues may produce a palpable bogginess. Changes in the quality of joint motion may be felt before they produce visible symptoms. Deeper palpation is used to search for masses, outline organ size and consistency, test muscle tone, and feel the impulse of the heart.

During palpation, the physician concentrates on the sensations received through the fingers and hands. The distribution and depth of receptor organs determine which part of the hand is most useful in specific tests. Since the heat receptors lie deep, the ulnar or dorsal aspect of the hand, where the skin is thinner than on the palms, should be used to test for temperature changes. Touch receptors such as Merkel's disks and Meissner's corpuscles are most numerous in the pads of the fingers, making these the most sensitive areas.

Observation is an important aid to palpation. The area being examined should be inspected for color changes (pallor) or erythema (redness). Increased erythema may indicate infection or inflammation and commonly occurs with acute somatic dysfunction. Pallor may occur with chronic somatic dysfunction. The physician should also look for signs of trauma, such as scars, bruises, lacerations, abrasions, and swelling. Blemishes or masses on the skin's surface should be noted.

Palpation
The following is an organized approach to the development of palpatory skills.

Temperature Changes
1. Palpate lightly. Pressure or friction causes vasodilation, creating temperature changes.
2. See which area of the hand is most sensitive to temperature: the back or side of the hand, the fingertips, the wrist. (Thinner skinned areas are most sensitive).
3. Palpate various areas of the back to discriminate temperature differences. The thoracic area is usually warmer, owing to the underlying heart and great vessels. Compare the skin temperature in several individuals.

Evaluation of Skin Drag
1. Slide fingertips lightly across the surface of the skin to see if any drag can be felt on the fingertips.
2. Increased drag may be due to a fine film of moisture.
3. A decrease in drag may be due to excessive moisture, oily skin, or abnormally atrophic skin.

Evaluation of Erythema
1. Rub the skin with the fingers in a firm stroke. Observe for blanching (whiteness) or erythema (redness). Note the length of time required for the skin color to return to normal.
   Note: Are both sides equally red? Does the redness fade equally? Does one side remain red longer than the other? Areas of acute somatic dysfunction tend to remain red longer.

Evaluation of Skin Texture
1. Palpate for roughness or smoothness. Compare individual skin differences.
2. Feel for sebaceous activity (oiliness).
3. Try palpating through cloth to get the feel of its effect on sensations.

Palpation of Fluid in Tissues
1. Excess fluid in tissues is called *edema*. Edema results in a spongy or boggy feel to the tissues. Edema of significant proportions may accumulate over the sacrum or anterior aspect of the lower legs and ankles. It is also found in hives or welts.

Turgor (Elastic Rebound of the Skin)
1. Pick up the skin, then release it.
2. Observe how it returns to its former tautness. If

the skin returns to its original state immediately, it has normal turgor. If the skin remains tented, it has poor turgor.

Lack of turgor is found in dehydration, aging, and certain metabolic diseases.

Tenderness
1. Tenderness is a subjective rather than an objective finding. Palpation of certain areas may cause the sensation of pain to the patient. This is known as tenderness. Because it is subjective, this finding is not as reliable as the objective findings of the physician.

LAYER BY LAYER PALPATION
During palpation, it is helpful to mentally visualize the depth of the palpation. A gradually increasing pressure of the fingertips gives the sensations and textures of structures deeper and deeper in the body.

Subcutaneous Tissues
Beneath the surface of the skin lie the subcutaneous tissues, consisting of various connective tissues, fascia, and fat. These tissues normally have a slightly spongy feel. Edema fluid may collect here and produce a "doughy" feel.

In these tissues lie some of the superficial blood vessels. Palpate veins over the back of the hand or in the antecubital fossa. Occlusion with a tourniquet makes the veins more prominent. Note the springy feel. Palpate the radial and carotid arteries. Note that they are much firmer than unoccluded veins. Palpate the back for any abnormal tensions in the subcutaneous tissues. This may indicate contracture or fibrous changes of the fascia.

Muscle
Muscle tissue consists of bundles of fibers arranged in parallel fashion.

1. Press more deeply into the tissues until you contact the firmer muscle tissues.
2. Select several large muscles (trapezius, biceps, sternocleidomastoid, deltoid) and follow the directions of their fibers to the muscle attachments.
3. Palpate the paraspinal muscles, feeling for the following:
   a. **Tone:** The normal feel of a resting muscle (if

palpation is too rough it may change the tone):
   i. *Hypertonic*—an increase in normal tone
   ii. *Hypotonic*—a decrease in normal tone
   iii. *Atonic*—no tone; a limp, flaccid muscle
   b. **Contraction:** Normal tension built up in muscle as it shortens
   c. **Contracture:** Abnormal fixing of a muscle in a shortened position with fibrous changes in the tissue
   d. **Spasm:** Abnormal contraction maintained beyond physiologic need
   e. **Bogginess:** Increased fluid in a hypertonic muscle; feels like a wet sponge
   f. **Ropiness:** Cordlike or ropelike feel to a muscle that has been chronically contracted
   g. **Stringiness:** A finer version of ropiness—the muscle feels as if it were made of tense strings

Tendons
Tendons are fibroelastic strands of connective tissue attaching muscle to bone.

1. Palpate the Achilles tendon at the heel and the biceps tendon at the elbow.

Ligaments
Ligaments are tough fibrous bands that connect bone to bone. Since they lie very deep, they are difficult to palpate. Some are not accessible to palpation.

1. The lateral collateral ligament of the knee may be palpated by asking the patient to cross his or her legs so that one ankle lies on the knee of the other leg. The knee should be flexed and the thigh externally rotated. The ligament may be palpated crossing the joint space laterally and slightly posteriorly.

References

Barry G. 1984. Lecture, Physiology. Old Westbury, New York: New York College of Osteopathic Medicine.

Becker FR. 1975. The meaning of fascia and continuity. Osteopath Ann 3:8–32.

Bullock J, Boyle J III, Wang MB, Ajello RR. 1984. The National Medical Series for Independent Study: Physiology. New York: John Wiley & Sons.

Cathie AG. 1966. Manual of Osteopathic Principles

and Practice—Second year, article C-17. Philadelphia: Philadelphia College of Osteopathy.

Ettlinger H. 1987. Myofascial Release. Osteopathic
Principles and Practice. Old Westbury, New York:
NYCOM.

Ganong WF. 1981. Review of Medical Physiology. Palo
Alto, Calif: Lange Medical Publications.

Guyton AC. 1986. Textbook of Medical Physiology,
7th ed. Philadelphia: W.B. Saunders Co.

Hollinshead HW. 1974. Textbook of Anatomy, 3rd ed.
Hagerstown, Md: Harper & Row.

Kandel E, Schwartz JH. 1985. Principles of Neural Science. New York: Science Publishing.

Langley LL, Telford IR, Christenson JB. 1980. Dynamic
Anatomy and Physiology. New York: McGraw-Hill
Book Co.

Moritan T, Moramatsu S, Neuo M. 1987. Activity of

the motor unit during concentric and eccentric contractions. Am J Physiol 66:338–350.

Nicholas AS. 1978. Palpation in osteopathic medicine. Osteopath Ann 67:36–42.

Sauer GC. 1980. Manual of Skin Diseases, 4th ed. Philadelphia: J.B. Lippincott Co.

Schiowitz S, DiGiovanna E, Ausman P. 1981. An Osteopathic Approach to Diagnosis and Treatment.

Smith PE, Copenhaver WM, eds. 1984. Bailey's Textbook of Histology. Baltimore: Williams & Wilkins
Co.

Taber W. 1970. Taber's Cyclopedic Medical Dictionary,
2nd ed. Philadelphia: F.A. Davis Co.

Upledger JE, Vredeboogd JD. 1983. Craniosacral Therapy, chap. 5. Seattle: Eastland Press.

Williams PL, Warwick R, eds. 1980. Gray's Anatomy,
36th ed. Philadelphia: W.B. Saunders Co.

3

Static Symmetry

STATIC SYMMETRY
Stanley Schiowitz

Any observation of a patient that can be used to differentiate normal from abnormal function is an asset in determining a differential diagnosis. Changes in skin color, gait, or regional motion restrictions are used daily to this end. This chapter describes ideal and variant postures of an immobile, upright patient as seen in the sagittal, anterior, and posterior planes. The technique of examination and common causes of abnormal findings are described in the next section.

Sagittal Plane Symmetry
In an ideal erect posture, a plumb line dropped from the ceiling along the body's midline would pass through the following points:

1. Slightly posterior to the apex of the coronal suture
2. Through the external auditory meatus
3. Through the bodies of most of the cervical vertebrae
4. Through the shoulder joint
5. Through the bodies of the lumbar vertebrae
6. Slightly posterior to the axis of the hip joint
7. Slightly anterior to the axis of the knee joint
8. Slightly anterior to the lateral malleolus

Any deviation from these relationships is considered a normal variant or an abnormal postural relationship.

PHYSIOLOGIC CURVES IN THE SAGITTAL PLANE
The adult has four normal sagittal curves, as follows:

1. In the cervical region, C1 to C7, convex forward, normal lordosis
2. In the thoracic region, T1 to T12, concave forward, normal kyphosis
3. In the lumbar region, L1 to L5, convex forward, normal lordosis
4. In the sacral region, the fused sacrum, concave forward

These curves are physiologic, biomechanical, and were created by the body's functional development. At birth, the cervical, thoracic, and lumbar vertebrae form one continuous kyphotic (concave forward) curve. As the cervical extensor muscles develop, allowing the head to stay raised, the normal cervical (convex forward) lordosis develops. As the child begins to stand and walk, the back muscles strengthen and normal lumbar lordosis (convex forward) is achieved. This process begins at about age three years and is fully developed by the tenth year. The thoracic spine retains its kyphotic posture, but the angle of the curve is usually decreased.

TRANSITIONAL ARTICULATIONS

The normal sagittal spinal curve changes from anterior convexity to anterior concavity and back at specific articulations: C7 on T1, T12 on L1, and L5 on the sacral base. These articulations have special osteologic constructions that assist in maintaining balance and reduce local mechanical stress. A transition in the curve at any other articulation causes local strain and dysfunction.

The sagittal spinal curves are interrelated in function. An increase in lumbar lordosis will result in increased thoracic kyphosis and increased cervical lordosis. In addition, the curves promote spinal flexibility and strength, allowing the spine to withstand stress. The spine has elastic properties under force, aiding the supporting function of the ligaments and muscles. A straight spine would transmit vector forces through the vertebral bodies, contributing to fracture.

SACRAL BASE RELATIONSHIP

The normal angle between the lumbar spine and the sacral base is 25 to 35 degrees. A greater or lesser angle will affect the lumbar curve and cause compensatory changes in the curves higher in the spine.

Flexion of the sacrum in the sagittal plane increases lumbar lordosis (anterior convexity). This will be accompanied by a similar increase in thoracic kyphosis and cervical lordosis. Extension of the sacrum reduces the lumbar anterior convexity, decreasing lumbar lordosis and providing a similar flattening of the thoracic and cervical curves.

COMMON VARIATIONS IN SAGITTAL POSTURES

1. **Kypholordotic posture** (Fig. 3-1)
   Head forward
   Cervical spine lordotic
   Thoracic spine kyphotic
   Scapulae abducted
   Lumbar spine lordotic
   Anterior pelvic tilt
   Hip joints slightly flexed

Figure 3-1. Kypholordotic posture, lateral view.

   Knee joints extended
   Plantar flexion of ankle joints in relation
      to angle of legs
   Anterior bulging of abdomen
2. **Swayback posture** (Fig. 3-2)
   Head forward
   Cervical spine lordotic, thoracic spine kyphotic
   Decreased lordosis of lumbar spine
   Posterior tilt of pelvis
   Hip and knee joints hyperextended
3. **Flat back posture**
   Head forward
   Cervical spine has slightly increased lordosis

Figure 3-2. Swayback posture, lateral view. Body is anterior to plumb line.

Thoracic spine slightly kyphotic in upper portion, then flattens in lower segments

Lumbar lordosis flattened

Hips and knees extended

4. **Military-bearing posture**

Created by drilling in "chest out, stomach in" position

Head tilted slightly posteriorly

Cervical curve and thoracic curve normal

Chest elevated, creating anterior cervical and posterior thoracic deviation from plumb line

Increased lordosis of lumbar curve

Anterior pelvic tilt

Knees extended

Ankles plantar flexed

5. **Anterior postural deviation**

Entire body leans forward, deviating anteriorly from the plumb line

Patient's weight supported by metatarsals

6. **Posterior postural deviation**

Entire body leans backward, deviating posteriorly from plumb line

Balance maintained by anterior thrust of pelvis and hips

Marked lordosis from midthoracic spine down

7. **Rotary posture**

Body rotated to right or left

Entire body may be involved, with rotation beginning from ankles and proceeding up

Lateral alignment appears completely different when viewed from right and left sides; in scoliotic posture, rotation primarily of thorax, in direction of scoliotic convexity

8. **Lumbar lordosis**

Number of variations, described by increase in lumbar curve and height of curve

Simple lordosis: lordotic curve increased but contained within the lumbar region

High lordosis: lumbar lordotic curve passes into thoracic region, including half to two thirds of thoracic spine in anterior convexity; apex of curve moves upward toward first lumbar vertebra

These described variations of posture are commonly created by changes in pelvic, hip, and knee angles, or by multiple combinations of muscle hypo- and hypertonicities.

LOCALIZED THORACIC FLATTENING

The examiner may find a localized area of thoracic spine, encompassing no more than three contiguous vertebrae, that exhibits severe flattening of the usual kyphotic pattern. This relationship can occur at an area of change of direction of a scoliotic curve, such as a right convexity becoming a left convexity. If rotation in both directions is severe, the spinous processes of the vertebrae involved will be rotated off the midline. Failure of these processes to point directly posteriorly causes the flattened appearance.

Localized thoracic flattening may also be due to chronic somatic dysfunction in two contiguous vertebrae. The examiner should look for a segmentally related visceral-somatic reflex pattern as the underlying cause. Chronic visceral pathology can cause this condition.

Posterior Plane Symmetry

In a completely symmetric posture (Fig. 3-3), a plumb line dropped from the ceiling to the floor would pass through the following points:

1. The inion
2. The midline of the vertebrae
3. The midline of the sacrum
4. The midline of the coccyx
5. A point midway between both medial malleoli

In addition, all the points of reference described for sequential observation in the next section (Technique of Static Symmetry Examination) should be level and symmetric.

SCOLIOSIS

Muscles and ligaments balance the spine bilaterally. A second group of muscles maintains the position and alignment of the scapular girdle with respect to the spine. A difference in function between muscles and ligaments on the two sides of the spine will pull the spine out of alignment. The spine is not rigid but is made up of multiple movable vertebral links. In response to asymmetric pull, one or more vertebrae will move from the position of symmetry. This vertebral motion can occur in three planes—the sagittal plane (flexion-extension), horizontal plane (rotation), or frontal plane (side bending)—and always represents a combination of multiple planar motions.

Scoliosis is defined as an appreciable deviation of a group of vertebrae from the normal straight vertical line of the spine, as viewed in the posterior plane. Scoliosis can be structural (organic) or functional. A structural curve is fixed: when the patient side bends into the convexity of the curve, it does not straighten out. A functional scoliotic pattern will correct with side bending. If an acute muscle contracture is causing a scoliotic appearance, placing the patient in the prone position will straighten the curve. A functional scoliotic curve that remains uncorrected for a number of years can give rise to musculoskeletal changes and become a fixed structural curve.

Figure 3-3. Posterior view of the body. An ideal plumb line alignment is shown.

Harrison Fryette in *Principles of Osteopathic Technique* discussed specific coupled motion patterns. Of relevance here, when the spine is at rest, normal lateral flexion in one direction will cause the vertebral body to rotate in the opposite direction. (This rule applies only to the thoracic and lumbar regions.) If a group of vertebrae side bends toward the right, the vertebral bodies will rotate to the left. If this vertebral position is fixed, the patient would have a scoliotic curve. The scoliosis is said to have a *left convexity*. The spinous

Figure 3-4. C-shaped curve due to sacral base unleveling, posterior view.

changes requires a thorough understanding of functional anatomy.

What happens to the spine when the sacral base is not level? In the frontal plane, sacral base unleveling will cause a lumbar scoliotic pattern convex in the direction of the caudal sacral side, if the spine is flexible. The convexity may continue up through the thoracic region to create one thoracolumbar C-shaped scoliotic curve (Fig. 3-4). The body tries to compensate for the imbalance created by the C curve by creating a secondary, compensatory curve above the first lumbar curve. The side of convexity of the second curve is opposite that of the primary curve, producing an S-shaped curve (Fig. 3-5). Additional compensatory scoliotic curves can develop higher in the spine, into the cervical region, with alternating convexities. Because the body always attempts to maintain the eyes on a level plane, the last compensatory maneuver may be side bending of the head. The body waist crease lines usually follow the pattern of the largest scoliotic asymmetry. The waist crease would have the most acute angle at the site and side of the greatest lateral flexion concave curve.

FACTORS THAT COMMONLY INFLUENCE OR CAUSE SCOLIOSIS (see Chap. 29)
1. Structural or organic scoliosis—all causes
2. Bone deformities caused by congenital etiology, trauma, or disease
3. Muscle tone changes due to hypo- or hypertonicity, hypertrophy, or atrophy
4. Postural changes created by habits or occupation
5. Unilateral structural changes: Short leg or unilateral flat foot or pronation. Tibial torsion, knee deformity, or hip deformity. Sacral torsion or pelvic torsion
6. Somatic dysfunctions

processes are deviated to the right of the midline and the left transverse processes are rotated posteriorly. If the thoracic region is involved, the rib cage will rotate and side bend with the vertebrae. The ribs will be more posterior and separated on the left side. The scapular girdle may follow the rib cage in its displacement.

Muscle imbalance, representing unilateral hypo- or hypertonicity, will create scoliotic patterns. The examiner must be aware of the line of force of the muscles involved, and of the complexity of multiple muscle actions at one region. The assignment of cause or effect to postural

Common Variations of Frontal Postures
1. **Right-handedness**
    a. Upper thoracic scoliosis, concave to right
    b. Right shoulder lower than left
    c. Right buttock deviated away from midline
2. **Left-handedness**
    a. Upper thoracic scoliosis, concave to left
    b. Left shoulder lower than right
    c. Left buttock deviated away from midline

Figure 3-5. S-shaped curve compensating for thoracolumbar scoliosis, posterior view.

4. **C-type compensated structural scoliosis**
   a. Thoracic and lumbar scoliotic convexity form one continuous curve in same direction
   b. Rib cage rotated posteriorly with thoracic convexity
   c. Buttocks not deviated away from midline
   d. Iliac crest heights may be level
5. **Lateral pelvic tilt functional curve, cephalad on right, C-type**
   a. Thoracic and lumbar curves continuous and convex to left
   b. Scapula lower on right
   c. Rib cage rotated posteriorly on left
   d. Waist crease has more acute angle on right
   e. Neck laterally tilted to left
6. **Lateral pelvic tilt functional curve, cephalad on right, S-type**
   a. If compensated, should act as described in item 3, except that iliac crest height is higher on right
7. **Unilateral erector spinal muscle hypertonicity**
   a. Side bending of spine in direction of hypertonic muscle
   b. Scoliotic convexity in opposite direction
   c. Elevated iliac crest on side of hypertonicity
   d. Placing patient prone should change above findings
8. **Unilateral upper trapezius muscle hypertonicity**
   a. Head tilted toward side of hypertonic muscle
   b. Shoulder girdle elevated on affected side
   c. Scapula on hypertonic muscle side rotated upward and slightly adducted

The patterns of asymmetry described in this chapter are not all-inclusive. The body exhibits various biomechanical responses to all factors that influence the musculoskeletal system.

3. **S-type compensated structural scoliosis**
   a. The lumbar and thoracic scoliotic convexities are in opposite directions
   b. The rib cage will rotate posteriorly with the thoracic convexity
   c. The shoulders may be level
   d. The iliac crest heights may be level
   e. The buttocks are not deviated away from the mid line

TECHNIQUE OF STATIC SYMMETRY EXAMINATION
Stanley Schiowitz

A postural examination begins with the patient and physician in a fixed, reproducible position, so that observations may be correlated with observations made on future examinations. The patient stands on a level surface, without shoes. All extremities should be in full extension. The feet are placed six to eight inches apart with the heels in the same frontal plane and the toes abducted about 15 degrees. The physician stands facing the aspect of the patient to be evaluated (front, back, or side) and at a sufficient distance to permit a complete body view. In the course of the examination the physician will step closer to observe local areas of interest. The examiner's eyes should be at the level of the part being viewed, which may entail crouching or kneeling during evaluation of lower body portions. Light palpation may be used to confirm anatomic landmarks or observations. Areas of observation are highlighted in Fig. 3-6.

Posterior View
For posterior inspection, a good method is to observe the patient in the following sequence:

Distant Evaluation, Posterior View
1. General observation of gross body symmetry and asymmetry
2. Achilles tendon
3. Medial malleoli
4. Popliteal lines
5. Gluteal creases
6. Greater trochanters
7. Posterior superior iliac spines
8. Heights of iliac crests
9. Thoracolumbar spines for deviations from midline symmetry, or flattening
10. Waist creases
11. Level of inferior angles of scapula, abduction-adduction
12. Rib cage rotation or scapular rotation
13. Level of shoulders
14. Level of fingertips

15. Deviation of cervical spine and skull from midline
16. Level of earlobes

Note the following factors:

1. Head
2. Earlobes
3. Neck
4. Shoulders
5. Shoulder girdles
6. Spine
7. Rib cage
8. Waist crease lines
9. Iliac crests
10. Gluteal creases
11. Fingertips
12. Popliteal creases
13. Achilles tendons
14. Heels

After gaining an overall impression, the examiner steps within arm's length of the patient and adds palpation to confirm visual observation. The sequence of observations is repeated.

Close Evaluation with Palpation, Posterior View
1. Is the head straight? Palpate the inion. Is it in the midline?
2. With one finger on the inion, place a finger of the other hand at the gluteal cleft. Are they in a line directly above each other?
3. Touch the earlobes; measure their heights. Touch the tips of the mastoid bones. Are they level?
4. Are the neck and head tilted?
5. Put one finger of each hand on the right and left trapezius muscles where the neck meets the trunk. Are they level?
6. Slide those fingers laterally to the top of each acromium process. Are they level?
7. Place one finger at the inferior angle of each scapula, about the level of the seventh thoracic vertebra. Are they level?

Figure 3-6. Points of interest on the static symmetry examination. (**A**) Posterior view. (**B**) Anterior view. (**C**) Sagittal view.

8. Move both fingers up the vertebral borders of the scapulae to their spinous processes. Are they level?

9. Place a palm flat on the posterior surface of each scapula, with your fingers resting on the superior scapular border. Are the scapulae rotated? Are they level?

10. Have the patient bend forward. Slide your palms over the angles of the ribs. Is there an exaggerated rib hump indicating scoliotic convexity?

11. Place one finger on the spinous process of the first thoracic vertebra. Slide it down the spine, one vertebra at a time, to the sacrum. Are the spinous processes symmetric with respect to each other in all three planes?
    a. *Frontal plane*—feel for deviation from the midline.
    b. *Sagittal plane*—feel for depression or prominence.
    c. *Horizontal plane*—feel the space between the tips of the spinous processes. Are they equal?
    d. Do areas of the spine seem flat?

12. Follow the waist crease lines. Are the angles equal? Does the more acute angle coincide with the concavity of a spinal scoliosis?

13. Measure the posterior superior iliac spines bilaterally. Place your thumb or index finger at each dimple in the lower back. Identify the most prominent (posterior) bony point. Bend down by flexing your knees, so that your eyes are at finger level. Note the following:
    a. Are they at the same height?
    b. Are they of the same depth?

14. Move these fingers up the iliac crest until they are resting on the uppermost portion of the ilium bilaterally. Are the crest heights level?

15. Place a finger of each hand at the gluteal lines. Move your eyes to that level. Are the lines level?

16. Bend down further and measure the heights of the popliteal lines. Are they level?
17. Measure the distance from the fingertips to the floor.
18. Trace each Achilles tendon to its insertion. Are they bowed or straight?

Anterior View

The sequences for anterior observation are as follow:

Distant Evaluation, Posterior View
1. General observation of gross body symmetry and asymmetry
2. Medial longitudinal arches
3. Medial malleoli
4. Patellas
5. Greater trochanters
6. Anterior superior iliac spines
7. Heights of iliac crests
8. Waist creases
9. Rib cage angle
10. Rib cage rotation
11. Nipple levels—males or children only
12. Level of shoulders
13. Level of fingertips
14. Deviation of cervical spine and skull from midline
15. Level of earlobes
16. Level of eyes

Note the following factors:

1. Head
2. Eyes
3. Neck
4. Chin
5. Shoulders
6. Clavicles
7. Chest wall
8. Rib angle
9. Nipples
10. Umbilicus
11. Iliac crests
12. Patellae
13. Finger tips
14. Medial malleoli
15. Medial arches

After completing the general evaluation, the examiner moves forward and adds palpation to confirm visual observations.

Close Evaluation with Palpation, Anterior View
1. Is the head straight? Palpate the earlobes.
2. Are eyes level?
3. Is the chin deviated from midline?
4. Palpate and measure the shoulder heights at the top of the acromium processes. Are they level?
5. Palpate and measure the clavicle heights. Are they level?
6. Note chest wall symmetry and rotation. If asymmetric, does it match the posterior view findings?
7. Note nipple heights.
8. Measure the rib cage angle and length of each angle arm.
9. Is the umbilicus at the midline? Are there scars on the abdomen?
10. Palpate the waist crease lines and note their length and angle.
11. Palpate the anterior superior iliac spines and note their heights and A-P orientation (examiner's eyes at that level).
12. Follow the iliac crests to their greatest heights and measure them (examiner's eyes at that level). Are they equal?
13. Palpate the superior aspect of both patellae and measure their heights (examiner's eyes at that level). Are they level? Do they point anteriorly, medially, or laterally?
14. Measure the heights of the tips of the fingers from the floor. Are they equal? Are the hands internally rotated?
15. Measure the heights of the lowest aspect of each medial malleolus from the floor. Are they equal?
16. Measure the height of each medial arch. Are they equal?

Sagittal Plane View

Distant Evaluation, Sagittal View
1. Head
2. Cervical curve
3. Cervical-thoracic junction
4. Thoracic curve
5. Thoracolumbar junction

6. Lumbar curve
7. Lumbosacral junction
8. Sacral curve
9. Shoulders
10. Hips
11. Knees
12. Ankles
13. Anterior silhouette, chest to abdomen

With these observations in mind, the examiner moves forward and adds palpation to confirm visual observations, reproducing the sequence of evaluation.

Close Evaluation with Palpation, Sagittal Plane View

1. Is the head displaced anteriorly?
2. Is the anteroposterior cervical curve exaggerated or flattened?
3. Is the transition from the cervical lordosis to thoracic kyphosis a smooth minimal curve?
4. Is the upper thoracic posterior convexity increased?
5. Is the thoracic posterior convexity a smooth curve? Is its kyphosis exaggerated? Do segments seem flattened?
6. Is the thoracolumbar junction at the articulation of the 12th thoracic and first lumbar vertebrae? Is the transitional curve smooth?
7. Is the lumbar anteroposterior curve smooth? Is it exaggerated or flattened?
8. Is the lumbosacral junction a smooth transitional curve? Does the lumbosacral angle appear normal?
9. Is there marked posterior angulation of the sacrum?
10. Look directly at the nearest shoulder. Is it forward, depressed, rotated? Can you see the other shoulder without moving your head?
11. Repeat the same examination with the scapula and rib cage. Are they rotated?
12. Is the body rotated?
13. Bend down and look at the hips. Are they rotated? Are they fully extended?
14. Look at the knees. Are they rotated? Are they fully extended? Are they hyperextended?
15. Look at the ankles. Are they rotated?
16. Look at the anterior silhouette. What is the shape and position of the chest? What is the shape and position of the abdomen? What is the relationship of the chest to the abdomen, in position and size?
17. Does the body seem displaced from the midline anteriorly or posteriorly?

FACTORS THAT COMMONLY INFLUENCE THE SAGITTAL CURVES

Osseous-Muscular Factors

1. Bone deformities, of which the most common result from:
   a. Congenital deformities of the vertebrae
   b. Trauma creating fracture or dislocation
   c. Diseases such as tumors, infections, and osteopenia
2. Ventral or dorsal muscle tone changes, commonly caused by:
   a. Muscle disuse or atrophy secondary to neurologic disease, immobilization, or age
   b. Obesity or pregnancy, creating abdominal muscle stretch
   c. Contracture of muscles due to burns, overdevelopment, injuries, or viscerosomatic reflexes

Structural-Mechanical Factors

1. Change in location of transitional areas of the sagittal curves, commonly caused by:
   a. Congenital vertebral formation
   b. Sacral base imbalance in the sagittal or frontal plane
   c. Localized regional scoliotic patterns
   d. Organic kyphoscoliosis
   e. Wearing high heels
   f. Habit or occupation
2. Endomorphic characteristics (usually increase the lordotic curve)
3. Hereditary characteristics (increase lordotic curve)
4. Foot defects such as pronation or calcaneal valgus (increase lumbar lordosis)
5. Genu valgus or varus (influences lumbar curve)
6. Hip joint changes such as femoral ante/retroversion or femoral valgus/varus (influence lumbar curve)
7. Localized somatic dysfunctions (flattened thoracic kyphosis)

General Considerations

In all close examinations, the examiner should use palpation whenever it can help confirm visual observations. The eyes should be at the level of the body part observed during close examinations. Looking up or down can distort the findings. The examiner may bend down by flexing the knees or sit in a suitable chair.

The first observations should be from a distance. The examiner first develops a sense of body symmetry, then uses closer observation and palpation to confirm or rule out initial impressions.

References

Basmajian JV. 1978. Muscles Alive, 4th ed. Baltimore: Williams & Wilkins Co.

Calliet R. 1975. Scoliosis. Philadelphia: F.A. Davis Co.

Fryette MM. 1954. Principles of Osteopathic Technique. Colorado Springs: Academy of Applied Osteopathy.

Heilig D. 1978. Some basic considerations of spinal curves. Osteopath Ann 311:318.

Kapandji IA. 1974. Physiology of the Joints, 2nd ed, vol 3. Edinburgh: Churchill Livingstone.

Kendall FP, McCreary EK. 1983. Muscles: Testing and Function, 3rd ed. Baltimore: Williams & Wilkins Co.

MacConaill MA, Basmajian JV. 1969. Muscles and Movements, 2nd ed. Huntington, New York: Robert E. Krieger Publishing Co.

Northup GW. 1972. Osteopathic lesions. J Am Osteopath Assoc 71:854–864.

Schiowitz S. 1980. Static symmetry and asymmetry. Osteopath Ann 8:9.

4

Spinal Motion

PHYSIOLOGIC MOTION OF THE SPINE
Dennis J. Dowling

In 1918, Harrison Fryette presented a paper on physiologic movements of the vertebral column at the American Osteopathic Association convention. What is now regarded by the osteopathic profession as important diagnostic theory was, by Fryette's account, not enthusiastically received. Much of his work was based on an earlier book by Robert Lovett, *Spinal Curvatures and Round Shoulders*. Before reading this work, Fryette experimented with radiographs and a spine mounted in soft rubber. He analyzed the movement of the vertebral column and developed several principles, now frequently referred to as Fryette's laws. They are not so much laws as guidelines for discriminating different types of dysfunction, determining diagnoses, and delineating treatment.

Physiology of Spinal Motion
In analyzing vertebral motion, it is useful to know the phylogeny involved. Humans were originally quadripeds with the spine in a basically horizontal state. In this position, all weight-bearing was carried by the articular facets (Fig. 4-1). The facets are hard, compact, and sturdy trabecular bone, as opposed to the more cancellous bone of the vertebral bodies.

In the vertical orientation, the articular bodies and intervertebral disks are subject to stresses that gradually compress the disks and further define the shape of the body. Humans are subject to stress fractures, herniations, and bulging disks, conditions virtually unknown in four-footed species. Gravity causes a further approximation of the superior and inferior facets while increasing the overall contribution of the vertebral body joints to spinal movement (Fig. 4-2).

Fryette credited Lovett with conceptualizing the backbone as consisting of two columns (Fig. 4-3). The anterior column is defined by the vertebral bodies and intervertebral disks. As this column is bent, the disks and bodies attempt to accommodate the distortion by moving away from the concave side (Figs. 4-4 through 4-6). The posterior or dorsal column is constituted by the facets, their capsules, and the ligaments. This column behaves as a flexible ruler with its edges oriented laterally. To induce side bending in this column, Lovett theorized, the region bent must also rotate away from the concave side and toward the convex side. Forward and backward bending can occur without a secondary rotary movement unless some restriction is present. Together the two columns act synergistically to produce total vertebral motion.

Forward and backward bending in a normal vertebral column occurs with the facets gapping in the first instance and approximating in the second instance (Fig. 4-7). In the nondysfunctional thoracic and lumbar spine, the actions of side bending and rotation are coupled and occur in opposite directions, owing to the flexible ruler action of the facets and their attachment.

An exception to coupled motion occurs in the cervical region and is caused by the extreme lordosis, planar relationship, and convergence of the facets. The mechanics in this region dictate that side bending and rotation are coupled and occur in the same direction (Figs. 4-8 and 4-9).

In the lumbar and thoracic spine, when one vertebra locks on another and a combination of extension-rotation-side bending or flexion-side bending-rotation occurs, then the rotation and side bending are in the same direction. In this situation, as the vertebra moves in any one plane, simultaneous movement is created along the other two component planes.

These observations are summed up in the three principles known as Fryette's principles I, II, and III.

PRINCIPLE I

When any part of the lumbar or thoracic spine is in neutral position, sidebending of a vertebra will be opposite to the side of rotation of that vertebra.

Figure 4-1. Weight-bearing in an animal with a horizontal spine (**A**) and in an animal (human) with a vertical spine (**B**).

Figure 4-2. Orientation of the vertebrae. *1*, spinous process; *2*, transverse process.

Figure 4-3. Lovett-Fryette conception of the backbone as consisting of two columns, the vertebral bodies and intervertebral disks (**A**) and the facets, capsules, and ligaments (**B**), which unite to form the spinal column (**C**).

Although this description applies chiefly to the lumbar and thoracic spine in neutral (normal resting) position, it also applies to moderate truncal flexion and extension. The facets must not be in a locked position, nor should there be single-sided tautness of ligaments. Therefore, on clinical examination of the vertebral column, the expected findings should be side bending and rotation in opposite directions (i.e., when side-bent to the right, the vertebral body will rotate counterclockwise to the left; Fig. 4-10).

Fryette's first principle is of use in analyzing dysfunctions that are most often initiated or maintained by muscle. Ideally the vertebral joints are free from restriction initiated by muscles. The vertebral column acts as a bow, with the muscles

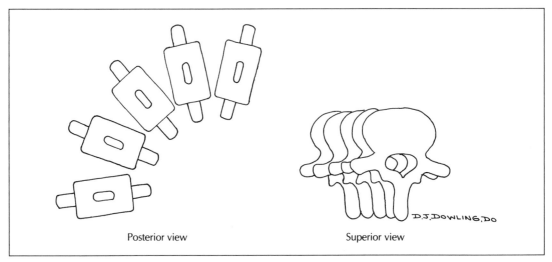

Figure 4-4. Pure (nonphysiologic) vertebral side bending without the influence of the facet joints.

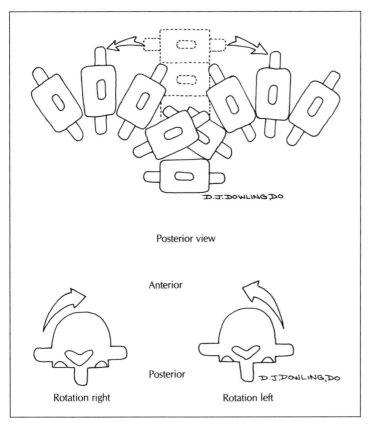

Figure 4-5. Pure (nonphysiologic) vertebral side bending, without the influence of the facet joints, to each side.

Figure 4-6. Orientation of rotation.

Figure 4-7. Flexion (forward bending) and extension (backward bending) of the spinal column, producing, respectively, gapping and approximation of the articular facets.

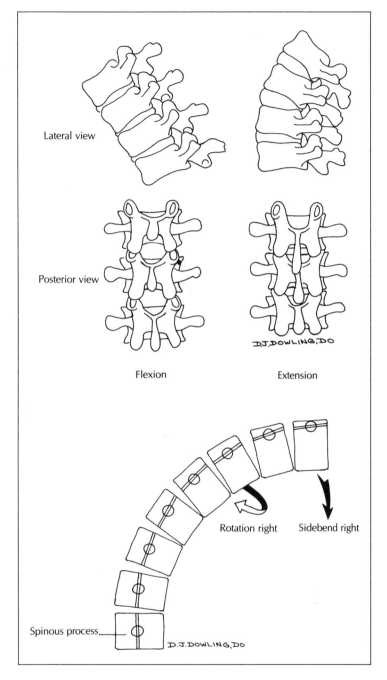

Lateral view

Posterior view

Flexion

Extension

D.J.DOWLING,DO

Figure 4-8. Pure (physiologic) cervical vertebral side bending. Side bending in the cervical vertebrae occurs in the same direction as rotation.

Rotation right

Sidebend right

Spinous process

D.J.DOWLING,DO

acting as a cord that induces a curve when single-sided contraction occurs (Fig. 4-11). The spinal segments compensate for this side bending by rotating in the opposite direction (Fig. 4-12), and the posterior facets or transverse processes are palpable on the convex side of the lateral curve. A curve of this sort may also represent a response to dysfunction occurring higher or lower in the spinal column (e.g., an unlevel sacral base), in which case it is generally more gradual in onset.

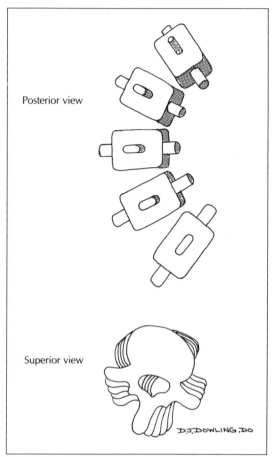

Figure 4-9. Normal cervical motion. Side bending and rotation occur in the same direction.

The shorthand notation for the lateral group curve is T3–8N Sr Rl. The 3 denotes the third thoracic segment at the top of the curve and the 8 denotes the eighth thoracic segment at the bottom of the curve. The S indicates the direction of side bending freedom, in this case to the right, with coupled rotation (R) to the opposite side (left) in the thoracic spine.

PRINCIPLE II
When any part of the spine is in a position of hyperextension or hyperflexion, the sidebending of a vertebra will be to the same side as the rotation of that vertebra.

A type II dysfunction (Fig. 4-13) is primarily a single-segment lesion. The movement has become pathologic and the segment is locked. Muscular involvement may occur but is second in importance to the restriction of the vertebral segment. Any attempt to move the segment along a single plane, whether sagittal, coronal, or horizontal (flexion-extension, side bending, and rotation, respectively), will produce motion in all planes, thereby initiating a helical movement (Fig. 4-14). The locked segment, rather than alleviating the compression by rotating away when side-bent or by side bending away when rotated, compensates by side bending and rotating to the same side.

This phenomenon can be observed when the region of the spine is side-bent with the locked region on the concave side of the curve and the whole spine is flexed or extended. With flexion and extension, the locked segment becomes more noticeable as it is moved in its direction of restriction (Fig. 4-15).

Table 4-1. Summary of Dysfunctions

	Type I Dynamics	Type II Dynamics
Number of segments	Multiple	Single
Rotation/side bending	Opposite side	Same side
Position of spine	Neutral	Flexion or extension
Clinical appearance	Lateral curve	Flattening or exaggeration of anteroposterior curve
Onset	Usually gradual	Usually abrupt
Site of pain	Either on concave side, owing to contracted muscle, or on convex side, owing to stretched muscles	Usually over posterior facet

Figure 4-10. Type I mechanics: the thoracic and lumbar vertebrae, when side-bent in one direction, will rotate in the opposite direction.

Spinous process

Posterior view

Figure 4-11. Bowing effect produced by contracted paravertebral muscles.

Figure 4-12. Side bending under the influence of the facets: side bending and rotation occur in opposite directions (Fryette's first principle).

Figure 4-13. Type II dysfunction at segment 4.

Palpation of single-segment somatic dysfunctions is important for localizing the area of involvement, but the sine qua non for diagnosis is the observation that it follows type II mechanics.

Pain, tenderness, and restricted motion are frequently noted at the site. The onset can be quite abrupt, with the patient aware of the time, duration, and direction of the precipitating event. Such situations may be brought about by unexpected or severe disruption, which may be initiated by sudden movement. Frequently the patient is at the extreme in one plane of the range of motion, then attempts to move in another plane(s) (e.g., the patient is fully flexed, then twists or turns to the side).

The single-segment aspect of type II dysfunction does not exclude the occurrence of a series of somatic dysfunctions that all behave in the prescribed manner. In fact, type II dysfunctions are often observed at the beginning, apex, and end of a type I group curve.

Fryette's observations on hyperflexion and hyperextension developed from his study of the movements of cadaver spines, which exhibit the biomechanics of a type II dysfunction when placed at extremes of motion. However, cadaver spines are significantly relaxed and not subject to the stresses of living spines.

The notation used to describe a type II somatic dysfunction indicates both the single-segment nature and the status of its freedom of movement. L3 E Sl Rl denotes a locking of L3 on L4 in which the top segment moves more easily into side bending and rotation to the left and extension.

PRINCIPLE III
Initiating motion of a vertebral segment in any plane of motion will modify the movement of that segment in other planes of motion.

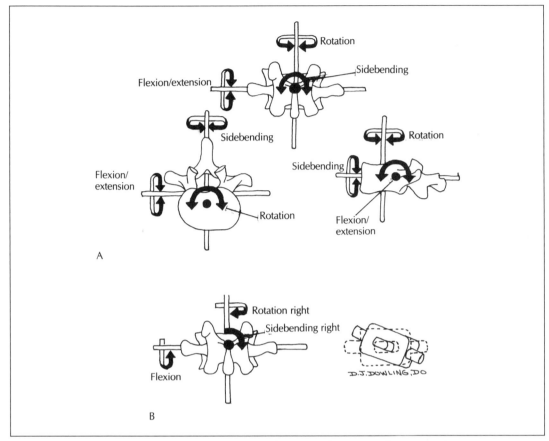

Figure 4-14. Helical axes of movement in type II mechanics. **B** shows a single-segment lesion, F Sr Rr.

Figure 4-15. Type II dysfunction. Segment marked by asterisk is side-bent and rotated in the same direction, whereas nondysfunctional segments side bend and rotate in opposite directions.

The third principle of coupled action alerts the clinician to spinal limitations. In type I dynamics, an example is the side-bent scoliotic curve. Normal coupled motion includes rotation to the opposite side. An attempt to induce further side bending is easier when bending is continued in the direction already established. Rotation is similarly modified. Movement in a direction opposite to the established direction is limited. The same observations apply to type II dynamics: movement produced in a direction opposite to the freedom of motion is restricted.

BIOMECHANICS OF JOINT MOTION
Stanley Schiowitz

All bones that have freedom of movement will move on other bones at their respective joints. Several factors influence these motions. Knowledge of why, when, and how joint motion is induced is essential for the understanding of functional anatomy and for the diagnosis and treatment of osteopathic somatic dysfunctions.

General Principles

None of the articulatory surfaces of the body are truly flat. They are ovoid or sellar (saddle-shaped) (Fig. 4-16). The joints that have evolved are an attempt at a mating of these forms: sella to sella, and ovoid convex to ovoid concave. The articulations thus formed are not truly congruent, permitting greater freedom of joint movement and geometrically created coupled and accessory motions.

Individual joint motions can be described in terms of spin, roll, and slide. *Spin* is defined as one bone rotating on its mechanical axis, in place, on another bone. *Roll* is defined as movement resulting from an increase or decrease in angle between the two articulating bones. *Slide* is a translatory motion of one bone sliding over the surface of another bone (Fig. 4-17).

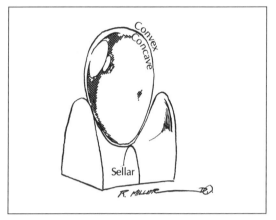

Figure 4-16. Bony shapes. At this articulation an ovoid shape sits in a sellar shape. Convex and concave surfaces are shown.

The curved articular surfaces, moving one upon another, develop complex patterns of motions. The coupled motions created by convex-concave mating articulations follow specific patterns. When a concave surface moves on a convex surface, the roll and slide motions are in the same direction.

Figure 4-17. (**A**) Spin, (**B**) roll, (**C**) slide.

Figure 4-18. Femoral extension on the tibia. Roll and slide occur in opposite directions.

However, when a convex surface moves on a concave surface, the roll and slide motions are in opposite directions.

Femoral extension on the tibia follows these patterns of motion. As the stance leg extends in gait, the femur rolls anteriorly with posterior slide on a fixed tibia (Fig. 4-18). However, the swing leg on extending creates tibial roll and slide anteriorly (in the same direction) on the distal femur (Fig. 4-19). Full femoral extension can be described as an anterior femoral roll with a posterior slide, accompanied at full extension by a medial femoral spin upon the tibia.

The fully extended knee undergoes another prescribed motion in its final stage of extension. This is a conjunct rotation created by the geometry of the articulating surfaces (see Chap. 20, The Knee Joint).

Motion is affected by ligamentous relationships. A "close-packed" joint position is one in which the ligaments have twisted, bringing the bones together into maximum congruence. The bones cannot be separated without first loosening the ligaments. Joint motion is lost, and forces are more easily transmitted through this joint into the next one. Tangential force will more likely cause fracture than sprain.

In weight-bearing joints, the close-packed position replaces muscle activity for maintenance of support. In the spine, motion is transmitted through the bodies of close-packed vertebrae into the first movable zygapophyseal articulation. Somatic dysfunction can result. The principle of transmittal of motion through close-packed joints is used therapeutically in high velocity, low amplitude thrusting techniques.

Articular stability is a combined function of the shape of the joint, its ligamentous and muscular attachments, the strength of its capsule, and the balance of joint pressure to atmospheric pressure. Variation in any of these factors may contribute to somatic dysfunctions.

Figure 4-19. Tibial extension on the femur. Roll and slide occur in the same direction.

It is usual to describe motion as occurring in cardinal planes about fixed axes. Shoulder abduction would be described as motion in a frontal plane about an anteroposterior axis. However, we know that the head of the humerus, a convex surface, moves on the concave glenoid fossa with an upward roll and downward slide. Since this is a coupled, continuous motion, it cannot be about a fixed axis. This type of motion is said to be about an *instantaneous axis of rotation*. This axis defines multiple motions, rotary and translatory, that occur simultaneously in the same plane. The abduction motion would require continuous determinations of its instantaneous axis as it moved. This would give a true pathway of the joint motion. This motion is still only in one plane.

In full extension the femur rolls, slides, and spins. The motion is multiplanar and involves more than one axis; it is said to occur on a *helical axis*. The helical axis completely defines a three-dimensional motion between two rigid bodies. Active functional motions, appendicular as well as vertebral, are usually motions about helical axes.

The addition of force to joint motions may bring into play accessory motions. Accessory motions cannot be performed voluntarily; they can only be activated against resistance or by an outside force. An example is long axis traction on the phalangeal articulations. The restriction of small accessory motions is a major factor in the creation of somatic dysfunctions, especially in the articulations of appendages.

Biomechanics of the Upper Extremities
SHOULDER GIRDLE

Five joints are primarily involved in shoulder girdle function. Three, the glenohumeral, acromioclavicular, and sternoclavicular, are true joints. The suprahumeral and scapulothoracic joints are pseudojoints (Fig. 4-20). These joints may be divided into two functional groups. Joints in the first group, the glenohumeral and suprahumeral joints, act in unison to produce the early motion of shoulder abduction. Joints in the second group, the scapulothoracic, sternoclavicular, and acro-

Figure 4-20. Shoulder girdle, anterior view.

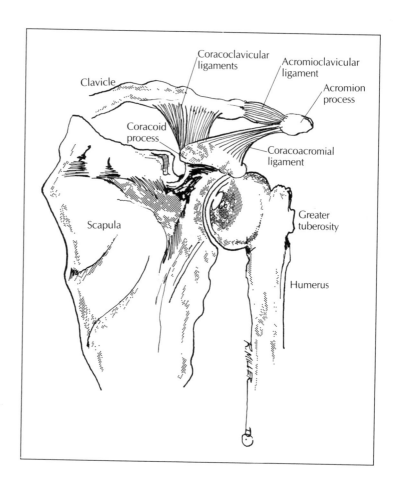

mioclavicular joints, act in unison to produce the mid to late motions of shoulder abduction.

The movements of the humerus on the glenoid fossa include the following:

1. Flexion and extension in the sagittal plane.
2. Abduction and adduction in the frontal plane. True adduction is absent owing to the presence of the trunk. Relative adduction is the return of the humerus toward midline from the position of abduction. Flexion adduction is humeral movement across the front of the body. Extension adduction is humeral movement across the back of the body.
3. Axial rotation: internal and external rotation of the humeral head.
4. Horizontal plane rotation: flexion plus adduction anteriorly or extension plus adduction posteriorly.
5. Circumduction: the conical motion of the distal end of the humerus as the shoulder moves through all planes.

Abduction-adduction and axial and horizontal rotations are coupled in that angular motions are accompanied by translatory slides. The caudal slide of the humeral head with abduction confers increased freedom of motion on the supraspinatous tendon beneath the coracoacromial ligament.

In addition to the slide motions, the joint exhibits the accessory motion of long axis extension.

The movements of the individual joints are as follows:

1. The glenohumeral joint has three degrees of cardinal motion: flexion and extension, abduction and adduction, and internal and external rotation.

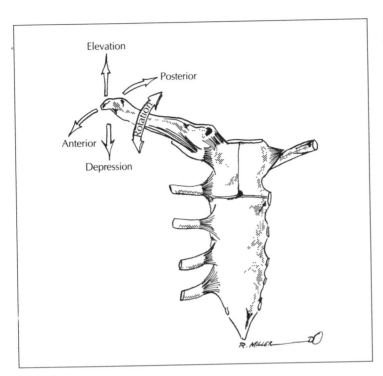

Elevation

Posterior

Rotation

Anterior

Depression

R. MILLER

Figure 4-21. Sternoclavicular joint motion.

2. The suprahumeral joint acts in concert with the glenohumeral joint.

3. The scapulothoracic joint movements are related to scapular motions. The motions are medial and lateral movements of the scapula on the thorax (abduction-adduction), elevation and depression of the scapula, upward and downward rotation of the scapula (tilt), all relative to the glenoid fossa.

4. The sternoclavicular joint moves cephalad and caudad in the frontal plane, ventrad and dorsad in the horizontal plane, and rotates on its mechanical axis (Fig. 4-21). All cephalad-caudad and ventrad-dorsad movements are accompanied by translatory slides.

5. The primary motion of the acromioclavicular joint is axial rotation.

The combined axial rotation of the sternoclavicular joint (30 degrees) and the acromioclavicular joint (30 degrees) allows the normal 60 degrees of rotation of the scapula on full abduction of the shoulder.

Total abduction of the shoulder joint can be divided into three phases. During the **first phase** (0 to 90 degrees), the supraspinatus and deltoid muscles are involved. At the beginning of the movement the supraspinatus is very efficient in abduction and in maintaining joint stability, while the deltoid is very inefficient and tends to produce superior dislocation. As abduction progresses, the deltoid's efficiency increases while that of the supraspinatus decreases. These actions are a direct result of the changes in position of the muscles' origins and insertions that accompany the motion.

In the **second phase** (90 to 150 degrees), upward rotation of the scapula causes the glenoid fossa to face upward. This is accomplished by concomitant rotations of the sternoclavicular and acromioclavicular joints. In the **third phase** (150 to 180 degrees) the spinal column is displaced laterally by the action of the contralateral spinal muscles. Bilateral abduction would require an exaggeration of the lumbar lordosis, since the spinal column would be otherwise synergistically balanced. These combined motions are known as the scapulohumeral rhythm.

Total flexion of the shoulder joint can also be divided into three phases. In the **first phase** (0 to 60 degrees), the muscles used are the anterior fibers of the deltoid, the coracobrachialis, and the clavicular fibers of the pectoralis major. Motion is limited by the tension of the coracohumeral ligament and by the resistance offered by the teres minor, teres major, and infraspinatus muscles.

In the **second phase** (60 to 120 degrees) the function is similar to the second phase of abduction, utilizing scapular rotation, with the glenoid facing upward and anteriorly. In the **third phase** (120 to 180 degrees), both unilateral and bilateral flexion require the same motion of the spinal column as for complete abduction.

In diagnosing somatic dysfunctions involving shoulder girdle motion, the clinician must be aware that dysfunctions limiting motion reflect involvement of multiple joints, muscles, tendons, ligaments, the synovium, and the joint capsules. Functional anatomic knowledge and diagnostic ability should include knowledge of the following:

1. The functioning of accessory and coupled motions
2. The origins and insertions of the shoulder muscles
3. The influence of these muscles on the entire spinal column
4. The relationship of the thorax and rib cage to all scapular motion
5. How the first rib, at its sternal attachment, is directly influenced by clavicular motion

The entire shoulder girdle, thorax, rib cage, and vertebral column must be evaluated for a comprehensive diagnosis of somatic involvement in shoulder girdle dysfunction. The plan for therapy should be similarly comprehensive.

ELBOW JOINT

The distal end of the humerus articulates with the ulna and radius, forming two articulations: the **humeroulnar,** between the trochlea of the humerus and the trochlear notch of the ulna, and the **humeroradial,** between the capitulum of the humerus and the head of the radius (Fig. 4-22).

The elbow joint has the composite motions of elbow flexion, with forearm supination, and elbow extension, with forearm pronation. Therefore, the superior radioulnar joint and its motions complicate, and are part of, elbow joint motion.

Humeroulnar articulation. The trochlea of the humerus consists of a central groove with a convex wing on each side. The central groove lies in

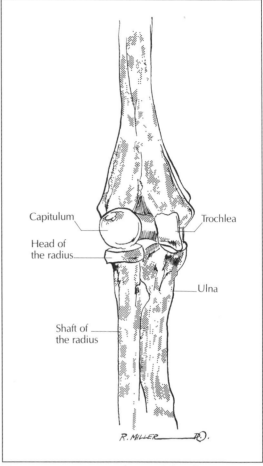

Figure 4-22. Bony articulation of the elbow joint.

an oblique sagittal plane. The obliquity creates the carrying angle of the arm. The trochlear notch of the ulna has a corresponding shape.

The major motion of the articulation is flexion-extension. However, extremes of supination and pronation create a rocking motion and the accessory motions of adduction with supination and abduction with pronation. Restrictions of these accessory motions influence normal flexion-extension and must be sought and normalized in elbow joint treatment.

Humeroradial articulation. This consists of the concave head of the radius articulating with the convex-shaped capitulum of the humerus. Motion of this articulation must accompany humeroulnar flexion-extension. This angular motion is accompanied by ventral and dorsal translatory

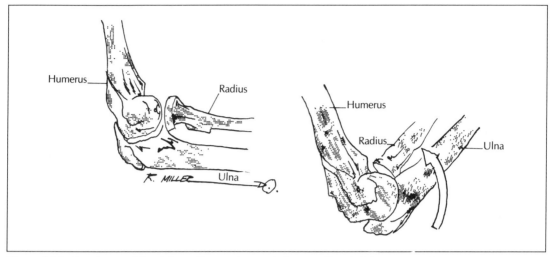

Figure 4-23. Translatory slide of the radius on the capitulum. Roll and slide occur in the same direction.

slide of the radius on the humerus: dorsal radial slide with extension, ventral radial slide with flexion (Fig. 4-23). Extension stress is the major cause of posterior radial head somatic dysfunction.

The proximal radioulnar articulation consists of the cylindric rim of the head of the radius articulating with the radial notch of the ulna. The annular ligament encompasses the head of the radius and is attached to the anterior and posterior margins of the radial notch. In conjunction with the distal radioulnar articulation, its main motions are supination and pronation. The axis of these motions is represented by a line drawn through the center of the head of the radius, with the distal end of the radius swinging around and in front of the ulna. The proximal end of the ulna moves backward and laterally during pronation and forward and medially with supination (Fig. 4-24). This means that the axis of rotation of the head of the radius does not remain constant. The accessory motions therefore consist of the previously mentioned dorsal-ventral radial slide on the capitulum, similar motion on the radial notch, and dorsal and ventral ulnar slide on the radius. All of these motions may contribute to somatic dysfunctions.

The motions of supination and pronation are also greatly influenced by the function of the interosseous membrane and the distal radial ulnar articulation.

WRIST JOINT

The wrist joint consists of 15 bones, each with multiple articulations. A good example is the capitate bone, which articulates with the second, third, and fourth metacarpals and with the lunate, scaphoid, trapezoid and hamate bones (Fig. 4-25). The wrist acts as a functional unit, exhibiting flexion, extension, adduction (ulnar deviation), abduction (radial deviation), and circumduction.

The articular complex of the wrist can be divided into three functional units:

1. The radiocarpal joint, consisting of the distal end of the radius articulating with the scaphoid and lunate
2. The midcarpal joint, consisting of the combined articulations between the proximal and distal rows of the carpal bones (Fig. 4-26)
3. The ulnomeniscotriquetral pseudojoint, consisting of the distal end of the ulna, the triquetrium, and the meniscus between the two

The movements that occur at the radiocarpal and midcarpal joints can be considered together because these joints act as a combined mechanism. Flexion involves the combined motion of both units, with midcarpal motion somewhat greater than radiocarpal motion. The roles are reversed in extension: radiocarpal motion is greater (Fig. 4-27). In adduction, most of the motion oc-

Figure 4-24. Supination to pronation. The radial head tilts downward and laterally.

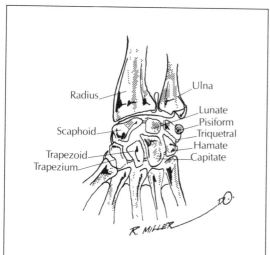

Figure 4-25. Bony articulation of the wrist.

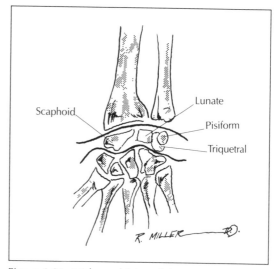

Figure 4-26. Midcarpal joint of the wrist.

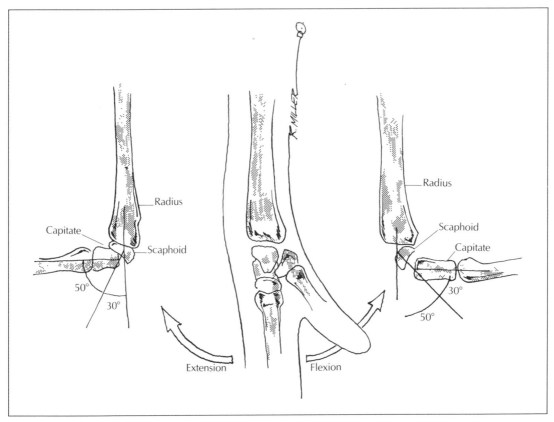

Figure 4-27. Major wrist joint motion.

curs at the radiocarpal and the ulnomeniscotriquetral joints. Abduction involves primarily the
midcarpal joint. There is a complex torsion movement of the carpal bones about their long axes
during abduction and adduction. Circumduction
of the hand is not axial rotation, but a series of
movements: flexion followed by adduction, extension, and abduction, or the same movements
in reverse order.

Accessory movements are greatest at the radio-
scaphoid and radiolunate articulations. These
movements are ventral-dorsal slide, axial rotation, slight side-to-side slide, and long axis traction. Similar accessory motions can be found at
all carpal articulations, but in greatly diminished
degree.

The close-packed position of the wrist is full
extension. Falling on the wrist in this position
will readily cause fracture. In a relaxed, loosely

packed position, the joints are relatively mobile.
For the performance of any task involving wrist
action, the articulations must enter into a combination of interdependent locked positions, creating a solid structure that can bear the strain of
torsional motion. In turning a doorknob, for example, the wrist joint changes from a sack of loose
bones into a solid functional unit for the transmission of force.

An infinite number of partially close-packed
positions of the wrist articulation can be created
by muscle contraction and tightening of the ligaments. The close-packed articulation transmits
force to the end of its total unit. Acting as a lever,
it produces maximum force impact at one end or
at one articulation. Somatic dysfunctions may
easily develop in this manner, without sustaining
direct trauma. The dysfunctions usually are loss
of accessory motions.

HAND

With the exception of the thumb, the movements of the carpometacarpal articulations consist of flexion-extension and abduction-adduction. The accessory motions are dorsal-ventral slide, axial rotation, and long axis traction. The thumb is a sellar articulation, permitting the motions of flexion-extension, abduction-adduction, rotation, and circumduction. The accessory motions are axial rotation and long axis traction.

The intermetacarpal joints are limited to slight gliding of one on another. The accessory motion is axial rotation. The metacarpophalangeal articulations have the following movements: flexion-extension, adduction-abduction, limited rotation, and circumduction. The accessory motions are axial rotation, dorsal-ventral slide, and long axis traction.

The interphalangeal joints are limited to flexion-extension motions. Flexion is usually accompanied by a conjunct rotation to assist in thumb-finger approximation. The accessory motions are dorsal-ventral slide, abduction-adduction, axial rotation, and long axis traction.

The early motion dysfunctions caused by arthritic involvement of the hands are manifested in loss of accessory motions.

Biomechanics of the Lower Extremities

HIP JOINT

The anatomic relationships of the hip joint are similar to those of the glenohumeral joint. It is a ball-and-socket articulation, allowing 3 degrees of motion plus circumduction (Fig. 4-28). The entire weight of the body is transmitted through the hip joints, which therefore must have a greater degree of stability than the shoulder joints. Increased stability is afforded by a deeper acetabulum, the acetabular labrum, and the strong supportive hip ligaments. The acetabulum is in the innominate bone and relates to spinal, sacral, and ilial movements.

During normal gait, the stance leg starts in hip flexion. At midstance, hip extension begins until a close-packed position is achieved. The vector force transmitted from the ground passes into the innominate bone and causes rotation of the ilium. Disturbances of gait will create iliosacral joint dysfunctions.

Movements of the hip joint include flexion-extension, abduction-adduction, internal and external rotation, and circumduction. The range of flexion depends on the action of the knee joint. Hip flexion is always greater with the knee flexed (Fig. 4-29). Greater hip flexion can be achieved

Figure 4-28. Bony anatomy of the hip joint.

Figure 4-29. Hip flexion. Shown are ranges of active motion with the knee in different positions.

120°

90°

R MILLER

passively than actively. Both hips can undergo full passive flexion when both knees are approximated to the chest. This is accompanied by a posterior pelvic tilt and lumbar flattening. The range of flexion motion is 90 degrees with the knee extended, 120 degrees with the knee flexed, and more than 120 degrees in passive flexion.

Hip extension is greater when the knee is in extension (Fig. 4-30). Passive extension is greater than active extension. Active hip extension is 10 degrees with the knee flexed and 20 degrees with the knee extended; passive extension can reach 30 degrees.

The gluteus maximus muscle is the major extensor muscle of the hip. Its ability to create extension depends on the planar relationships of its origin and insertion. According to the rule of muscle detorsion, all muscles attempt to align their origins and insertions into the same plane when contracting. Therefore, as the pelvis is tilted anteriorly, the origin of the gluteus maximus changes its planar relationship, allowing for femoral extension in an attempt to align the origin and insertion of the muscle into one plane. Maximum extension (anterior dance splits) creates marked anterior pelvic tilt accompanied by lumbar lordosis. The abduction of one joint is accompanied by pelvic tilt to the weight-bearing side and bilaterally equal abduction of the legs in relation to the pelvis. Maximum abduction creates a 90-degree angle between the two legs (45 degrees for each limb in abduction).

Figure 4-30. Hip extension.

True adduction is not possible because of the midline interference of the other limb. Relative adduction is the return from abduction. As in shoulder motion, there can be adduction-flexion and adduction-extension motions. A complex motion of adduction of one hip accompanied by abduction of the other hip is achieved by a pelvic tilt in the frontal plane to the abduction side, with accompanying increased lumbar convexity.

Internal and external hip rotation can be easily measured with the patient prone and the knee flexed to 90 degrees. From the true vertical position, moving the foot laterally causes internal rotation (30 to 40 degrees). Moving the foot medially causes external rotation (60 degrees). The same test can be performed with the patient sitting on a table with the feet dangling. The position of greatest hip instability is in sitting with the legs crossed (abduction, flexion, and external rotation).

The accessory hip motions consist of slide with abduction-adduction and internal-external rotation and long axis traction.

Of major importance in function and dysfunction, many large hip joint muscles involve the function of both the hip and the knee. Muscle contraction always involves an attempt at motion of both joints. Limiting the motion to one joint requires stabilization of the other joint by other muscles.

Pure extension of the hip joint would require the synergistic actions of the gluteus maximus, gluteus medius and minimus, the hamstrings, the rectus femoris, and the adductor magnus muscles. The gluteus maximus and hamstrings, along with the iliopsoas and erector spinae, are major factors in maintaining the stability of the pelvis and the lumbar lordosis.

The somatic dysfunctions related to hip joint dysfunction may involve the lower spine, sacrum, ilium, ischium, acetabulofemoral joint, femoral shaft, and the knee joint.

KNEE JOINT

The knee joint is the largest appendicular articulation. In function it resembles a hinge joint. However, it is a compound articulation within one joint cavity. It consists of two condylar joints between the corresponding condyles of the femur and tibia, with convex-concave relationships, and an additional sella-shaped joint between the patella and the femur.

The knee joint is one of the few joints of the body that have menisci. Menisci contribute to stability, weight-bearing, and mobility of the joint.

The patella's articulation allows it to slide up and down on the femur and act as a pulley for its musculotendinous attachments. The joint has an intricate ligamentous network to create stability while still permitting joint mobility.

The major movements of the knee joint are flexion and extension. These motions are a classic example of coupled roll and slide. The passive range of motion is 0 degrees at extension and 135 degrees at flexion.

With the foot on the ground, the final 30 degrees of femoral extension is accompanied by a conjunct medial femoral rotation (Fig. 4-31). This conjunct rotation results from the geometry of the articulating surfaces and the action of the ligaments. In full extension, the knee is in close-packed position, which confers greater stability and strength on the joint. As in all close-packed joints, trauma can more easily cause fracture. However, the more common ligamentous tears occur in mid- or loose-packed positions. With the foot off the ground, extension is associated with conjunct lateral rotation of the tibia.

The voluntary movements of axial internal and external rotation also occur in the knee. These motions are best observed with the knee in a flexed position. Passive internal and external rotation are each about 10 degrees.

The accessory motions of the femorotibial joint consist of passive internal and external rotation, conjunct rotation, dorsal and ventral tibial slide, abduction, adduction, and long axis traction.

Besides the possibility of multiple soft tissue dysfunctions, the major somatic dysfunctions of joint motion affect abduction and adduction, or dorsal and ventral slide.

Figure 4-31. Tibial-femoral extension accompanied by conjunct rotation of the tibia.

The patella, with the knee semiflexed, can be passively moved in the dorsal-ventral, cephalic-caudal, and side-to-side directions.

TIBIOFIBULAR JOINTS

The superior tibiofibular joint is a plane oval articulation. The tibial facet lies on the posterolateral aspect of the rim of the lateral tibial condyle. It faces obliquely posteriorly, inferiorly, and laterally.

The inferior tibiofibular joint is a syndesmosis. The tibial facet is a rough concave notch into which the convex fibular facet fits. This fibular facet continues below as the fibulotalar articulation.

Dorsiflexion and plantar flexion of the ankle automatically create motion in both tibiofibular joints. Dorsiflexion causes the lateral malleolus to move laterally, vertically in a caudal direction, and to rotate medially. This causes the superior tibiofibular joint to move in an upward posterior direction while rotating medially. The reverse occurs in plantar flexion.

The most common somatic dysfunction found in this area is a posterior fibula at the superior tibiofibular joint. This may be secondary to ankle dysfunction and marked dorsiflexion. To resolve the superior tibiofibular dysfunction, it is important to evaluate the ankle joint and treat any dysfunctions found in that region.

FOOT AND ANKLE

The foot and ankle joints constitute a complex unit of 28 bones that must be strong enough to bear the body's weight yet elastic enough to allow adaptation to terrain, walking, jumping, or the stress of additional weight (Fig. 4-32).

The patient must be examined both in the static position and while walking, with the shoes on and off. Static examination is conducted with and without weight-bearing to determine changes in arch as well as bony relationships.

Pediatric examination of the feet prior to weight-bearing is very important. The early diagnosis of congenital deformities may allow a nonoperative therapy while increasing the quality of the results obtained.

The distal end of the tibia, along with the lateral malleolus, forms a concave surface into which is fitted the body of the talus. This is the ankle mortice articulation (Fig. 4-33). This hinge joint per-

Figure 4-32. Bony anatomy of the foot.

mits the major motions of dorsiflexion and plantar flexion of the foot on a transverse axis. The tibial malleolus extends about one third of the way down the medial surface of the body of the talus and is anterior to the lateral malleolus. The fibular malleolus extends down the entire lateral aspect of the talus.

The body of the talus is wedge-shaped, with its anterior portion larger. Dorsiflexion creates a close-packed position with medial rotation and elevation and separation of the fibula in relation to the tibia (Fig. 4-34).

The active motions of this articulation are dorsiflexion and plantar flexion. With the articulation in the loose-packed position, accessory motions of the side-to-side slide, internal and ex-

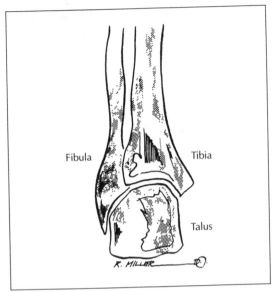

Figure 4-33. Bony anatomy of the ankle mortice articulation.

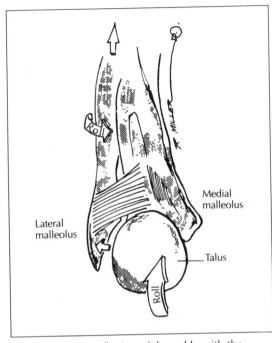

Figure 4-34. Dorsiflexion of the ankle with the accompanying motions.

ternal rotation, abduction and adduction, and long axis traction are permitted. Somatic dysfunction involving joint motion restriction usually occurs in abduction or adduction, as evidenced by the large number of inversion and eversion ankle sprains encountered.

The posterior portion of the foot consists of the talocalcaneal, talonavicular, and calcaneocuboid articulations. The calcaneus can move into abduction (valgus) or adduction (varus) in relation to the talus (Fig. 4-35). The other motions are best described as combined talocalcaneal-navicular-cuboid efforts. Inversion in relation to a stable talus can be described as a medial rotation of the calcaneus and navicular bone, increasing the height of the medial arch, accompanied by the cuboid rotating downward on the calcaneus (Fig. 4-36). Motion of the anterior tarsus and plantar flexion will increase this movement. Eversion is the reverse of the above.

With weight-bearing, the distal tarsus and metatarsals become involved, creating the combined motions of pronation and suppination. *Pronation* of the foot consists of a combination of calcaneal abduction (valgus), eversion, foot abduction, and dorsiflexion. In reverse order, these motions produce *supination*.

The accessory motions of these articulations are slide and conjunct rotations.

Somatic dysfunction restricting joint motion will affect the motions of slide and conjunct rotation. An example is the conjunct rotation of the cuboid on the calcaneus with eversion and inversion of the foot.

The movements of the cuneiforms, cuboid, and navicular bone in relation to each other are primarily gliding and conjunct rotations. Accessory motions of increased glide and rotation can be created, especially if accompanied by long axis traction.

The primary motions of the tarsometatarsal joints are flexion and extension. The axis of flexion and extension of the fourth and fifth metatarsals is oblique. This raises and lowers the transverse metatarsal arch with flexion and extension movements of these metatarsals. The intermetatarsal joint movement is primarily that of slide. Accessory motions of the tarsometatarsal and intermetatarsal joints consist in exaggeration of all sliding motions, especially when accompanied by long axis traction. The metatarsopha-

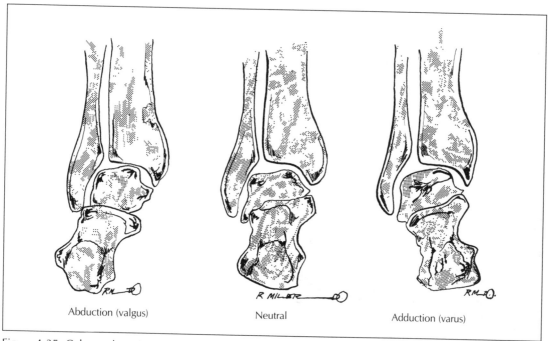

Abduction (valgus)   Neutral   Adduction (varus)

Figure 4-35. Calcaneal motion on the talus as viewed from the rear.

Figure 4-36. Forefoot inversion creating medial rotation of the cuboid bone (*Cu*) on the calcaneus (Ca) and navicular bone (*N*) on the talus (*T*).

Figure 4-37. Lateral longitudinal arch of the foot.

Figure 4-38. Medial longitudinal arch of the foot and its associated torsion.

langeal articulations allow active motions of extension-flexion and adduction-abduction. Accessory motions are sliding, axial rotation, and long axis traction.

The active interphalangeal motions are flexion and extension. The accessory motions are abduction and adduction, axial rotation, and long axis extension.

Biomechanical and functional relationships of the foot. To perform its weight-bearing and elastic mobile activities, the longitudinal arch is constructed in two different anatomical forms. The *lateral longitudinal arch* is a firm osseous structure consisting of the calcaneus, cuboid, and the fourth and fifth metatarsals. It resembles the classical architectural definition of an arch, having a keystone (the cuboid) with a flank stone (calcaneus and metatarsal) on each side. It is low, of limited mobility, and built to transmit weight and thrust to and from the ground (Fig. 4-37).

The *medial arch* is higher, without firm osseous support, and can be increased or reduced to meet the needs of motion or terrain. MacConaill describes the subtalar area as functioning as a twisted plate. It is flattened transversely along the

line of the metatarsal heads and vertically at the calcaneus. It can be elongated or untwisted in pronation, dropping the medial "arch," or, with supination, become more twisted, raising the medial arch (Fig. 4-38).

The medial arch is controlled by the rotation of the calcaneus on a longitudinal axis (calcaneal valgus-varus). Extreme adduction of the standing feet (crossing one foot over the other) causes posterior clockwise rotation of the calcaneus (varus) and a high medial arch. Extreme abduction of the standing foot with dorsiflexion of the ankle causes counterclockwise rotation of the calcaneus (valgus) with a dropping of the medial arch.

Therefore, the structure and motions of this area of the foot can be said to twist and untwist the foot in various positions.

If on examination the foot arch changes in conformity with these principles, the feet are not structurally flat. Calcaneal valgus can have far-reaching structural and mechanical effects. It can reduce the medial arch, exaggerating foot pronation and increasing toe abduction and the tendency for eversion. This is very evident when observing gait. Calcaneal valgus also increases genu valgus, anterior pelvic tilt, and lumbar lordosis. The evaluation and treatment of foot imbalance is an integral part of the osteopathic examination.

Biomechanics of Intervertebral Joint Motion

The general rules of motion discussed with regard to appendicular articulations pertain as well to spinal synovial articulations. The vertebral articulations, however, have a tripod arrangement, which further complicates their motions. This tripod consists of an anterior synarthrosis, the vertebral bodies with intervertebral disks, and a pair of matched posterior synovial articulations. These three articulations are involved simultaneously in every vertebral motion.

A functional unit of the vertebral column is composed of two segments: an anterior segment that consists of two neighboring vertebral bodies separated by an intervertebral disk, and a posterior segment consisting of the two neural arches, their pedicles, laminae, superior and inferior articulations, transverse processes, and a spinous process (Fig. 4-39).

The main functions of the anterior segment are supportive, weight-bearing, shock absorbing, and, in combination with the posterior segment, protection of the spinal cord. The posterior segment primarily effects directional guidance of joint motion. In the upright position it is almost non-weight-bearing.

Common factors that influence segmental motion include the design and spatial relationships of the individual facets; the vertebral ligamentous and muscular attachments and their function; the size and health of the intervertebral disks; the osteology of the vertebra; and the age, sex, and health of the patient. In addition, preload, gravity, and tone, and the amount and direction of applied load and stress must be taken into account.

DESIGN AND SPATIAL RELATIONSHIPS OF FACETS

The facets of the typical cervical vertebrae, C3 through C7, are flat and oval. Their average spatial orientation is a 45-degree angle between the horizontal and frontal planes. The superior facets face backward and upward (Fig. 4-40). They therefore have great freedom of motion in all planes. Because of the 45-degree spatial planar relationship, the coupled motions of rotation and lateral flexion always occur in the same direction.

The thoracic articular facets are flat, with the superior facets facing backward, upward, and laterally. The spatial orientation is a 60-degree angle from the horizontal to the frontal plane, and a 20-degree rotation from the frontal to the sagittal plane in a medial direction (Fig. 4-41). Without the rib attachments, the coupled motions of lateral flexion and rotation would be excellent. Flexion is greatly reduced by the 60-degree angle toward the frontal plane. Combined lateral flexion with rotation can be in the same or opposite directions.

Figure 4-39. Functional unit of the vertebral column.

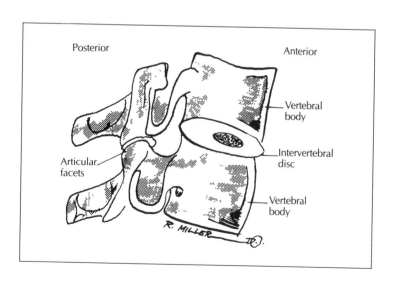

The lumbar facets have curved surfaces. The superior facets are concave and face backward and medially. The inferior facets mirror them by being convex, facing forward and laterally. The rules of concave-convex relationship are evident with joint motion. Lateral flexion is a coupled roll and slide motion. This creates a slight rotary movement. As in the thoracic region, lateral flexion and rotation can be in the same or opposite directions.

The average lumbar facet spatial orientation is a 45-degree angle from the frontal to the sagittal plane, turning in the lateral direction (Fig. 4-42). The greatest motion is found in flexion-extension; some lateral flexion is present with slight rotation. The described typical motion patterns may vary segmentally if other factors intervene.

The motion found at transitional intervertebral segmental levels is unpredictable. The additional stress created by changes in curve directions, and the osseous shape variations, create a climate for the development of somatic dysfunctions.

The anterior and posterior longitudinal ligaments respectively limit extension and flexion. Posteriorly they are joined by the interspinous and supraspinous ligaments and the ligamentum flavum. Collectively they create a firm connection, linking all the vertebrae together. This supports and limits excessive motion. Dysfunction can develop when degenerative disks allow a loosening of the supportive ligaments, and posterior or anterior spondylolisthesis occurs.

The muscular attachments are commonly described as bilaterally symmetric. Unfortunately this is not the case. Everyone has asymmetric development. This causes unstable hypo- or hypertonic muscular development. Even simple spinal motions would become imbalanced, but for the synergistic or stabilizing assistance of other groups of muscles. All motions are susceptible to dysfunction because of these factors. The greater the imbalance, the greater is the tendency for the development of somatic dysfunction.

When evaluating muscle function or using muscle contractive force therapeutically, the clinician must be cognizant of the differences in strength and action between the superficial, powerful muscles and the deep, weaker muscles. The deep muscles, owing to their vertebral attachments, create localized intervertebral balancing movements. The clinician uses the localized but lesser strength of the deep muscles in muscle energy therapy.

Figure 4-40. Cervical vertebral facet orientation at the level of C4.

INTERVERTEBRAL DISKS

The intervertebral disks influence joint motion in a number of ways. The annulus consists of layers of fibroelastic fibers that are attached to the superior and inferior vertebral end-plates. These fibers intertwine in oblique patterns that permit rolling, rotation, and translation of one vertebra on another. The relative size of the disk with reference to its attached veretebrae is proportional to the motion allowed.

Disk degeneration, with a reduction in height, creates an imbalance of the articular facet relationship. The possible ligamentous effect was discussed earlier.

Figure 4-41. Thoracic vertebral facet orientation at the level of T6.

Figure 4-42. Lumbar vertebral facet orientation at the level of L3.

Osteology

The various shapes and structures of the vertebrae may also affect their motions. The cervical vertebral bodies are sella-shaped, which encourages freedom of motion. The joints of Lushka modify the translatory lateral motion of the cervical vertebral bodies. The shingle effect created by the thoracic spinous processes can restrict extension. A similar restriction can occur in the lumbar region if the spinous processes are elongated. The rib cage restricts lateral flexion and unilateral joint rotation.

The fifth lumbar vertebra is subject to a greater number of congenital abnormalities than any other bone. These abnormalities affect motion and create the tendency for dysfunction. A very common abnormality of this region, usually not reported radiologically, entails a change in the fifth lumbar vertebra-sacral base articular facet relations. It is common to find atypical bilateral horizontal articulations or one horizontal and one vertical facet articulation in this region. This creates an imbalance that develops into low back dysfunction.

Preload and Gravity
Normally, the effects of preload (gravity, weight, and muscle tone) are greater at the fifth lumbar vertebra than at the fifth cervical vertebra in the upright subject. However, the cervical muscles of a patient who has been living with constant stress may be chronically contracted, with a marked increase in tone. The disks would be subjected to a constant increased preload. Slight force can create great dysfunctions. The effect of scoliosis at any level creates an imbalance in muscle tone, with increased preload on one side of the disk. One-sided muscular overdevelopment, a common occurrence over time in most humans, can produce dysfunction in this manner.

Normal gravitational force directly affects the functional spinal unit. A gravitational force that is not directed toward the center of gravity of an object creates a secondary rotary force vector. None of the functional spinal units are completely horizontal to the earth. There are normal or abnormal lateral physiologic spinal curvatures, and multiple compensatory scoliotic patterns. Thus, spinal muscles are in a constant state of hypertonicity, trying to maintain an upright stature against gravity's rotary force. All of these factors affect articular motion and function.

Vertebral Motion at the Functional Spinal Unit
Coupled motions are normally present in a functional spinal unit. **Flexion** is the rotary motion of anterior vertebral approximation coupled with ventral translatory slide. **Extension** is the rotary motion of anterior vertebral separation coupled with dorsal translatory slide.

Rotation right is the turning of the anterior aspect of the body of the vertebra toward the right, coupled with a diminution of intervertebral disk height, described as vertical translatory compression (Fig. 4-43).

Rotation left is the turning of the anterior aspect of the body of the vertebra toward the left, coupled with the previously described vertical translatory compression. As the vertebra turns back toward the midline, either from right or left rotation, the intervertebral disk returns to its usual height.

Lateral flexion right or left is a rotary motion that causes the side of upper vertebral body to approximate the one below it, right or left, accompanied by a contralateral translatory slide (Fig. 4-44).

Each of these described coupled motions occurs in a single plane and on an instantaneous axis of rotation. If these motions are again coupled, lateral flexion with rotation, then multiple planes are involved and the motion occurs on a helical axis of rotation.

When the somatic dysfunction diagnosis is T4 ESr Rr, the motion of the fourth thoracic vertebra on the fifth thoracic vertebra is greater in the directions of extension, right lateral flexion, and right rotation. These three coupled motions occur in three planes simultaneously on a helical axis

Figure 4-43. Coupled rotation and translatory motion in the horizontal plane.

Figure 4-44. Coupled rotator and contralateral translator motions in the frontal plane that occur during lateral flexion.

Lateral flexion

Figure 4-45. Fourth thoracic vertebra, right side bending, right rotation with extension.

T_4

T_5

Neutral

$T_4ES_RR_R$

of rotation (Fig. 4-45). The barriers to freedom of the described motion would all be in the opposite directions, but on the same helical axis of rotation.

Many osteopathic diagnostic and therapeutic approaches can be explained by combining the laws of physiologic motion, vertebral biomechanics, and the kinetic principle of the effect of resistance to linear motion. The effect of resistance to linear motion can be described as follows: If an object in linear motion encounters an obstacle or resistance, it will turn about its point of contact with the interfering factor.

Example: On palpation, the transverse process of the fourth thoracic vertebra is more prominent posteriorly on the right. Is it part of a somatic dysfunction complex involving three planes and six motions on a helical axis? The vertebra is placed into a position of flexion. The right transverse process becomes more prominent posteriorly. It is assumed that this has happened because there is a barrier present to the motion of flexion, and the vertebra is responding according to the rule of the effect of resistance on linear motion. That is, on meeting this flexion barrier, the vertebra turns away from and around it in the direction of allowable freedom of motion, or right rotation.

Two parts of the diagnosis are now available. Freedom of motion in extension (flexion barrier),

and right rotation. According to the laws of physiologic motion, if flexion or extension is involved in the motion diagnosis, then lateral flexion is in the same direction as the motion of rotation. Therefore, the diagnosis is T4 ESr Rr, moving on a helical axis.

To treat this dysfunction, the vertebra is placed in a position duplicating its helical axis. This allows it to move into or away from the barriers of motion. A force is then applied along this same helical axis of rotation in the direction desired, depending on whether direct or indirect treatment procedures are used.

MOTION TESTING
Donald E. Phykitt

The diagnosis of somatic dysfunctions of the axial skeleton includes assessment of symmetry of spinal motion. This assessment occurs on a number of levels, ranging from evaluation of movement of a complete section of the spine (regional motion testing) to evaluation of movement of a single spinal functional unit (rotoscoliosis testing, intersegmental motion testing). This section describes the goals, theories, and interpretation of these techniques. The techniques themselves are described in later chapters.

Regional Motion Testing
The goal of regional motion testing is to assess the overall motion of a section (cervical, thoracic, lumbar) of the axial skeleton. Gross motion of the spine is modified by numerous conditions, including osseous deformities (e.g., structural scoliosis), ligamentous imbalances, muscle spasm (acute or chronic), articular disease (e.g., degenerative joint disease), somatic dysfunction, and pain, usually due to one or more of the preceding conditions. These conditions limit both the degree and the quality of motion. Limitations can occur in one (or more) of three planes. Limitation of flexion-extension occurs in the sagittal plane, limitation of rotation occurs in the horizontal plane, and limitation of lateral flexion occurs in the frontal plane.

Regional motion testing is used as a screening procedure to:

1. Determine a region to be more closely evaluated.
2. Provide a measurement with which a patient's progress can be assessed.
3. Identify regions that could benefit from general techniques such as myofascial treatment.

The evaluation of regional motion entails evaluation of the *degree* of motion, the *symmetry* of motion (e.g., right rotation vs. left rotation), and the *quality* of motion (restrictions may be due to one or more of the conditions listed in the section on the biomechanics of joint motion in this chapter).

Assessment of Group Curves (Type I Somatic Dysfunctions)
The goal of assessment of group curves is to identify groups of adjacent vertebrae (usually three or more) that are dysfunctional in such a way that they obey Fryette's first law of vertebral motion.

Lateral group curves can occur in any region of the axial skeleton. They are most often caused by (1) asymmetric muscle contraction or contracture producing a "bowstring" effect on the spine, (2) structural asymmetries elsewhere in the body (e.g., short leg), for which they are compensating (functional or physiologic scoliosis), and (3) structural scoliosis secondary to known or idiopathic etiologies.

As a result of the prevailing conditions, the vertebrae in a group curve exhibit type I motion (side bending and rotation occur to opposite sides). The techniques involved in diagnosing group curves address both the side bending and rotational components of the dysfunction. These techniques are:

1. **Observation of the standing patient.** Lateral deviation of a group of vertebra from the midline can be observed when the patient is examined from behind. The rotational component can be observed as posterior prominence of the paravertebral musculature, scapula, or ribs on one side of the body. This prominence is usually located on the side opposite to the direction of side bending (on the same side as the convexity of the curve). This is a result of side bending and rotation occurring in opposite directions. The prominence is more obvious if the patient is asked to bend forward.

2. **Rotoscoliosis testing.** This technique evaluates the rotational component of group curves when the spine is in the neutral position. Vertebrae involved in a group curve display rotation opposite to their direction of side bending. This is detected by palpating the transverse processes, which should be more prominent on the side of the direction of rotation of the involved vertebrae. Flexion or extension of the individual vertebrae should not alter this rotation factor. From Fryette's first law of vertebral motion it can be inferred that the group is laterally flexed to the opposite side. It should be noted that the biomechanics of the cervical region are such that rotoscoliosis testing cannot be used to evaluate group curves. Static symmetry examination of landmarks of the skull and evaluation of range of motion are the best means of diagnosing group curves in this region.

3. **Interpretation.** A group curve in the thoracic or lumbar spine in which the vertebrae are side-bent left and rotated right would display the following features: a lateral curve with its convexity facing right; more prominent musculature, ribs, or scapula on the right; and posterior transverse processes on the right when palpated in neutral position.

Individual Vertebral Motion Testing
ROTOSCOLIOSIS TESTING

The goal of rotoscoliosis testing is to detect somatic dysfunctions of single vertebral functional units, by comparing the rotational position of vertebrae when they are in flexion to that when they are in extension. Somatic dysfunctions usually involve restrictions in three planes: the sagittal plane (restriction noted on flexion-extension), the horizontal plane (noted on rotation), and the frontal plane (noted on lateral flexion). These restrictions affect static position as well as motion. A vertebra's position is always away from its restriction (i.e., toward its freedom of motion) in all three planes.

A principle of physics states that when a moving object encounters a barrier, it will change direction to follow the path of least resistance. Similarly, when a vertebra encounters a barrier in one plane, it tends to move further in the direction of its freedom of motion in the other two planes. A three-dimensional example is a box that is pushed along the floor. If the front of the box (the vertebra) hits a pole (barrier), it has encountered restriction to motion. If the portion of the box that contacts the pole is away from the midline (as is usually the case in a somatic dysfunction), pushing the box further (moving it into its barrier) causes the box to rotate around the pole. In contrast, pulling the box back away from the pole allows straight sliding (no rotation).

Rotoscoliosis testing is based on the assumption that placing a vertebra into its flexion-extension barrier results in rotation of the vertebra in the direction of its freedom of motion. For example, in T4 ERr Sr, T4 is extended on T5. The barriers to motion are flexion, left side bending, and rotation. Placing T4 into flexion would further accentuate the restrictive forces (the box hits the pole). In an attempt to follow the path of least resistance, T4 would rotate and flex laterally to the right.

By palpating the transverse processes or articular pillars, the clinician can detect the rotational position of a vertebra. Noting whether rotation to a certain side is greatest in flexion or extension allows discrimination of the freedom of motion in the sagittal plane (i.e., the position opposite to that in which the greatest rotation was noted). The freedom of motion in the frontal plane (side bending) is deduced from Fryette's second law of vertebral motion, according to which rotation and lateral flexion occur in the same direction when either flexion or extension barriers are present.

Of aid in rotoscoliosis testing are the following observations:

1. The position (flexion-extension) in which rotation is the greatest is the barrier of motion.
2. The side on which the transverse process is more posterior denotes the direction of rotational freedom of motion.
3. Since, in single somatic dysfunctions, rotation and side bending occur in the same direction, the side bending component is named for the same direction as the rotational component. For example, the left transverse process of T3 is most prominent when it is placed in flexion. The dysfunction is designated as T3 E Rl Sl.

DIRECT INTERSEGMENTAL MOTION TESTING

The goal of direct intersegmental motion testing is to dynamically diagnose somatic dysfunction of single vertebral functional units by directly assessing the symmetry of motion in all three planes.

The clinician localizes motion to a single vertebral level, then induces motion in all three planes. Symmetry of motion may be noted in flexion versus extension, rotation right versus rotation left, and right lateral flexion versus left lateral flexion. The somatic dysfunction is named for the directions of freedom of motion. This method can be used in the cervical, thoracic, and lumbar regions. The somatic dysfunction is named for the directions of freedom of motion, using the accepted nomenclature, e.g., T3 E Rr Sr.

INDIRECT INTERSEGMENTAL MOTION TESTING WITH TRANSLATORY MOTION

The goal of this form of testing is to dynamically detect somatic dysfunctions of single vertebral functional units (usually in the cervical region) by indirectly assessing asymmetry of lateral flexion.

The method incorporates the principle that lateral flexion of a vertebra to one side is accompanied by translation of that vertebra to the opposite side in the frontal plane (see the first section on palpation in this chapter). This is interpreted to mean that asymmetric lateral flexion will be accompanied by asymmetric translation to the opposite side. Furthermore, asymmetry of transla-

tion (and therefore of lateral flexion) is most noticeable when the vertebra is placed into its barrier in the sagittal plane (flexion or extension). This latter point can be explained by the fact that placing a vertebra into its barrier of motion in one plane of motion enhances the restrictive forces to motion in the other two planes. Finally, as previously mentioned, side bending and rotation occur to the same side. Therefore, by determining in which direction asymmetry of translatory motion is present, by determining if the asymmetry of translation is greatest in flexion or extension, and by applying knowledge of cervical vertebral biomechanics, the clinician can diagnose a somatic dysfunction in the cervical region in all three planes. As a nomenclatural example, C3 translates easier from right to left when placed in flexion, so the dysfunction is named C3 E Sr Rr.

References

Basmajian JV. 1978. Muscles Alive, 4th ed. Baltimore: Williams & Wilkins Co.

Cailliet R. 1968. Foot and Ankle Pain. Philadelphia: F.A. Davis Co.

———. 1981. Neck and Arm Pain. Philadelphia: F.A. Favis Co.

Ealton WJ. 1970. Textbook of Osteopathic Diagnosis and Technique Procedures, 2nd ed. Colorado Springs, Colo: American Academy of Osteopathy.

Fryette HH. 1918. Physiologic movements of the spine. J Am Osteopath Assoc 18:1. Reprinted in 1950 Yearbook of Selected Osteopathic Topics, pp 91–92. Ann Arbor, Michigan: Academy of Applied Osteopathy.

———. 1954. Principles of Osteopathic Technique. Kirksville, Mo: American Academy of Osteopathy.

Fujiwara M, Basmajian JV. 1975. Electromyographic study of two joint muscles. Am J Phys Med 54:234–242.

Hoag JM, Kosok M, Moser JR. 1960. Kinematic analysis and classification of vertebral motion. J Am Osteopath Assoc 54:894, 982.

Hoover HV, Nelson CR. 1950. Basic physiologic movements of the spine. In: 1950 Yearbook of Selected Osteopathic Topics, p 63. Ann Arbor, Michigan: Academy of Applied Osteopathy.

Jones L. 1955. The Postural Complex. Springfield, Ill: Charles C Thomas, Publisher.

Kapandji IA. 1974. The Physiology of the Joints, 2nd ed, vols 1, 2, 3. Edinburgh: Churchill Livingstone.

Kraus H. 1970. Clinical Treatment of Back and Neck Pain. New York: McGraw-Hill Book Co.

MacConaill MA. 1949. The movements of bones and joints. J Bone Joint Surg [Am] (31B)1:100–104.

———, Basmajian JV. 1977. Muscles and Movements. Huntington, New York: Robert E. Krieger Publishing Co.

Mitchell FL Jr, Moran PS, Pruzzo MT. 1979. An Evaluation and Treatment Manual of Osteopathic Muscle Energy Procedures. Valley Park, Mo: self-published.

Moore KL. 1980. Clinically Oriented Anatomy. Baltimore: Williams & Wilkins Co.

Project on Osteopathic Principles Education. 1982. Glossary of Osteopathic Terminology. Chicago: Educational Council on Osteopathic Principles.

Rasch PJ, Burke RK. 1978. Kinesiology and Applied Anatomy, 6th ed. Philadelphia: Lea & Febiger.

Schiowitz S, DiGiovanna EL, Ausman PJ, eds. 1983. An Osteopathic Approach to Diagnosis and Treatment. Old Westbury, NY: New York College of Osteopathic Medicine.

Warwick R, Williams P. 1973. Gray's Anatomy, 35th British ed. Philadelphia: W.B. Saunders Co.

Wells KF, Luttgens K. 1976. Kinesiology, 6th ed. Philadelphia: W.B. Saunders Co.

White AA, Panjabi MM. 1978. Clinical Biomechanics of the Spine. Philadelphia: J.B. Lippincott Co.

5

Principles of Osteopathic Manipulative Techniques

MYOFASCIAL TECHNIQUES
Toni Murphy

Myofascial techniques are a group of specific maneuvers that, in general, achieve the same goals. They can be used as the primary modality of treatment or in combination with other methods.

The term *myofascial* comes from the root words *myo*, meaning "muscle," and *fascia*, which is self-explanatory. Myofascial techniques are among the soft tissue techniques. Muscle and fascia are most commonly thought of as the tissues treated by these techniques, but all of the fibroelastic connective tissues as well as skin, tendons, ligaments, cartilage, blood, and lymph may be affected.

Because of the great overlap in function among manipulative techniques, it is difficult to delimit myofascial techniques from other soft tissue techniques. Therefore, the present discussion addresses myofascial techniques in general. Specific techniques are discussed in detail in later chapters.

The musculoskeletal system comprises a large percentage of the human body, and myofascial techniques can and do have significant effects on the body. Dysfunction of musculoskeletal and neuromuscular components can be as disabling as infectious organ diseases or metabolic disorders. Myofascial techniques aid in achieving the primary goal of the human body—homeostasis, or the restoration and preservation of optimal bodily function. The effects of myofascial techniques on homeostasis include, but are not limited to, the following:

1. Relaxation of contracted muscles, which decreases the oxygen demand of the muscle, decreases pain, and allows normalized range of motion across a joint
2. Increased circulation to an area of ischemia, therefore supplying blood carrying oxygen and nutrients to the tissues and removing harmful metabolic waste products
3. Increased venous and lymphatic drainage, thereby decreasing local swelling and edema
4. A stimulatory affect of the stretch reflex in hypotonic muscles

The schematic diagram in Figure 5-1 explains the tissue changes that lead to impaired mobility, function, pain, and soft tissue changes seen and felt in the human body at various stages. The initiating insult or trauma may be subtle or quite dramatic. Cailliet defines *trauma* as "a wound or injury with implication of a force applied exter-

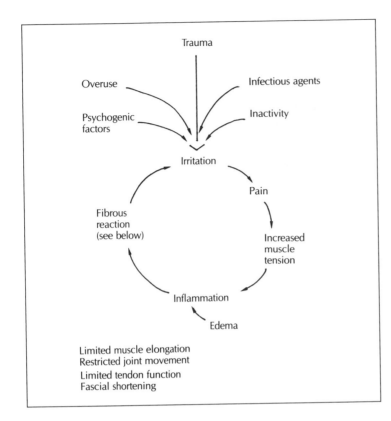

Figure 5-1. Cycle of soft tissue changes/pain/soft tissue changes following traumatic insult.

nally or internally causing a tissue reaction. Pain is the resultant which has varying degrees of intensity and effective interpretation with numerous avenues of transmission."

The initiating trauma may be anything that causes soft tissue irritation. The irritation is interpreted as pain. The body's usual reaction to pain is an increase in muscle tension. A vicious cycle ensues: a positive feedback mechanism informed by pain leads to increased muscle tension, which leads to increased pain, and so on. The increase in muscle tension plays an important role in tissue ischemia. The cycle continues, with tissue ischemia hindering provision of nutrients to the tissue and permitting buildup of waste products in the tissues. These waste products act as noxious stimuli, causing further irritation of the tissues, pain, and inflammation.

To this point the process can be thought of as acute. If the process continues, it may become chronic. The next step is fibrous tissue reaction. If this occurs, it is believed to be permanent, which makes the soft tissue damage less reversible. An effect of the fibrous reaction is limited muscle elongation or stretch, which allows muscle shortening to develop, which in turn may limit movement across a joint. Other effects are limitation in tendon function and fascial shortening. All lead to a decrease in the functional ability of the body part and person.

Myofascial techniques are useful in breaking the pain-muscle tension-pain cycle. Increasing the circulation to and drainage from the tissues may aid in diminishing the inflammatory response.

Some of the physiologic principles applied in myofascial techniques include the following:

1. **Extensibility of the connective tissues:** Connective tissue placed under prolonged mild tension shows plastic elongation.
2. **Stretch reflex:** The stretch of a muscle excites the muscle spindle, resulting in reflex contraction of that muscle. This is to be avoided when applying passive myofascial techniques to contracted or contractured muscles. It can be avoided by applying slow, even force and releasing that force slowly and evenly. However,

the stretch reflex is to be used during active myofascial techniques for the purpose of stimulating muscle tone in hypotonic muscles.

3. **Heat:** Heat applied to a muscle usually results in an increase in elastic response of the muscle to stretch.

4. **Muscle spindle reflex:** This is utilized in active resistive myofascial techniques. If the extrafusal fibers contract less than the intrafusal fibers, the muscle spindle will maintain a stretch reflex, further exciting the extrafusal fibers.

5. **Golgi tendon organ reflex:** This is utilized in active myofascial techniques. When the tension on the tendon becomes extreme, the inhibitory effect from the Golgi tendon organ can cause sudden relaxation of the entire muscle.

6. **Reciprocal inhibition:** This is utilized in active myofascial techniques with or without resistance. When a stretch reflex stimulates one muscle it simultaneously inhibits the antagonist muscle; e.g., if the stretch reflex excites the biceps, reciprocal inhibition inhibits the triceps.

7. **Crossed extensor reflex:** This is utilized in active myofascial techniques with resistance. When a stretch reflex excites one muscle it simultaneously excites the contralateral antagonist muscle. Motion is created that crosses from one side of the spine to the other in an X pattern; e.g., the stretch reflex excites the right biceps, the crossed extensor reflex excites the left triceps.

Passive and Active Techniques

Passive techniques are used by the physician with the patient relaxed. Passive techniques entail application of a manual traction force in one of four directions:

1. Linear pull at either end of the muscle
2. Linear pull at both ends of the muscle at the same time
3. Pushing the muscle in a direction perpendicular to the long axis of the muscle fibers, thus creating stretch
4. Pulling the muscle in a direction perpendicular to the long axis of the muscle fibers, thus creating stretch

In **active** techniques the patient assists the physician by actively contracting certain muscles under the guidance of the physician. There are two forms of active myofascial techniques. **Active direct** techniques are those in which the patient is asked to contract the involved muscle. These techniques utilize the Golgi tendon organ reflex to relax the involved muscle(s). In these techniques the physician applies isometric resistance to the contraction. (*Isometric resistance:* The physician applies resistance to the patient's contraction such that little shortening of the muscle is permitted but a great increase in muscle tension results.)

Active indirect techniques are those in which the patient is asked to contract the muscles antagonistic to those being treated. This method uses the reciprocal inhibition reflex to relax the muscles being treated. In these techniques the physician applies isokinetic resistance to the patient's contraction. (*Isokinetic resistance:* The physician applies a resistive force such that the muscle contraction increases very little with the gradual decrease in muscle length; i.e., the joint is allowed to move and the resistance is gradually increased.)

General Considerations

There are a few general rules to follow when applying myofascial techniques.

1. The patient should be in a position of comfort and be relaxed.
2. The physician should be in a position of comfort and be at ease.
3. The physician should minimize energy expenditure and use body weight whenever possible instead of upper arm strength.
4. The force must be of low intensity, is slowly applied and maintained for 3 to 4 seconds, and is slowly released.
5. The force applied must not create pain.
6. Always push or pull muscle away from bone, as it is painful to push into bone.
7. Push or pull muscle in a direction perpendicular to the long axis of the muscle fibers.
8. Avoid rubbing or irritating the patient's skin by the friction of your fingers or hands.
9. Use leverage whenever possible.
10. When treating muscles with myofascial techniques, the physician's fingertips and the thenar and hypothenar eminences are used to apply pressure.

11. When a transverse force (push or pull) is applied across a muscle body, a counterforce may also be applied to maintain the patient's position.
12. Muscle stretch may also be achieved by applying traction in a lengthwise direction of the muscle fibers at the insertion or attachment of the muscle, thus lengthening the distance between the two.
13. Compression may be used in areas of multiple muscle layers in order to reach the deeper tissues.

MUSCLE ENERGY TECHNIQUES
Sandra D. Yale

Muscle energy therapy is a modality of osteopathic treatment that was designed by Fred L. Mitchell, Sr, and later expanded by his son Fred L. Mitchell, Jr, and others. The techniques use active muscle contraction to mobilize specific articulations. The patient participates actively by contracting muscles statically in a situation controlled by the physician. Muscle energy techniques are direct techniques because the barriers to motion are engaged.

Muscle energy techniques can be directed toward a single-segment somatic dysfunction. The physician positions the area of dysfunction into its barriers to motions (flexion-extension, side bending, and rotation). The patient is then asked to move the joint back toward its unrestricted or free motions. The movement is a gentle, controlled contraction of less than one pound of force, which is completely resisted by the physician.

The static contraction is maintained for 2 to 3 seconds and is followed by a relaxation period of about 2 seconds. The joint is then moved to its new physiologic motion barriers and the procedure is repeated three to four times.

Several principles should be followed to achieve the most benefit from muscle energy treatment:

1. The positioning of the somatic dysfunction into its physiologic motion barriers should be specific in all three planes (flexion-extension, side bending, rotation).
2. The patient statically contracts muscles toward the freedoms of motion of the somatic dysfunction.
3. The patient relaxes between muscle-contracting efforts.
4. The physician reengages the joint into its new motion barriers.

Precisely why muscle energy techniques are effective is unclear. According to one prominent theory, the effectiveness of muscle energy techniques depends on the function of the Golgi tendon organ. The Golgi tendon organ is located in the area of the muscle where the fibers insert into the tendon. It responds to changes in tension (see Chap. 2, Neurophysiology Relevant to Osteopathic Manipulation). When the muscle contracts or is stretched, the tendon is also stretched. The Golgi tendon organ responds by relaxing and resetting the tendon at its new length.

With muscle energy treatment, the Golgi tendon organ is subjected to increased tension during the active as well as the passive phase. It resets the muscle to a longer length, allowing more motion at the area of somatic dysfunction.

Muscle energy techniques are particularly effective in patients who have severe pain from acute somatic dysfunction, such as a patient with a whiplash injury from a car accident, or a patient with severe muscle spasm from a fall. Muscle energy techniques are also an excellent treatment modality for the hospitalized or bedridden patient. They can be used in older patients who may have severely restricted motion from arthritis or who have brittle, osteoporotic bones.

COUNTERSTRAIN
Eileen L. DiGiovanna

Perhaps the newest form of osteopathic manipulation is counterstrain. It became popular in the 1970s, and the number of practitioners is increasing. The technique was devised by Lawrence Jones, an osteopathic practitioner in Oregon. He spent many years perfecting the technique before introducing it to the profession.

In *Strain and Counterstrain*, Jones offers two definitions of the technique.

1. "Relieving spinal or other joint pain by passively putting the joint into its position of greatest comfort."
2. "Relieving pain by reduction and arrest of the continuing inappropriate proprioceptor activity. This is accomplished by markedly shortening the muscle that contains the malfunctioning muscle spindle by applying mild strain to its antagonists."

Figure 5-2. Muscular activity. Bar gauge represents extent of muscle fiber stretch; circular gauge indicates impulses from muscle stretch receptors. (**A**) Arm flexed. (**B**) Arm hyperflexed. (**C**) Arm extended. (**D**) Arm hyperextended.

Figure 5-3. Etiology of tender point. (**A**) Both flexors and extensors are in easy normal position. (**B**) Force is suddenly exerted counter to the flexors, forcing the arm into extension. (**C**) Fibers and stretch receptors indicate that a danger point has been reached. Extensor fibers are hypershortened. (**D**) Arm is relatively flexed, exciting the muscle stretch receptors. (**E**) Rapid rate of flexion overstimulates extensor stretch receptors. (**F**) Arm is in same position as in **A**, but stretch receptors continue to respond as if muscle were being rapidly stretched.

The theory of counterstrain is based on the belief that somatic dysfunction has a neuromuscular basis (Fig. 5-2). With trauma or muscle effort against a sudden change in resistance, or with muscle strain incurred by resisting the effects of gravity (e.g., bending over) for a period of time, one muscle at a joint is strained and its antagonist is hypershortened. When the shortened muscle is suddenly stretched the annulospinal receptors in that muscle are stimulated, causing a reflex contraction of the already shortened muscle. The proprioceptors in the short muscle now fire impulses as if the shortened muscle were being stretched. Since this inappropriate proprioceptor response can be maintained indefinitely, a somatic dysfunction has been created. The joint is restricted, within its physiologic range of motion, from achieving full range of motion by this shortened muscle. It is therefore an active process rather than a static injury such as is usually associated with strain (Fig. 5-3).

In counterstrain, the diagnosis is made by finding reflex "tender points". Each involved joint has its own specific tender points, either anterior or posterior. The point may lie in the shortened muscle or in a more distant area to which it has been referred reflexly. It is about the size of a dime and can be palpated as tissue change—a tense, slightly fibrotic area. It is tender to an amount of pressure that would not normally cause pain. The tender points may be related to myofascial trigger points (Travell points) and acupuncture points; there are similarities in distribution.

The treatment technique is positional. According to Jones, positioning the joint in the exactly opposite position to the one that produces the pain will relieve the pain and dysfunction. In treatment, therefore, the joint is positioned in such a manner that pressure on the tender point

no longer elicits tenderness. The physician may be able to palpate a softening of the tissues.

To position the joint, the physician makes a gross adjustment toward the position of comfort and then fine-tunes. For example, the joint may require flexion to reduce the degree of pain, and then a little rotation or side bending to remove the remaining tenderness. Jones refers to the final position as the mobile point. The position is held for 90 seconds, the amount of time required for the proprioceptive firing to decrease in frequency and amplitude.

The next step is important. The joint is returned *slowly* to its neutral position. The slow motion prevents reinitiation of the inappropriate proprioceptive firing. The patient is cautioned that some muscle soreness may result, but since this is not a somatic dysfunction, the muscle will return to normal quickly.

Counterstrain treatment is an extremely effective and nontraumatic treatment. It is especially good for elderly or hospitalized patients, and any others for whom gentleness is desirable. Patients who have experienced an acute strain respond well.

THRUSTING TECHNIQUES
Eileen L. DiGiovanna

Most thrusting techniques are direct techniques, in that the dysfunctional unit is placed into at least one of its barriers to motion and the physician thrusts through that barrier. The techniques are considered passive because the physician provides the treating force and the patient remains passive.

High Velocity, Low Amplitude Techniques

The best known of all manipulative techniques are the high velocity, low amplitude techniques. In these techniques, the physician positions the patient in such a way that the restricted joint is placed into its barriers to motion. The physician

then quickly applies a small amount of force to the joint in such a way as to move it through the barriers. Improved joint motion should result.

To achieve the best results with as little pain as possible, the surrounding tissues should be relaxed before the thrusting force is applied. Myofascial (soft tissue) techniques or other nonthrusting techniques may be used for this purpose. When the muscles and soft tissues are relaxed, less force is needed to move the joint and the treatment will be less painful.

High velocity, low amplitude techniques may have been the first type of manual medicine ever devised. They are the therapeutic maneuvers most commonly used by chiropractors and many osteopathic physicians, as well as other practitioners of manual medicine.

Low Velocity, High Amplitude Techniques

In some thrusting techniques a large force is applied slowly with the goal of moving the joint through the barrier. Care must be taken to avoid joint or soft tissue damage. These techniques when applied skillfully are quite useful, but the force must be carefully controlled. Again, relaxation of the soft tissues before force is applied makes the procedure safer and less painful.

Springing Techniques

Springing techniques are similar to high velocity, low amplitude techniques except that a full force is not applied. The joint is positioned as before, then gently sprung several times into its barriers. This maneuver gently nudges the joint motion through its barrier. The springing force is much less than that applied in high velocity, low amplitude techniques.

With repeated springing thrusts against the barrier, the joint may be moved as effectively as with high velocity, low amplitude thrusting but with less danger of trauma. Springing techniques are useful in more painful joints, older persons, children, and whenever a stronger force is contraindicated.

General Principles of Thrusting Techniques

1. Prepare the joint to be treated by relaxing the soft tissues so that the joint may be moved more easily.
2. Place the joint into its barriers of motion. If only one barrier is to be engaged, it is essential that all other joint motions be "locked" out.
3. Once a joint has been placed into its barriers of motion, this position must be held firmly by the physician and the "locking" thus created not lost as the force is applied.
4. The force must be controlled by the physician. Maximum force should not be applied in the hope that the joint will move. Only force sufficient to create the motion desired should be used.
5. Treatment must be localized and applied to the specific restricted joint. A "shotgun" approach to an entire area of the spine is inappropriate and harmful.

Pops and Cracks

Particularly with high velocity, low amplitude techniques, a popping or cracking sound may be heard, similar to the sound made by cracking the knuckles. Some observers believe the sound is due to the breaking of a vacuum in the joint, others that it is caused by release of a nitrogen bubble. Whatever its cause, eliciting this noise is not essential to the correction of a dysfunction. Feeling the joint move is more important than hearing it pop.

Many patients feel the treatment is successful only if they hear this sound. Others are frightened by it, fearing bones may be breaking. The patient must be assured that the sound is harmless.

EXERCISE THERAPY
Stanley Schiowitz

The average physician, before prescribing a specific drug, will have arrived at a working diagnosis and a therapeutic plan. The physician is expected to know the appropriate drug dosage, its side effects, its compatibilities with other drugs, and its effects on other clinical entities that the patient might have.

These minimal requirements of physician capability hold equally true in the prescription of exercise as a therapeutic modality. All physicians encounter patients who are voluntarily pursuing some form of exercise or for whom an exercise program should be prescribed. This chapter addresses the primary care physician's use and prescription of exercise therapy for musculoskeletal dysfunctions.

Biomechanics of Muscle Function

Muscle tissue has the properties of extensibility, elasticity, and contractility. *Extensibility* is the ability of muscle fiber to lengthen, usually to an additional 50% of its resting size. As one bends forward to touch the toes, the back muscles lengthen to accommodate the stretch.

Elasticity is the ability of muscle fiber to return to its original length. When one straightens up after touching the toes, the back muscles return to their former length.

Contractility is the ability of muscle fiber to shorten its length up to 50%. Only muscles have this capability, and it is the muscle property that is usually acknowledged.

In the example of forward bending, inability to touch the toes has no relationship to the contractile property of the abdominal muscles. Loss of extensibility of the hamstrings might be the culprit. Therefore, exercises would be directed toward increasing the extensibility of the hamstrings, and not toward strengthening the abdominals.

In daily usage, "tight, shortened, hypertonic" muscles need restoration of extensibility. "Flaccid, stretched, atonic" muscles have lost their elasticity, and "weak, hypotonic" muscles require increased contractility. The type of exercise, massage, and myofascial therapy prescribed is different for each of these dysfunctions.

MOMENT OF FORCE

Muscle power is used to move one part of the skeletal system around another part, with their articulation acting as a fulcrum. This creates a torque or *moment of force*. The torque around any point equals the product of the amount of force and its perpendicular distance from the direction of force to the axis of rotation (*moment arm*). If one were to hold a 5-pound weight in the palm, with the elbow flexed at a 90-degree angle, and if the distance from the elbow joint to the weight were one foot, then 5 foot-pounds of flexor muscle effort would be needed to maintain this position. If the elbow were flexed at a 45-degree angle, the force, the 5-pound weight, would stay the

same but the moment arm would be reduced. Less than 5 foot-pounds of flexor muscle effort would be needed to maintain this position.

LEVER ACTION

The use of the joint as a fulcrum brings into play Newton's laws of levers.

1. A first class lever has the fulcrum placed between the point of effort and resistance.
2. A second class lever has the resistance placed between the fulcrum and the point of effort.
3. A third class lever has the point of effort between the fulcrum and resistance.

Of the three levers, the second class lever is most efficient with regard to minimizing effort needed to move a resistance. A wheelbarrow is an example of such a lever. Most of our long muscles act as third class levers. The biceps muscle's flexion effort in moving the forearm is an example of such a lever action. The triceps' action causing forearm extension is an example of a first class lever. First class lever action usually requires less effort for motion than third class lever action.

An interesting demonstration of lever action is afforded by the brachialis muscle in flexion. Simple forearm flexion represents a third class lever action, but with a weight in the palm, lowering the forearm from a position of flexion to one of extension reverses the designations, in that gravity becomes the effort or moving force, while the insertion of the brachialis becomes the resistant force. This creates a second class lever action.

SPURT AND SHUNT ACTION

MacConaill defines the spurt and shunt action of muscles as follows. When a muscle contracts it creates two vector forces with regard to the articulation. One is a swing (rotation) force around its axis (spurt action). The second is transarticular motion into the joint in relation to its axis (shunt action). Both of these motions are present simultaneously, but in different proportions in all muscles. A large spurt to shunt ratio permits greater rotary motion with diminished joint stability. The reverse is true with an increased shunt to spurt ratio.

The biceps flexion motion of the forearm is primarily a spurt action at the elbow, but contraction of the long head of the biceps is a stabilizing, shunt action at the glenohumeral articulation.

A third motion is created by muscle contraction—spin motion. The amount of spin will depend on the difference in the planes of the origin and insertion of the muscle. Spin motion plays a part in the second law of myokinematics, described below.

LAWS OF MYOKINEMATICS

According to the first law of myokinematics (MacConaill and Basmajian, 1977), the law of approximation, states that, "when a muscle contracts it tends to bring its attachments (origin and insertion) closer together." In most activities the effect of this law is modified by using other muscle activity or resistant force to stabilize either the insertion or origin end of the muscle. This creates motion at one end of the muscle only.

The second law, the law of detorsion, states that "when a muscle contracts it tends to bring its line of origin and its line of insertion into one and the same plane." A simple example is sternocleidomastoid action. Unilateral contraction creates ipsilateral side bending, extension, and contralateral rotation of the head.

A less commonly recognized application of this principle is in hip extension. Pure gluteus maximus contraction tightens the hip joint and raises the femur somewhat toward the ilium in the frontal plane. To achieve hip extension, the pelvis rotates anteriorly in the sagittal plane. This rotation changes the planar relationships of the origin and insertion of the muscle. The law of detorsion is activated, and the insertion will try to match the plane of muscle origin. The more the pelvis is rotated, the greater will be the hip extension.

Gravity

Gravitational force is the attraction of each mass-particle in the universe for every other mass-particle. Gravitational force has three unique characteristics:

1. It is applied constantly.
2. It is applied in one direction only.
3. It acts on each mass-particle of the body.

This force is constantly exerted on all parts of the musculoskeletal system. Its effects, however, can be modified by body position. In the upright, anatomic position, gravity assists in stabilizing the hip, knee, and ankle joints. At the same time it creates instability of the glenohumeral articulation. In the supine position, gravitational force on all these joints is markedly different. The physician must be aware of the action of gravity when using exercise therapy. Bending the head forward in the upright position does not use the cervical flexor muscles. Gravity is the primary force involved. Extensor muscles are brought into play if control of the speed of forward bending is desired. In the supine position, forward bending or bringing the chin to the chest would necessitate use of the neck flexors.

An important aspect of all exercises is the patient's position, and its relationship to gravitational force.

Muscle Contraction Definitions

1. **Concentric contraction.** The muscle shortens, using the property of contractility to perform the task.
2. **Eccentric contraction.** The muscle lengthens, using extensibility to perform the task.
3. **Static contraction.** The muscle is in partial or complete contraction without changing its length. There is no rotary joint motion.

Note: In the previous example of forward bending of the head:

1. In the upright position, the eccentric contraction (lengthening) of the extensor muscles controls the speed of forward bending. These muscles are exercised.
2. In the supine position, the concentric (shortening) contraction of the flexor muscles lifts the head off the floor. These muscles are exercised.
3. In the prone position, the patient may try to bend forward, but the floor will prevent the motion. This will create static contraction of the neck flexors, which are exercised.

Classification of Exercise

1. **Isotonic.** A dynamic exercise with a constant load. The resistance is the product of the load and the resistance arm (moment arm), and therefore is not constant.

2. **Isokinetic.** A dynamic exercise in which the speed of motion is controlled by varying the resistance.
3. **Isometric.** A static exercise in which the muscle contracts with little or no shortening (static contraction).

Note: The previous example of elbow flexion by contraction of the biceps with a weight held in the palm can be described as follows:

1. As flexion proceeds from a position of 90 degrees, the moment arm lessens; therefore, the resistance lessens. If the contraction force of the biceps is maintained constant, then the speed of flexion will correspondingly increase. This is an example of isotonic exercise.
2. If, as the moment arm lessens, the weight in the palm correspondingly is increased, then the resistance continually increases with flexion. The speed of flexion will remain constant. This is an example of isokinetic exercise, which can only be performed by using machines designed for this purpose.
3. If the weight in the palm were too heavy to be moved, then, as the biceps contracted, flexion would not be created, the muscle would not change its length, and the moment arm and resistance would be constant. This is an example of isometric exercise.

Isokinetic exercise increases the work a muscle can do more rapidly than either isometric or isotonic exercise. It is more efficient. *Isometric* exercise should be used when motion of the joint is contraindicated or creates pain. For skill training, the best form of exercise is isotonic repetition of the motions needed in performing those skills.

Indications for Exercise Therapy

1. To develop a sense of good postural alignment
2. To relax or lengthen contracted or shortened musculature
3. To achieve flexibility of joint motion within its normal range of motion
4. To increase muscle strength as needed to attain and maintain proper function.

Other chapters of this book describe methods for determining if these indications exist: static

symmetry scan, regional motion testing, joint motion testing, palpation, and intersegmental motion testing. The only dysfunction testing not yet described is that used for muscle strength.

Testing for Muscle Function (Strength-Contractility)

The general procedure for strength testing is to direct the patient to concentrically contract the muscle to be tested, and then quantitatively measure the results and classify the findings.
1. Procedure for strength testing
   a. Place the segment in a completely relaxed position with minimal influence of gravity.
   b. Position the segment of the body involved so that the motion being tested can occur.
   c. Have the patient contract the involved muscle in an attempt to achieve concentric contraction and joint motion.
   d. Evaluate results.
2. Classification
   a. No contraction at all—paralysis—Grade 0.
   b. Contraction felt by examiner's fingers, but no motion—Grade 1.
   c. Contraction with motion achievable only on elimination of gravity—poor—Grade 2.
   d. Contraction with motion against gravity—fair—Grade 3.
   e. Contraction with motion against resistive force—good—Grade 4.

Inactivity and Hypokinetic Disease

Kraus and associates reported on studies performed to measure strength and flexibility of the trunk and leg muscles in children. Whereas only 8.7% of European children failed this test, 57.9% of American children failed. The poor American showing may be explained by the high degree of mechanization available.

In addition to mechanization, civilization has inhibited the "fight or flight" response. Urbanized man lives in an almost constant alert reaction phase. This imbalance in our lives—excessive unresolved stimulation—combined with insufficient exercise keeps us living in a potentially pathogenic environment.

The terms "tension neck," "tension headache," and "tension back pain" are common to the primary care physician. These syndromes are diffi-

Figure 5-4. Test of upper abdominal–psoas muscle strength.

Figure 5-5. Test of upper abdominal muscle strength without psoas involvement.

cult to diagnose and even more difficult to treat. A multifactorial approach, incorporating behavior modification with relaxation and lengthening exercises, is advisable. Prevention by means of universal relaxation and lengthening exercises and stress modification techniques should begin in childhood and continue throughout life.

Kraus-Weber Test (Modified)

The modified Kraus-Weber test is a scanning procedure for evaluating groups of muscles acting together to perform specific body motions. Tests 1 through 5 primarily evaluate muscle strength. As the primary agonist muscles are contracted, the antagonist muscles are stretched. Contracture of these antagonist muscles might lead to a false interpretation of agonist muscle weakness. Tests 6 and 7 primarily test for muscle shortening (loss of extensibility).

Physicians treating musculoskeletal dysfunctions should use some form of screening to assist in prescribing effective exercise therapy. Numerous other tests are available, in addition to the one described here.

Test 1 tests upper abdominal-psoas muscle strength (Fig. 5-4):

1. **Patient position:** Supine, with hands folded across chest, and legs fully extended.
2. **Physician position:** At foot of table holding patient's feet down.

3. Patient is instructed to curl head and body up, off the table. If the back is elevated 30 degrees or more off the table, the upper abdominal muscles are functioning adequately. If the back is elevated more than 60 degrees to the fully upright position, psoas muscle strength is being used and tested.

Test 2 tests upper abdominal muscle strength without psoas involvement (Fig. 5-5):

1. **Patient position:** Supine, with hands folded across chest, hips and knees flexed, with feet flat on table.
2. **Physician position:** Holding patient's feet down flat on table.
3. Patient is instructed as before to curl the body up to a seated position.
4. Measure degree of compliance.

Test 3 tests lower abdominal muscle strength (Fig. 5-6):

1. **Patient position:** Supine with hands behind neck and both legs extended.
2. **Physician position:** At head of the table, holding patient's shoulders to the table.
3. Patient is instructed to lift both feet off the table, with legs extended, to a height of 10 inches, and to hold this position for 10 seconds.
4. Measure degree of compliance.

Figure 5-6. Test of lower abdominal muscle strength.

Figure 5-7. Test of upper back muscle strength.

Test 4 tests upper back muscle strength (Fig. 5-7):

1. **Patient position:** Prone, with pillow under abdomen, legs fully extended, hands clasped behind back.
2. **Physician position:** At foot of table, holding patient's hips and legs down to table.
3. Patient is instructed to raise his chest and abdomen off the table, and hold this position for 10 seconds.
4. Measure degree of compliance.

Test 5 tests lower back muscle strength (Fig. 5-8):

Figure 5-8. Test of lower back muscle strength.

1. **Patient position:** Prone, with pillow under abdomen, legs fully extended, hands clasped behind neck.
2. **Physician position:** At head of table holding patient's shoulders down.
3. Patient is instructed to raise both legs off the table, without bending the knees, and to hold this position for 10 seconds.
4. Measure degree of compliance.

Test 6 tests hamstring extensibility (Fig. 5-9):

1. **Patient position:** Upright, completely erect, feet together, hands at sides.
2. Patient is told to bend forward, trying to touch the floor, without bending the knees.
3. Physician measures the distance of the fingertips from the floor to determine degree of compliance.

Figure 5-9. Test of hamstring extensibility.

Figure 5-10. Test of hamstring extensibility.

3. Evaluate the effect of exercising two joint muscles on both joints.
4. Start with relaxing (postural) exercises, then add mild corrective exercise, gradually increase to strenuous corrective exercises, specifically planned and to patient's tolerance.
5. Do not stop exercising abruptly. Return to mild exercises and relaxing exercises, gradually tapering off.
6. Instruct patient to relax between individual exercises.
7. Change position of patient and vary the exercises.
8. Multiple repetitions of identical movements should be avoided. Perform only two or three of the same exercise in one session.
9. All exercises are performed slowly and smoothly.
10. Avoid patient fatigue.
11. Perform regimen regularly.

Test 7 tests hamstring extensibility (Fig. 5-10):

1. **Patient position:** Supine, both legs fully extended.
2. **Physician position:** At side of hamstrings to be tested.
3. Physician places one hand under the patient's heel. The physician's other hand is at the ipsilateral anterior superior iliac spine.
4. Physician passively raises the fully extended leg off the table until rotary motion is felt at the anterior superior iliac spine.
5. Measure the degree of hip flexion. Less than 60 degrees of flexion is considered loss of hamstring extensibility.
6. Flexion of 80 to 90 degrees indicates good extensibility of the gluteus maximus muscle. More than 90 degrees of flexion indicates good extensibility of the erector spinae muscle.
   Note: The interpretation of this test can be invalidated by the presence of radiculitis or hip joint restriction.

Planning an Exercise Program— General Principles
1. Do not perform if exercise causes pain.
2. Evaluate the gravitational force and patient's position.

General Precautions
These precautions should be taken into account when writing exercise prescriptions.

1. Protect one body segment from strain while exercising another part.
2. Be aware of the needs, expectations, and limitations of the older patient.
3. Be aware of the needs, expectations, and limitations of debilitated patients.
4. Patients may have illness that may be worsened with active exercises.
5. Always prescribe specific therapy for specific purposes.
6. Avoid overdose of exercise therapy.
7. Do not cause pain by movement.
8. Prescribe supportive medications as indicated.
9. Prescribe follow-up treatments.
10. Prescribe home therapy and exercise as you would prescribe drug therapy.

Relaxing Exercises
There are many variations and styles of relaxing exercises. The one described here uses static muscle contraction.

Patient position: Supine, legs extended and arms at sides. Instruct patient as follows:

1. Bring your ankles and toes into full dorsiflexion; now try to push the foot and toes into further dorsiflexion. Hold for a count of 4, relax.
2. Contract your calf muscles statically, hold for a count of 4, relax.
3. Contract your buttocks statically, hold for a count of 4, relax.
4. Bend your hips and knees and place your feet on the floor. Push your low back to the floor as firmly as possible, hold for a count of 4, relax.
5. Raise your back off the floor so that you are supported by your feet, upper spine, and shoulders. Push down on your upper spine and shoulders. Hold for a count of 4, relax.
6. Contract your hands, making a firm fist. Hold for a count of 4, relax.
7. Contract your forearm muscles statically. Hold for a count of 4, relax.
8. Contract your biceps muscles statically. Hold for a count of 4, relax.
9. Shrug your shoulders up toward your ears, as far as possible. Hold for a count of 4, relax.
10. Bring your shoulders forward, trying to meet in the midline. Hold for a count of 4, relax.
11. Tuck your chin in, then push your neck firmly backward toward the floor. Hold for a count of 4, relax.

Writing an Exercise Prescription

The exercise prescription must do the following:

1. Be specific for musculoskeletal dysfunctions.
2. Take into account the patient's physical and mental condition.
3. Take into account the patient's muscle function:
   a. Ability to shorten—*contractility*
   b. Abilty to lengthen—*extensibility*
   c. Ability to return to normal size—*elasticity*

Patient's Name: _____

Date: _____

Goals: _____

_____

Procedures to follow:

1. Patient position: perform the following relaxing exercises:

   a. _____   time _____

   b. _____   time _____

   c. _____   time _____

   d. _____   time _____

2. Rest; change position; perform the following mild exercises (specific for goals):

   a. _____   time _____

   b. _____   time _____

   c. _____   time _____

3. Rest; change position; perform the following more difficult exercises, without pain (specific for goals):

   a. _____   time _____

   b. _____   time _____

   c. _____   time _____

4. Rest, repeat item 2.

5. Rest, repeat item 1.

You have completed this set of exercises. It should have taken _____ minutes to complete them.

Repeat this set of exercises _____ times daily.

You are to continue these exercises until your next appointment at this office on

_____(date).

Warning: *Do not perform any of the prescribed exercises if they create pain. Call my office for advice before continuing with this program.*

References

Ashmore EF. 1981. Osteopathic Mechanics. London: Tamor Pierston Publishers.

Bove AA, Lowenthal DT. 1983. Exercise Medicine. New York: Academic Press, Inc.

Cailliet R. 1977. Soft Tissue Pain and Disability. Philadelphia: F.A. Davis Co.

Daniels L, Worthingham C. 1972. Muscle Testing, 3rd ed. Philadelphia: W.B. Saunders Co.

———, Worthingham C. 1977. Therapeutic Exercise, 2nd ed. Philadelphia: W.B. Saunders Co.

De Lateur B, Lehmann J, Stonebridge J. 1972. Isotonic versus isometric exercise. Arch Phys Med Rehabil 53:212–217.

Gowitzke BA, Milner M. 1980. Understanding the Scientific Basis of Human Movement. Baltimore: Williams & Wilkins Co.

Greenman PE. 1987. Models and mechanisms of osteopathic manipulative medicine. Osteopath Med News IV:11–14, 20.

Guyton AC. 1986. Textbook of Medical Physiology. Philadelphia: W.B. Saunders Co.

Hoag JM, Cole WV, Bradford SG. 1969. Osteopathic Medicine. New York: McGraw-Hill Book Co.

Hutton RS, Nelson DL. 1986. Stretch sensitivity of Golgi tendon organs in fatigued gastrocnemius muscle. Med Sci Sports Med 18(1):69–74.

Jones LH. 1981. Strain and Counterstrain. Colorado Springs: American Academy of Osteopathy.

Kendall FP, McCreary EB. 1983. Muscles: Testing and Function, 3rd ed. Baltimore: Williams & Wilkins Co.

Kraus H. Clinical Treatment of Back and Neck Pain. New York: McGraw-Hill Book Co.

———, Hirschland RP. 1954. Minimum muscular fitness tests in school children. Res Q 25(2):178–188.

———, Prudden B, Hirschorn K. 1956. Role of inactivity in production of disease: A hypokinetic disease. J Am Geriatr Soc 4(5).

MacConail MA, Basmajian JV. 1977. Muscles and Movement. Huntington, New York: Robert E. Krieger Publishing Co.

Mitchell FL Jr, Moran PS, Pruzzo NA. 1979. An Evaluation and Treatment Manual of Osteopathic Muscle Energy Procedures. Valley Park, Missouri: Mitchell, Moran, and Pruzzo Assoc.

Moffroid M, Whipple R, Hofkosh J, et al. 1969. A study of isokinetic exercise. Phys Med Ther 49:735–746.

Rasch PJ, Burke RK. 1978. Kinesiology and Applied Anatomy, 6th ed. Philadelphia: Lea & Febiger.

Spulman JM, Hauffer EK. 1986. Morphological observations of motor units connected in-series to Golgi tendon organs. J Neurophysiol 55(1):147–162.

Stauffer EK, et al. 1986. Responses of Golgi tendon organs to concurrently active motor units. Brain Res 375:157–162.

Stiles EG. 1984. Manipulation: A tool for your practice? Patient Care 18:137–189.

Thistle HG, Hislop HJ, Moffroid M. 1967. Isokinetic contraction: A new concept of resistive exercise. Arch Phys Med Rehabil 48:279–282.

Wells KF, Luttgens K. 1976. Kinesiology, 6th ed. Philadelphia: W.B. Saunders Co.

6 Evaluation of the Cervical Spine

FUNCTIONAL ANATOMY AND BIOMECHANICS
Jonathan Fenton

The cervical spine is made up of the seven cervical vertebrae. Functionally it is divided into two areas: the articulations between the occiput, atlas, and axis, and the articulations between the third through seventh cervical vertebrae.

Occipitoatlantal Joint

The occipitoatlantal articulation consists of the superior articular facets of the atlas and the two occipital condyles. The superior facets of the atlas face backward, upward, and medially and are concave in both anteroposterior and transverse diameters. The surfaces of the occipital condyles match the facets of the atlas, and the joint is best thought of as a sphere (the occiput) gliding on the articular surfaces of the atlas (Fig. 6-1). The freely movable occiput is limited by its muscular and ligamentous attachments, which make flexion-extension the primary motion, producing a small-amplitude nodding of the head. Flexion of the occiput on the atlas is accompanied by a posterior translatory slide of the occiput, extension is accompanied by an anterior translatory slide.

Side bending and rotation of the occipitoatlantal joint always occur in opposite directions, in part because of the position of the lateral atlanto-occipital ligament. When the occiput rotates left on the atlas, the lateral atlanto-occipital ligament causes the occiput to slide (translate) to the left and therefore side bend to the right (Fig. 6-2). Somatic dysfunctions of the occipitoatlantal joint most often involve the minor motions of side bending and rotation.

Atlantoaxial Joint

The atlantoaxial articulation is specially adapted for (nearly) pure rotation. In addition to the inferior articular facets of the atlas and the superior articular facets of the axis, movement other than rotation is limited by the anteriorly located odontoid process (dens) of the axis. The odontoid process is held close to the anterior arch of the atlas by the transverse ligament of the atlas, which allows only a slight amount of flexion of the atlas on the axis.

There is no true lateral flexion at the atlantoaxial joint, only a wobble created by the articulation of the superior axial and inferior atlantal articular facets. Unlike most facets, these four facets are all convex in shape (Fig. 6-3). During rotation of the atlas on the axis to the right, the left articular facet

Figure 6-1. Bony anatomy of the occipitoatlantal joint, posterosuperior view. *OC*, occipital condyle; *SF*, superior facet; *IF*, inferior facet; *TP*, transverse process.

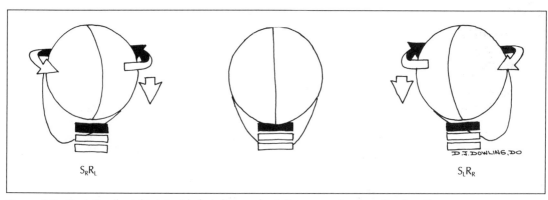

Figure 6-2. Occipitoatlantal joint: side bending and rotation occur in opposite directions.

Figure 6-3. Atlantoaxial articulation. *AT,* anterior tubercle; *PT,* posterior tubercle; *TF,* transverse foramen; *SP,* spinous process; *IFa,* inferior facet of atlas; *IFax,* inferior facet of axis; *SFa,* superior facet of atlas; *SFax,* superior facet of axis.

of the atlas in effect slides uphill on the left articular facet of the axis, while on the right the atlas slides downhill on the axis. This wobble motion is not true lateral flexion.

Somatic dysfunction at the atlantoaxial joint occurs in rotation.

The complex of the occipitoatlantal plus the atlantoaxial joints is known as the *suboccipital articulation.* Its range of motion makes it function as a universal (swivel) joint. Many consider the suboccipital articulation the final compensator of the spine, by which the body adjusts to any dysfunctions occurring below. Compensatory adjustment is needed to keep the eyes level in two planes, to promote binocular vision.

The articulation between the second (C2) and third (C3) cervical vertebrae sustains tremendous stress, owing to its position between the final compensator above and the rest of the spine below. Therefore, it is a common location for chronic somatic dysfunction.

Third to Seventh Cervical Vertebrae (C3–C7)

This portion of the cervical spine allows for a great deal of motion, with special adaptation to meet the demands of mobility and stability placed upon it. The cervical intevertebral disks are the relatively thickest of the spinal disks; the ratio of disk height to vertebral body height in this section of the spinal column is 2:5. The disks are wedge shaped and thicker anteriorly than posteriorly (Fig. 6-4). In conjunction with the anteroposterior convexity of the vertebral end-plates, the wedge shape maintains the flexible cervical lordosis.

The facet joints in this area are located posterolaterally. Two articulating facets, one superior and one inferior, form the palpable articular pillars. The superior articular facets face backward and upward. The plane of the facet joints lies midway between the horizontal and frontal planes in normal lordosis (Fig. 6-5). This orientation causes rotation and side bending to be coupled motions,

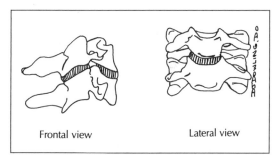

Frontal view   Lateral view

Figure 6-4. Cervical intervertebral disk between C3 and C4.

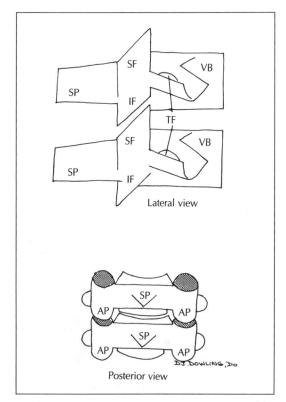

Lateral view

Posterior view

Figure 6-5. Orientation of articular facets of C3 and C4 vertebrae. *SP,* spinous process; *SF,* superior facet; *IF,* inferior facet; *VB,* vertebral body; *AP,* articular pillar; *TF,* transverse foramina.

Joints of Lushka

Figure 6-6. Location of the joints of Luschka (unciform joints), anterior view.

always occurring in the same direction. When the cervical spine is placed in a more backward bending position, the facets are more oriented in the frontal plane, where side bending is the primary motion. When the neck is brought into a forward bending position, the plane of the facets becomes more horizontal, and rotation is the major motion.

The cervical vertebrae C3 to C7 move least in flexion-extension. In flexion the inferior articular facets of the upper vertebrae must slide up the superior articular facets of the lower vertebrae, up a 45-degree incline. The normal lordotic curve in this area places the cervical spine in partial extension; the cervical spine has no neutral position.

To assist in maintaining some measure of stability in the face of the large amounts of motion possible in the midcervical spine, a specialized set of synovial joints has developed as an adaptation for upright posture in humans. These joints, known as the unciform joints or the joints of Luschka, are located on the lateral edges of the cervical vertebral bodies (Fig. 6-6). The lateral lips of two adjacent vertebrae articulate and are contained within a small synovial capsule. These joints develop at age eight to ten years.

The unciform joints (joints of Luschka) act as guide rails for the motions of flexion-extension. They also limit the lateral translatory motion (side slip) that occurs simultaneously with the coupled motions of side bending and rotation. When one vertebra side bends and rotates on another, that vertebra will translate laterally in the opposite direction. In the cervical spine this lateral translatory motion would be excessive to the point of subluxation were it not for the unciform joints.

Somatic dysfunctions in the C3 to C7 joints occur in the coupled rotary motions of side bending and rotation, and in lateral translation. Dysfunctions of translatory motion that accompany rotary dysfunctions create a complicated dysfunction, side slip.

Seventh Cervical-First Thoracic Joint (C7-T1)

The anatomy of the seventh cervical vertebra is transitional, resembling cervical vertebral anatomy superiorly and thoracic vertebral anatomy inferiorly (Fig. 6-7). At the cervicothoracic (C7-T1) junction, cervical lordosis normally ends and thoracic kyphosis begins. As a result, the forces

Figure 6-7. Seventh cervical vertebra. Note anatomic similarity superiorly to sixth cervical vertebra and inferiorly to first thoracic vertebra.

placed on this area are quite complex, and of a different nature from forces sustained higher or lower in the spine. Somatic dysfunction of the cervicothoracic junction is quite common and difficult to treat.

MOTION TESTING
Sandra D. Yale

Gross motion testing
FORWARD BENDING
1. Patient position: seated.
2. Physician position: standing at side of patient.
3. **Technique:**
   a. Place one hand on the occiput and the other hand on the cervicothoracic junction (Fig. 6-8).
   b. Gently push the patient's head forward until you feel motion at the cervicothoracic junction (between C7-T1).
   c. Note the angle of displacement from the upright position. This is usually 80 to 90 degrees, or until the patient's chin touches the manubrium.

BACKWARD BENDING
1. Patient position: seated.
2. Physician position: standing at side of patient.
3. **Technique:**
   a. Place one hand on the patient's forehead and the other hand on the cervicothoracic junction (Fig. 6-9).
   b. Gently push the patient's head backward until you feel motion at the cervicothoracic junction.

Figure 6-8. Gross motion testing of the cervical spine, forward bending.

Figure 6-9. Gross motion testing of the cervical spine, backward bending.

Figure 6-10. Gross motion testing of the cervical spine, lateral flexion.

c. Note the angle of displacement from the upright position. This is usually 80 to 90 degrees, or until the patient looks directly at the ceiling.

LATERAL FLEXION (SIDE BENDING)
1. Patient position: seated.
2. Physician position: standing behind patient.
3. **Technique:**
    a. To flex the patient's spine laterally to the right, place one hand on left parietal. Use the other hand to monitor left shoulder elevation (Fig. 6-10).
    b. Apply gentle pressure with the hand to bend the patient's neck to the right.
    c. Reverse hands for left side bending. Repeat step b to the left.
    d. Note the angle of displacement from the midline. This is usually 40 to 45 degrees in either direction.

ROTATION
1. Patient position: seated.
2. Physician position: standing behind patient.
3. **Technique:**
    a. To evaluate right rotation, place your right hand on the patient's left frontal area and use the left hand to monitor shoulder rotation or motion at C7-T1.
    b. With your left hand, gently turn the

patient's head to the right until you feel motion at the cervicothoracic junction (Fig. 6-11).
    c. Note the displacement from the midline. This is usually 80 to 90 degrees, or until the patient's chin is over his shoulder.
    d. Reverse hands to evaluate left rotation. Repeat steps b and c.

Intersegmental Motion Testing
OCCIPITOATLANTAL JOINT
1. Patient position: supine.
2. Physician position: seated comfortably at the head of the table with forearms resting on the table.
3. **Technique:**
    a. Tissue texture changes and asymmetry
        i. Slide fingers downward and laterally from inion to sulcus, between occiput and atlas (Fig. 6-12).
        ii. Note changes in tissue texture.
        iii. Slide fingers slightly laterally toward mastoid processes and note the depth of the sulcus.
    b. Motion testing technique
        i. Keep the palpating fingers in the occipitoatlantal sulcus.
        ii. Have the patient slowly flex his head, occiput on atlas only.

Figure 6-11. Gross motion testing of the cervical spine, rotation.

Figure 6-12. Intersegmental motion testing of the occipitoatlantal joint.

Figure 6-13. Intersegmental motion testing of the atlantoaxial joint.

iii. Note the symmetry of flexion bilaterally. Increased sulcal depth on one side may indicate a lateral flexion dysfunction on the other side.

iv. Keep your fingers in the occipitoatlantal sulcus.

v. Have the patient slowly extend his head over your fingers.

vi. Note the symmetry of extension bilaterally. Unilaterally increased sulcal depth indicates a lateral flexion dysfunction on the other side.

ATLANTOAXIAL JOINT

1. Patient position: supine.
2. Physician position: seated at head of table with forearms resting on table.
3. **Technique:**
   a. Tissue texture changes
      i. Slide fingers laterally along the occipitoatlantal sulcus until they are resting behind and near the tips of the mastoid processes bilaterally, and behind the transverse processes of the atlas (Fig. 6-13). *Note* tissue texture changes and changes in symmetry.
      ii. Move fingers anteriorly between the mastoid processes and the mandible to palpate the tips of the transverse processes of the atlas. *Note* any changes

in symmetry. One tip more prominent posteriorly may be an indication of a rotation dysfunction in that direction.

   b. Motion testing technique
      i. Place your fingers behind the transverse processes of the atlas.
      ii. Have the patient flex the occiput on the atlas (flex head) and maintain this locked position.
      iii. Rotate the patient's head bilaterally until motion is felt at each transverse process.
      iv. Note the degree of freedom of rotation. A decrease in rotation indicates restriction on that side and freedom in other direction.

C2–C7

1. Patient position: supine with head and neck relaxed.
2. Physician position: seated at the head of the table with forearms resting on the table.
3. **Technique:**
   a. Tissue texture changes
      i. Palpate the spinous processes and ligaments in the midline and slightly caudad to the occipitoatlantal sulcus.
      ii. Move your fingers slightly laterally and palpate the cervical paravertebral muscles.
      iii. Palpate the articular pillars in the

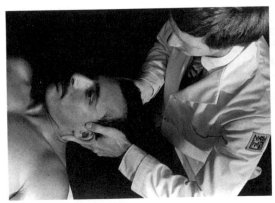

Figure 6-14. Intersegmental motion testing of C2 through C7, lateral flexion.

following manner. Slide your fingers slightly more laterally until they are in the groove between cervical paravertebral muscle masses. Then gently press your fingers medially until you palpate the bones beneath the muscles. C2 on C3 should be approximately 1 cm below the occipitoatlantal sulcus. To test your position, have the patient laterally flex slightly to one side. You should be able to feel the sliding motion with your palpating fingers.

  iv. Slide your fingers caudad bilaterally and palpate each pair of articular pillars. *Note* changes in tissue texture and in bony symmetry. When one articular pillar is more prominent posteriorly, it may indicate a rotation toward that side.

b. Motion testing technique—lateral flexion (Fig. 6-14)
  i. Keep the palpating fingers on the articular pillars.
  ii. Introduce lateral flexion until you feel motion at your fingertips.
  iii. Note the displacement of the patient's head from the midline.
  iv. Greater motion to one side than the other indicates a lateral flexion restriction on the side of the decreased motion.
  v. Feel the fluidity of motion at your fingertips.

c. Flexion-extension (Fig. 6-15)

  i. With your fingertips on the articular pillars, flex the patient's neck until you feel motion at the articular pillars.
  ii. Return the patient's head to neutral position. Introduce extension up to your palpating fingers at the articular pillars. Use your palpating fingers as fulcrums.
  iii. Feel the fluidity and amount of motion.
  iv. Note any asymmetry of motion. Decreased motion in extension indicates a flexion dysfunction. Decreased motion in flexion indicates an extension dysfunction.

Rotoscoliosis Motion Testing

When a cervical vertebra laterally flexes, it also rotates to the same side. A type II somatic dysfunction will exhibit restrictions in side bending and rotation in the same direction, as well as in flexion or extension.

C2–C7
1. Patient position: supine.
2. Physician position: seated at head of table.
3. **Technique:**
  a. Place your palpating fingers on the articular pillars bilaterally. Note the bony symmetry of articular pillars. If one side is more posterior than the other, the vertebra may be rotated to that side.
  b. Flex the patient's head to the palpating fingers (see Fig. 6-15)
    i. If the posteriorly rotated vertebra becomes more posterior, the vertebra has restricted motion in flexion. This also confirms freedom of rotation.
    ii. The posteriorly rotated vertebra will stay the same or improve in extension. This is considered an *extension dysfunction.*
  c. Extend the patient's head to the palpating fingers.
    i. If the posteriorly rotated vertebra becomes more posterior, the vertebra has restricted motion in extension.
    ii. The posteriorly rotated vertebra will stay the same or improve in flexion. This is considered a *flexion dysfunction.*

    Example: The C4 articular pillar is posterior on the left. The posterior articular pillar becomes more posterior

Figure 6-15. Intersegmental motion testing of C2 through C7, flexion-extension.

Figure 6-16. Rotoscoliosis motion testing of the atlantoaxial joint.

in flexion and less posterior in extension. The somatic dysfunction is designated C4 E Rl Sl. This is a type II somatic dysfunction.

ATLANTOAXIAL MOTION TESTING

The atlantoaxial joint never leaves the neutral position, because extension is limited by bony apposition and flexion is limited by the odontoid ligament. Therefore, the major motion of the atlantoaxial joint is rotation.

1. Patient position: supine.
2. Physician position: seated at head of table.
3. **Technique:**
   a. Cradle the patient's occiput in your hands.
   b. Fully flex the patient's neck, locking all the cervical vertebrae in flexion. This maneuver prevents motion of the vertebrae below the atlantoaxial joint.
   c. Maintain flexion and rotate the head from one side to the other until the physiologic barriers to motion are reached (Fig. 6-16).
      i. Note the symmetry of motion to each side.
      ii. If the motion on one side is greater than on the other, there is restriction on the side of limited motion.

      Example: If rotation is greater to the right, the somatic dysfunction would be designated AA Rr (atlantoaxial rotation right).

Translatory Motion Testing

Rotoscoliosis motion testing evaluates the rotation of the vertebra. Translatory motion testing evaluates side bending motion. Side-to-side translatory motion is coupled with individual vertebral side bending toward the opposite direction. Translatory motion of C4 toward the right is coupled with side bending of C4 to the left. For most cervical vertebrae, side bending and rotation are coupled and occur in the same direction.

C2–C7
1. Patient position: supine.
2. Physician position: seated at head of table.
3. **Technique:**
   a. Place palpating fingers on the articular pillars of the affected vertebra bilaterally.
   b. Push the pillar in a left to right direction, using the palpating fingers alternately. This translatory motion creates side bending to the left. Then push right to left, creating side bending to the right. *Note* any asymmetry of motion. If there is better translation to the left, the vertebra side bends better to the right side.
   c. Flex the neck to the area of palpation and apply a translatory force toward one side and then toward the other side (Fig. 6-17).
      i. Note any asymmetry of motion.
      ii. Compare the motion with the translatory motion that occurs in the neutral position.

Figure 6-17. Translatory motion testing of C2 through C7.

Figure 6-18. Translatory motion testing of the occipitoatlantal joint.

iii. If translatory motion is increased to one side in flexion, the restriction is exaggerated in flexion; therefore, flexion is restricted. This is designated an *extension dysfunction.*

d. Extend the neck to the area of the palpating fingers and apply the same type of translatory force.
   i. Note any asymmetry of motion.
   ii. Compare this motion with the translatory motion that occurs in the neutral position.
   iii. If translatory motion is decreased to one side in extension, the restriction is exaggerated in extension; therefore, extension is restricted. This is designated a *flexion dysfunction.*

OCCIPITOATLANTAL JOINT

1. Patient position: supine.
2. Physician position: seated at head of patient.
3. **Technique:**
   a. Flex the patient's neck slightly to the monitoring fingers in the sulcus.
   b. Stabilize the top of the head against your waist.
   c. Cup the occiput in your hands.
   d. Move the head on the neck by translating the occiput to the left. Translation to the left is coupled with side bending to the right (Fig. 6-18).
   e. This is coupled with rotation to the left. *Note* any asymmetry of motion.
   f. Extend the neck slightly.
   g. Repeat steps b through d.

Interpretation: Since rotation is opposite to side bending at the occipitoatlantal joint, there are four possible designations for the somatic dysfunction: OA F Sr Rl, OA F Sl Rr, OA E Sr Rl, OA E Sl Rr.

Example: If there is normal translation to the left in flexion and decreased translation to the left in extension, the somatic dysfunction is designated OA F Sl Rr (occiput restricted in right side bending while in the extended position; its free motions are flexion, side bending to the right, and rotation to the left).

References

Fryette H. 1954. Principles of Osteopathic Technique. Colorado Springs: Academy of Applied Osteopathy.

Kapandji IA. 1974. The Physiology of the Joints. Vol 3. The Trunk and the Vertebral Column. Edinburgh: Churchill Livingstone.

Schiowitz S, DiGiovanna E. 1981. An Osteopathic Approach to Diagnosis and Treatment. Old Westbury, New York: New York College of Osteopathic Medicine.

Warwick RW. 1973. Gray's Anatomy, 35th British ed. Philadelphia: W.B. Saunders Co.

White A, Panjabi MM. 1978. Biomechanics of the Spine. Philadelphia: J.B. Lippincott Co.

7

Treatment of the Cervical Spine

MYOFASCIAL TECHNIQUES
Toni Murphy

This section describes passive, indirect active, and direct active myofascial techniques used to treat dysfunction in the cervical region. Most of these techniques entail a linear stretch of the neck muscles or an active stretch of the suboccipital and paravertebral muscles.

Passive Techniques
Passive techniques are performed by the physician on a relaxed patient. The patient does no work. The purpose of the passive techniques described below is to place a linear stretch on the posterior extensor muscles of the cervical region.

LINEAR STRETCH ON THE MUSCLES OF THE OCCIPITOATLANTAL REGION
1. Patient position: supine.
2. Physician position: standing at the head of the table.
3. **Technique:**
   a. The physician cradles the patient's occiput in her hands.
   b. The physician's fingers are placed in the occipitoatlantal sulcus bilaterally.
   c. The occiput is cupped in her palms.
   d. For best results, the patient's neck should be straight or bent slightly forward.
   e. The physician's arms should be in near or

full extension, so that they can be used as long levers. This position allows the physician to use her weight as the force of traction, by rocking backward on her feet, rather than relying on upper body strength (Fig. 7-1).
   f. The force of traction is slowly and uniformly applied, maintained for a few seconds, and slowly released.
   g. The technique may be repeated without repositioning of the physician's fingers or feet.
4. Hints for performing technique:
   a. The physician's feet should be placed far enough from the table so that she may apply traction without changing her stance.
   b. To use her weight as the force of traction, the physician need only rock backward on her feet and maintain a slightly arched back while slowly applying the force.
   c. The physician should avoid creating friction by rubbing the patient's skin.
   d. The patient is relaxed throughout the procedure.
   Seated technique. In the seated technique, linear traction is applied to the posterior extensor neck muscles with the physician seated at the head of the table (Fig. 7-2). The technique is similar; however, the lever action is shorter, involv-

ing only the forearms. Therefore, the physician should keep her elbows close to her body while applying traction. The physician may still use body weight as the applied force, but with less efficiency because both the arms and body levers are shorter. Linear traction is applied by the physician slowly rocking backward on her buttocks. As in the original technique, traction is slowly and uniformly applied, maintained for a few seconds, and released. The maneuver may be repeated without repositioning.

Suboccipital technique. A similar technique can be used in the suboccipital region. In this technique, the physician's fingers rotate in the occipitoatlantal sulcus while linear traction is applied.

1. Patient position: supine.
2. Physician position: seated at the head of the table.
3. **Technique:**
   a. The physician cradles the occiput with her index and middle fingers placed in the occipitoatlantal sulcus bilaterally but medially so that middle fingers meet at the midline.
   b. The occiput is cupped in the physician's palms.
   c. The patient's neck is maintained in a straight or slightly forward bent position.
   d. The physician applies linear traction slowly and uniformly by rocking backward on her buttocks.
   e. Maintaining linear traction, the physician rolls her fingers laterally away from the midline. With the longitudinal axis of the forearm as the rotational axis, the fingers remain in the occipitoatlantal sulcus but gradually roll out laterally.
   f. The physician's wrist, forearm, hand, and fingers are maintained in straight alignment and maneuvered as a single unit. Rotational movement around the longitudinal axis causes the fingers to move laterally in the occipitoatlantal sulcus.
   g. The technique may be repeated.

LINEAR TRACTION APPLIED TO
THE LOWER NECK
1. Patient position: supine.
2. Physician position: standing or sitting at the head of the table.

Figure 7-1. Linear stretch with the physician standing.

3. **Technique:**
   a. The physician places her fingers on the patient's posterior neck muscles bilaterally at any cervical level, as long as she grasps the muscles at the same cervical level bilaterally.
   b. The physician applies a linear traction force to the musculature, slowly and uniformly, by rocking backward on her feet, or buttocks if sitting.
   c. The patient's neck is held straight or bent slightly forward as traction is applied.
   d. Release is accomplished by the physician slowly rocking forward.

LINEAR TRACTION APPLIED TO LOWER
NECK, WITH ADDED PERPENDICULAR
STRETCH OF THE MUSCLE FIBERS
1. Patient position: supine.
2. Physician position: standing or sitting at the head of the table.
3. **Technique:**
   a. The physician places her fingers on the patient's posterior neck muscles at the same cervical level bilaterally.
   b. The physician applies linear traction by rocking backward.
   c. A perpendicular stretch to the muscle fibers is added by pushing the fingers ventrally while maintaining the linear traction.
   d. Traction is slowly released. The maneuver may be repeated if necessary.

Figure 7-2. Linear stretch with the physician seated.

Figure 7-3. Linear stretch of posterior extensor neck muscles, cupping the chin.

Figure 7-4. Unilateral perpendicular stretch.

LINEAR STRETCH OF POSTERIOR EXTENSOR NECK MUSCLES

1. Patient position: supine.
2. Physician position: sitting at the head of the table.
3. **Technique:**
   a. The physician cradles the occiput in one hand and cups the patient's chin with the other hand (Fig. 7-3).
   b. The physician applies a linear traction force along the longitudinal axis of the cervical spine with the hand cradling the occiput. The hand cupping the chin is primarily used to stabilize the neck and hold it slightly bent forward. The main force of traction is applied by the hand cradling the occiput.
   c. The maneuver may be repeated as necessary.

PERPENDICULAR STRETCH OF THE MUSCLE FIBERS

1. Patient position: supine.
2. Physician position: standing at the patient's side opposite the side to be treated.
3. **Technique:**
   a. The physician places one hand on the patient's forehead and rotates the patient's head approximately 45 degrees away from herself (Fig. 7-4). This position is maintained and used as a stabilizing counterforce.
   b. The physician places her other hand across the patient's body and grasps the posterior cervical muscles of the opposite side.
   c. A gentle stretch is applied to the muscle body by pulling it away from the spinous processes and ventrally.
   d. The stretch is maintained for a few seconds, then slowly released. The maneuver is repeated.
   e. Hints for performing technique: The force used is smallest in the suboccipital region and gradually increased as the physician moves more caudad. This is because the smaller neck muscles are located higher up, and the muscle bulk increases lower down.
4. Modification
   When applying the perpendicular stretch to the muscle body, the physician may rotate the patient's head and neck into the stretch. This is achieved by rotating the patient's head more than 45 degrees while applying the perpendicular stretch.

Figure 7-5. Crossed arms technique.

Figure 7-6. Unilateral linear stretch.

BILATERAL LINEAR STRETCH APPLIED TO BOTH ENDS OF THE MUSCLE

1. Patient position: supine.
2. Physician position: standing at the head of the table.
3. **Technique:**
   a. The physician crosses her forearms under the patient's occiput so that the patient's head is fully supported on the physician's forearms and the physician's hands are on the patient's contralateral shoulders (Fig. 7-5).
   b. The physician gently and slowly lifts her forearms, creating a lever-fulcrum effect that puts linear traction on both ends of the muscles.

      Note: The patient's neck should be bent forward to a comfortable position of maximum stretch. When applying the force, the physician must avoid injuring the muscles, arteries, veins, and nerves, as well as the structures of the anterior neck.
   c. This position is held for a few seconds and slowly brought back to neutral.
   d. When repeating this technique, the physician should bend the neck forward a bit more than the previous time. Each repetition of the technique should increase the range of motion.
4. Modification: Active direct technique
   a. While the physician is fully supporting the head at maximal linear stretch, she may ask the patient to push back into her arms.
   b. The physician resists this motion with an isometric counterforce.
   c. The patient is allowed to push for 3 seconds, then told to relax.
   d. The physician allows the patient 3 to 6 seconds of relaxation, then bends the neck forward to the new point of maximal stretch.

UNILATERAL LINEAR STRETCH APPLIED TO BOTH ENDS OF THE MUSCLE

1. Patient position: supine
2. Physician position: standing at the head of the table
3. **Technique:**
   a. The physician places one forearm under the patient's head with the hand on the patient's contralateral shoulder, on the side of the neck to be treated. The patient's head should be fully supported.
   b. The physician places her other hand on the parietotemporal region of the patient's head.
   c. The physician slowly and gently lifts the patient's head up, causing the cervical spine to bend forward (Fig. 7-6).
   d. As the neck bends forward, the physician rotates the patient's head toward her elbow.
      Note: This technique is used to treat the

Figure 7-7. Linear stretch of
suboccipital muscles.

Figure 7-8. Active direct
myofascial technique applied to
suboccipital muscle region.

muscles on the side opposite to the rotation
of the head. The technique may be applied
to either side of the neck.

SUBOCCIPITAL MUSCLE TREATMENT
1. Patient position: supine.
2. Physician position: standing at the side of the
   table facing the patient.
3. **Technique:**
   a. The physician places one forearm under the
      patient's neck in the suboccipital sulcus so
      that the patient's neck rests on the forearm.
4. The other hand is placed on the patient's
   forehead and gentle pressure is applied
   downward toward the table. This maneuver
   stretches the occipitoatlantal sulcus (Fig. 7-7).

Active Direct Techniques

Active direct techniques use the Golgi tendon reflex to cause relaxation. These techniques are described for the suboccipital muscle region and for
unilateral occipital and paravertebral muscles.

SUBOCCIPITAL MUSCLE REGION
1. Patient position: supine.
2. Physician position: seated at the head of the
   table with her forearms resting on the table,
   the palms facing up.
3. **Technique:**
   a. The physician places her fingertips in the

patient's occipitoatlantal sulcus, allowing
the occiput to rest in her palms.
   b. The patient gently pushes his head into the
      physician's palms, with the physician's
      fingertips used as a fulcrum, avoiding neck
      extension.
   c. As the patient pushes into her palms, the
      physician resists this motion with an
      isometric counterforce (Fig. 7-8).
      The muscles involved in this technique
      include the bilateral suboccipital muscles,
      the rectus capitis posterior major, rectus
      capitis posterior minor, obliquus capitis
      inferior, and obliquus capitis superior.
4. Modification:
   a. The same technique can be applied to the
      lower extensor muscles of the cervical
      region. The physician places her fingers
      more caudally bilaterally.
   b. The patient may push his head into the
      physician's palms with slightly greater force
      the lower down the neck one is treating,
      because of the increased muscle bulk.

UNILATERAL SUBOCCIPITAL
MUSCLE TREATMENT
1. Patient position: supine.
2. Physician position: seated at the head of the
   table with his forearms resting on the table,
   palms facing up.
3. **Technique:**
   a. The physician places her fingertips in the

patient's occipitoatlantal sulcus on the side to be treated.

b. The physician's other hand guides the patient's head into lateral flexion (side bending) over the fulcrum of her fingers.

c. The patient tries to side bend his head farther into the freedom of motion (toward the dysfunctional side).

d. The physician resists this motion by applying an isometric counterforce with her palm.

4. Modification:

The physician may instruct the patient to push his head gently backward toward the table. This motion is similarly resisted with an isometric counterforce.

UNILATERAL SINGLE PARAVERTEBRAL MUSCLE TREATMENT—SIDEBENDING AND ROTATION

1. Patient position: supine.
2. Physician position: seated at the head of the table with her forearms resting on the table, palms facing up.
3. **Technique:**
   a. The physician places her index or middle finger on the midportion of the involved muscle. This is the palpating or monitoring finger.

b. With her other hand, the physician grasps the patient's head under the occiput and bends it backward, sidebends and rotates it ipsilaterally until motion of the involved muscle is felt by the palpating finger.

c. The patient attempts to push his head into further backward bending and ipsilateral side bending and rotation.

d. The physician resists this further motion with an isometric counterforce for no more than 2 seconds. Relax and repeat the process.

Active Indirect Techniques

Active indirect techniques use the crossed extensor reflex, a specialized form of reciprocal inhibition that crosses the spinal cord and involves multiple motions. Active indirect techniques are described for the paravertebral muscles.

1. Patient position: supine with his head off the end of the table.
2. Physician position: seated at the head of the table, fully supporting the patient's head.
3. **Technique:**
   a. The physician places the palm of one hand on the patient's ipsilateral parieto-occiput so that the patient's head is fully supported.

Figure 7-9. Active indirect stretch of the paravertebral muscles. (**A**) Starting position. (**B**) Midway through the maneuver, with the patient attempting to reverse the motions applied by the physician. (**C**) A passive stretch ends the technique.

A
B
C

b. The palm of the physician's other hand is placed on the other side of the patient's head. No pressure is placed on the patient's ear.

c. The physician places the patient's head in a position of backward bending, lateral flexion (side bending), and rotation toward the side of the hand on the occiput (Fig. 7-9A).

d. The patient tries to reverse the motions that the physician has just engaged by bringing his neck into flexion and touching his chin to the opposite shoulder (Fig. 7-9B).

e. The physician applies isokinetic resistance to this motion with her hand on the patient's temporoparietal region.

f. The patient will stop this motion because of a restricting contracted muscle or pain.

g. The physician then gently applies a passive stretch of the patient's neck, manually increasing the desired muscle stretch (Fig. 7-9C).

h. The patient relaxes. The physician returns to the starting position and repeats the maneuver.

MUSCLE ENERGY TECHNIQUES
Nancy Brous

This section describes muscle energy techniques used to treat type II dysfunctions of the occipitoatlantal joint, rotational dysfunctions of the atlantoaxial joint, and type II dysfunctions of a typical cervical vertebral joint. Unless the dysfunction is severe, the techniques are repeated two or three times, with the motion barrier engaged at each repetition.

Occipitoatlantal Dysfunction
DYSFUNCTION IN FLEXION
Example OA F Sr Rl
1. Patient position: supine.
2. Physician position: seated at the head of the table.
3. Hand position: The physician's monitoring hand cradles the patient's occiput. Two fingers of the monitoring hand are in the patient's occipital sulci (medial and inferior to mastoid). The physician's other hand is placed on the inferior aspect of the patient's chin.
4. **Technique:**
   a. The physician extends the patient's head back over his monitoring hand until motion is felt at the occipitoatlantal joint (Fig. 7-10).
   b. With the monitoring hand, the physician side bends the occiput left and rotates it

right until motion is felt at the occipitoatlantal joint.

c. The patient is instructed to push his chin down against the isometric resistance of the physician (into the freedom of motion) for about 3 seconds. *Ounces* of force are used to achieve the desired results.

d. The patient relaxes for 3 seconds.

e. The physician repeats steps a through d twice more, reengaging the motion barrier each time.

f. The patient's head is returned to neutral and the lesion is reassessed for change.

DYSFUNCTION IN EXTENSION
Example: OA E Sr Rl
1. Patient position: supine.
2. Physician position: seated at the head of the table.
3. Hand position: The physician's monitoring hand cradles the patient's occiput. Two fingers of the monitoring hand are in the patient's occipital sulci. The physician's other hand is placed on the superior aspect of the patient's chin.
4. **Technique:**
   a. The physician bends the patient's head forward until he feels motion at the monitoring hand (Fig. 7-11).
   b. With his monitoring hand, the physician

Figure 7-10. Muscle energy technique for a dysfunction in flexion of the occipitoatlantal joint.

Figure 7-11. Muscle energy technique for dysfunction in extension of the occipitoatlantal joint.

Figure 7-12. Muscle energy technique for atlantoaxial rotation restriction.

side bends the patient's neck left and rotates it right until motion is felt at the occipitoatlantal joint.

c. The patient is instructed to push his chin up against the isometric resistance of the physician for about 3 seconds. *Ounces* of force are used to achieve the desired result.

d. The patient relaxes for 3 seconds.

e. The physician repeats steps a through d twice more, reengaging the motion barrier each time.

f. The patient's head is returned to neutral and the lesion is reassessed for change.

Atlantoaxial Dysfunction

Example: AA Rr

1. Patient position: supine.
2. Physician position: seated at head of table.
3. **Technique:**
   a. Since the motion at the atlantoaxial joint involves primarily rotation, the physician need address only the motion barrier of rotation.
   b. The physician supports the back of the patient's head with his palms.

c. The physician bends the patient's neck and head forward until motion is palpated only at the atlantoaxial joint and until locking occurs below that segment.

d. Keeping the patient's neck bent forward, the physician rotates the head toward the side of the restricted rotation and engages the motion barrier (left).

e. The physician then places the palm of his hand opposite the side of the restriction, on the patient's cheek and temple (Fig. 7-12).

f. The patient turns his head with a pure rotary force against the isometric resistance provided by the physician's hand on the patient's cheek.

g. After 3 seconds the patient relaxes and the physician simultaneously stops applying the counterforce.

h. Once the patient has completely relaxed, the physician increases the rotation into the restriction, engaging a new motion barrier.

i. Steps f through h are repeated two or three times. Symmetry of motion at the atlantoaxial joint is rechecked.

j. The patient's head is returned to neutral position and the lesion is reassessed for change.

A

Figure 7-13. Muscle energy technique for dysfunction in extension of a typical cervical vertebra. (**A**) Note position of monitoring finger. (**B**) Rotation is introduced into barrier to motion of a typical cervical vertebrae.

B

Typical Cervical Vertebral Dysfunctions (C2–C7)

Example: C4 E Sr Rr

1. Patient position: supine.
2. Physician position: seated at the head of table.
3. **Technique:**
   a. The physician places the fingertip of the index finger of the monitoring hand against the posterior facet at the level of the involved segment (left side) (Fig. 7-13A).
   b. The physician introduces flexion to treat an extension dysfunction, or extension to treat a flexion dysfunction. The motion is monitored and localized at the particular level being treated. The first motion barrier has now been engaged.
   c. Side bending is introduced by placing a medial translatory force on the side of the restricted segment, resulting in side bending into the barrier (left).
   d. Rotation is introduced by rotating the patient's head and into the restriction (left) until motion is felt at the monitored

segment (Fig. 7-13B).
   e. The physician then asks the patient to move into the freedom of motion by having the patient bring his ear to his shoulder, causing a side bending away from the barrier. (The physician could also ask the patient to rotate his head toward the freedom.) These actions are performed against isometric resistance provided by the physician's hand against the patient's cheek.
   f. The patient relaxes and the physician simultaneously stops applying the counterforce.
   g. Once the patient is completely relaxed, the physician engages the new motion barriers, increasing the side bending, rotation, and flexion or extension further into the restriction.
   h. Steps e through g are repeated two or three times.
   i. The patient's head is returned to neutral and the lesion is reassessed for change.

COUNTERSTRAIN TECHNIQUES
Lillian Somner

The treatment of tender points by the Jones counterstrain method requires that the patient be comfortable and relaxed. All treatment positions are held for 90 seconds, then released slowly without the help of the patient.

1. Patient position: supine.
2. Physician position: seated at the head of the table. The physician supports the patient's head with one hand and monitors tissue changes at the tender point with the other hand.

Anterior Tender Points
In general, the anterior tender points are located on the tip of the transverse processes and are treated in flexion, with side bending and rotation added to increase the softening of the tender point. Figure 7-14 shows the location of the anterior cervical tender points.

Figure 7-14. Cervical anterior tender point location. *TP*, transverse process; *AC7*, anterior C7; *AC8*, anterior C8; *PC8*, posterior C8.

1. C1: posterior edge of the ascending ramus of the mandible.
   C2: anterior surface of the transverse process.
   Technique: Head is rotated and slightly side bent away from the tender point (Fig. 7-15).
2. C1 tender point: inner table of the mandible anterior to the angle.
   C3 tender point: tip of the transverse process.
   Technique: Marked flexion, side bending toward, and rotation are induced away from the point.
3. C4 tender point:
   Technique: Neck is extended slightly. Side bending and rotation are away from the tender point (Fig. 7-16).

Figure 7-15. Treatment of tender point on the right side of C1. The head is rotated and bent laterally away from the tender point.

Figure 7-16. Treatment of tender point on the left side of C4. Side bending and rotation are induced in the direction away from the tender point.

Figure 7-17. Treatment of anterior tender point on the left side of C6.

Figure 7-18. Treatment of anterior tender point on the left side of C7.

4. C5 and C6:
   Technique: Flexion, with side bending, and rotation are away from the point (Fig. 7-17).
5. C7: posterosuperior surface of the clavicle, 3 cm lateral to the medial end.
   Technique: Marked flexion is induced to the level of C7, with the neck supported at mid-neck for the comfort of the patient. The technique entails slight rotation away and marked side bending toward the point (Fig. 7-18).
6. C8 tender point: medial end of the clavicle.
   Technique: Marked flexion, marked rotation, and marked side bending are induced. The side bending and rotation are away from the point.

Posterior Tender Points

In general, the posterior points are treated with the neck in extension to the level of the segment being treated. Side bending and rotation are away from the tender point. Figure 7-19 shows the location of the posterior tender points.

1. a. Inion C1: medial side of the muscle mass that attaches to the occiput about 3 cm below the inion.
   b. C2: lateral side of the muscle mass and the upper surface of the spinous process.
   c. C3: lateral side of the muscle mass and the upper surface of the spinous process.
   d. C3: side of the spinous process of C2.
   Technique: All four tender points are

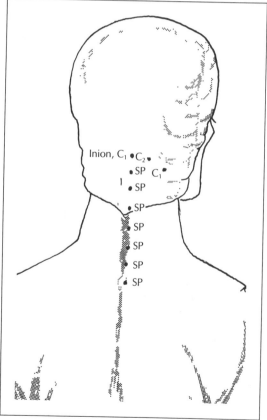

Figure 7-19. Posterior cervical tender point locations. *SP*, spinous process.

Figure 7-20. Treatment of posterior C_3 tender point on the right side.

Figure 7-21. Treatment of posterior transverse process tender points, requires placing the neck in slight extension.

Figure 7-22. Treatment of posterior spinous process tender point at C6. For treatment of the C1 to C7 spinous processes, the neck is placed in extension.

treated in flexion with side bending and rotation away from tender point (Fig. 7-20).

2. Posterior transverse processes.
   Technique: Slight extension, rotating and sidebending away (Fig. 7-21).

3. C1–C7 spinous processes:
   Technique: Extension of the neck to the segment to be treated. Side bending and rotation, when needed, are away from the tender point (Fig. 7-22).

HIGH VELOCITY, LOW AMPLITUDE THRUSTING TECHNIQUES

Barry Erner

The principles of thrusting techniques were discussed in Chapter 5. This section describes the application of high velocity, low amplitude thrusting techniques to correct dysfunctions of the cervical spine. The veterbra is first placed into its barrier to motion. The physician applies a rapid, brief force to pass through the barrier.

Occipital Joint Dysfunction

1. Patient position: supine.
2. Physician position: at the head of the table, on the same side as the freedom of rotation.
3. **Technique:**
   a. The physician grasps the patient's head

with his nonthrusting hand, holding the lateral cheek (and chin, if desired) steady.

b. The physician places the metacarpo-phalangeal joint of the index finger of his thrusting hand at the junction of the occiput and the cervical spine. His thumb rests on the patient's cheek.

c. The patient's occiput is sidebent and rotated into its barriers to motion. Minimal extension is added.

d. The physician exerts a simultaneously coupled rotation and side-bending thrust, with the vector of force passing through the patient's uppermost eye (Fig. 7-23).

Figure 7-23. High velocity, low amplitude thrusting technique for somatic dysfunction of the occipitoatlantal joint.

Figure 7-24. High velocity, low amplitude thrusting technique for somatic dysfunction of the atlantoaxial joint.

Figure 7-25. High velocity, low amplitude thrusting technique for somatic dysfunctions of the cervical spine, C3 to C7.

Atlantoaxial Joint Dysfunction

1. Patient position: supine.
2. Physician position: standing at the head of the table.
3. **Technique:**
   a. The physician cups the lateral aspect of the patient's chin (and/or side of the jaw).
   b. The patient's head is rotated into its rotation barrier.
   c. The physician's thrusting hand is positioned so that the lateral aspect of the second metacarpal joint is firmly over the atlantoaxial joint. His thumb is placed over the angle of the jaw for stability.
   d. The physician exerts a rapid rotary thrust with his second metacarpal joint (Fig. 7-24).

C3 to C7 Dysfunction

1. Patient position: supine.
2. Physician position: standing at head of the table
3. **Technique:**
   a. The physician cups the lateral aspect of the patient's chin (and/or side of the jaw) in his nonthrusting hand.

b. The patient's head is slightly extended over the physician's index finger and then is rotated into the motion barrier, keeping the head in the midline.
   c. The physician's thrusting hand is positioned so that the lateral aspect of the second metacarpal joint is firmly behind the posteriorly rotated transverse process.
   d. The patient's neck is side-bent up to the monitoring finger, away from the table.
   e. The physician exerts a rapid rotary thrust with his metacarpal joint (Fig. 7-25).
      Note: In the described technique, the barrier to rotation is engaged and corrected. The technique can be modified so that all three barriers to motion are engaged before the thrusting force is added.

Cervical Somatic Dysfunction: Alternative Technique

1. Patient position: supine.
2. Physician position: standing at the head of the table.
3. **Technique:**
   a. The physician places the lateral aspect of

the second metacarpal joint of the thrusting hand on the side opposite the posteriorly rotated transverse process.

b. The other hand is placed along the opposite side of the patient's head.

c. Engage the barriers of extension/flexion, rotation, and sidebending.

d. The physician exerts a rapid lateral flexion thrust through the dysfunctional vertebra (Fig. 7-26).

Figure 7-26. An alternative high velocity, low amplitude technique for the treatment of somatic dysfunctions of the cervical spine.

EXERCISE THERAPY

Stanley Schiowitz
Albert DeRubertis

The exercises described can be used to increase regional cervical motion (muscle stretch, extensibility), to increase regional strength (muscle contractility), or to restore structural symmetry. Many cervical muscle functions and structural changes involve the thoracic region. It is suggested that the physician review the section in Chapter 9, Exercises for the Thoracic Region, when writing an exercise prescription.

Regional Stretch

FORWARD BENDING

1. Patient position: seated or standing, with the back erect.

2. **Instructions:**

a. Drop your head forward; let its weight (gravity) pull it down.

b. Add anterior (flexor) muscle contraction to bring your chin to your chest.

c. Place both hands behind your head and passively pull your head down, chin to

chest (Fig. 7-27). Do not create pain.

d. Hold this position for 5 to 15 seconds. Relax, rest, and repeat.

BACKWARD BENDING

1. Patient position: seated or standing, with the back erect.

2. **Instructions:**

a. Drop your head backward; let its weight pull it back.

b. Add posterior (extensor) muscle contraction to increase the backward bending.

c. Place both hands on your forehead and passively push your head back (Fig. 7-28). Do not create pain.

d. Hold this position for 5 to 15 seconds. Relax, rest, and repeat.

SIDE BENDING

1. Patient position: seated or standing, with the back erect.

2. **Instructions:**

Figure 7-27. Exercise therapy for the cervical spine: forward bending.

Figure 7-28. Exercise therapy for cervical stretch: backward bending.

Figure 7-29. Exercise therapy for cervical stretch: side bending.

Figure 7-30. Exercise therapy for cervical stretch: rotation.

a. Without moving your shoulders, drop your head to the right; let its weight pull your right ear toward the right shoulder.

b. Add right-sided muscle contraction to increase the side bending.

c. Place your right hand over your head, palm on the left side of your head, and passively pull your head down to the right (Fig. 7-29). Try not to introduce rotation motion. Do not create pain.

d. Hold this position for 5 to 15 seconds. Relax, rest and repeat. For left side bending, reverse the instructions.

ROTATION

1. Patient position: seated or standing, with the back erect.

2. **Instructions:**

a. Without moving your shoulders, turn your head to the right as far as you can, using right rotation muscle contraction.

b. Place your right hand in front of your forehead with the palm on the left side of your head. Passively pull your head to the right as far as possible (Fig. 7-30). Do not create pain.

Note: In steps a and b, keep the chin in one horizontal plane. Avoid adding lateral bending motion.

c. Hold this position for 5 to 15 seconds. Relax, rest, and repeat. For left rotation, reverse directions.

Regional Strength

The exercises for promoting cervical strength use static contraction. Exercises are described for flexor muscles, extensor muscles, side bending muscles, and rotation muscles.

FLEXOR MUSCLES

1. Patient position: seated or standing, with the back erect.
2. **Instructions:**
   a. Place both your palms on your forehead.
   b. Push your head forward against your palms. Resist the forward push so as to prevent all head motion (Fig. 7-31).
   c. Hold for 4 seconds, then relax.
   d. Repeat the exercise, gradually increasing the strength of the contracting force and hand resistance. Do not create pain. Do not hold static contraction beyond 5 seconds.

Figure 7-31. Cervical strengthening exercise: flexor muscles.

EXTENSOR MUSCLES

1. Patient position: seated or standing, with the back erect.
2. **Instructions:**
   a. Place both hands behind your head.
   b. Push your head backward against your resisting hands (Fig. 7-32). Prevent all head motion.
   c. Hold for 4 seconds, then relax.
   d. Repeat the exercise, gradually increasing the strength of the contracting force and hand resistance. Do not create pain. Do not hold a static contraction for more than 5 seconds.

Figure 7-32. Cervical strengthening exercise: extensor muscles.

SIDE BENDING MUSCLES

1. Patient position: seated or standing, with the back erect.
2. **Instructions:**
   a. Place your right hand on the right side of your head, above the ear.
   b. Push your head to the right against your resisting right hand (Fig. 7-33). Prevent all head motion.

Figure 7-33. Cervical strengthening exercise: side bending muscles.

Figure 7-34. Cervical strengthening exercise: rotator muscles.

Figure 7-35. First exercise for cervicothoracic asymmetry.

c. Hold for 4 seconds, then relax.
d. Repeat the exercise, gradually increasing the strength of the contracting force and hand resistance. For left side bending, reverse directions. Do not create pain. Do not hold a static contraction for more than 5 seconds.

ROTATOR MUSCLES
1. Patient position: seated or standing, with the back erect.
2. **Instructions:**
   a. Place your right hand on the right side of your forehead.
   b. Turn your head to the right against your resisting right hand (Fig. 7-34). Prevent all head motion.
   c. Hold for 4 seconds, then relax.
   d. Repeat the exercise, gradually increasing the strength of the contracting force and hand resistance. For left rotation, reverse directions. Do not create pain. Do not hold a static contraction for more than 5 seconds.

Cervicothoracic Asymmetry

Exercises for cervicothoracic asymmetry are designed to reduce excessive cervical lordosis and upper thoracic kyphosis (dowager's hump). Three exercises are described.

Exercise 1
1. Patient position: supine on solid flat surface.
2. **Instructions:**
   a. Tuck in your chin.
   b. Try to push your neck down, flattening your neck against the surface (Fig. 7-35).
   c. Hold for 4 seconds, relax, and repeat.

Exercise 2
1. Patient position: seated in a chair with back pressed firmly against the back of the chair. A pillow may be used to maintain a low back lordotic curve if necessary.
2. **Instructions:**
   a. Tuck in your chin.
   b. With one hand, push your chin toward the back of your neck, trying to flatten the neck. Your chin must be kept in one horizontal plane (Fig. 7-36).
   c. Hold for 4 seconds, relax, and repeat.

Figure 7-36. Second exercise for cervicothoracic asymmetry.

Figure 7-37. Third exercise for cervicothoracic asymmetry.

Exercise 3
1. Patient position: standing.
2. **Instructions:**
   a. Stand straight with your back and neck stretched as tall as possible.
   b. Tuck in your chin.
   c. Place both hands on top of your head.
   d. Push your head up toward your hands, lengthening your neck. Keep your chin in horizontal plane (Fig. 7-37).
   e. Hold for 4 seconds, relax, and repeat.
      Note: Do not increase your lumbar lordosis. Once this procedure has been mastered, keep your hands down and practice standing and walking with your chin and neck in this position, as often as possible.

8   Evaluation of the Thoracic Spine

FUNCTIONAL ANATOMY AND BIOMECHANICS

Jonathan Fenton
Donald E. Phykitt

The thoracic spine is a relatively immobile area, compared with the cervical or lumbar spine. The immobility has two anatomic causes. First, considerable stability is provided by the intimate connection of the thoracic spine to the thoracic cage, the ribs and sternum, via the costovertebral articulations. Second, the ratio of intervertebral disk height to vertebral body height is small (1:5), which greatly reduces intersegmental motion. By contrast, the disk height-vertebral body height ratios in the cervical and lumbar regions are 2:5 (permitting greatest motion) and 1:3, respectively.

The thoracic spine normally displays a gentle kyphosis, a C-shaped curve, convex posteriorly. This is mainly due to the wedge shape of the vertebral bodies, which are slightly higher at the posterior edge than at the anterior edge. The degree of kyphosis can vary with age and postural habits as well as with pathologic conditions, such as osteoporosis.

Although the thoracic spine has characteristic features that distinguish it from the cervical and lumbar spinal regions, it is mainly a transitional zone between the cervical and lumbar regions, as evidenced by the steady increase in height of the vertebral bodies from T1 to T12. Moreover, the inferior articular facets of T12 correspond to those in the lumbar area to allow proper articulation with L1. The different forms of articulation play a considerable role in the amplitude of various physiologic motions in the thoracic spine.

Osteology

VERTEBRAL BODY

The transverse diameter of the thoracic vertebral body is approximately equal to its anteroposterior diameter. The vertebral body is slightly higher at the posterior edge than at the anterior edge, contributing to normal kyphosis in the area. The anterior and lateral edges of the body are hollow.

The posterolateral corners of the superior and inferior vertebral plateaus bear the costal articular facets. These facets are oval, set into the body at an oblique angle, and lined by cartilage. They articulate with the heads of the ribs. Of the thoracic vertebrae, only T12 has costal articular facets only at the superior plateau.

ARTICULAR FACETS

The superior articular facets face backward, upward, and laterally. They are rotated approximately 60 degrees from the horizontal plane and 20 degrees from the frontal plane. In the transverse dimension they are convex.

125

The inferior articular facets face forward, downward, and medially. In the transverse dimension they are concave. The inferior articular facets of T12 resemble those of a lumbar vertebra in that they face laterally and anteriorly and are convex transversely.

TRANSVERSE AND SPINOUS PROCESSES
The transverse processes of the thoracic vertebrae face laterally and slightly posteriorly; they are easily palpated. They bear costal articular facets at the anterior aspects of their bulbous tips, the point of articulation with the costal tubercles of the corresponding ribs.

THE SPINOUS PROCESS
The spinous process faces posteriorly and inferiorly, the degree of inferior angulation varying with the area of the thoracic spine. The "rule of 3's" is used to locate a vertebra's spinous process in relation to its transverse process.

RULE OF 3'S
1. The upper three thoracic vertebrae (T1, T2, T3) have spinous processes that project directly posteriorly; therefore, the tip of the spinous process is in the same plane as the transverse processes of that vertebra.
2. The next three vertebrae (T4, T5, T6) have spinous processes that project slightly downward; therefore, the tip of the spinous process lies in a plane halfway between that vertebra's transverse processes and the transverse processes of the vertebra below it.
3. The next three vertebrae (T7, T8, T9) have spinous processes that project moderately downward; therefore, the tip of the spinous process is in a plane with the transverse processes of the vertebra below it.
4. The last three thoracic vertebrae (T10, T11, T12) have spinous processes that project from a position similar to T9 and rapidly regress until the orientation of the spinous process of T12 is like that of T1. That is, the spinous process of T10 is near the plane of the transverse processes of the vertebra below it, the spinous process of T11 is halfway between its own transverse processes and the transverse processes of the vertebra below it, and the spinous process of T12 projects directly posteriorly in the plane of its own transverse processes.

Rib Articulations
COSTOVERTEBRAL ARTICULATION
The articular facets on the vertebral bodies are really demifacets (i.e., partial facets). The entire facet consists in the demifacet on the superior aspect of one vertebra and the demifacet on the inferior aspect of the vertebra above it.

The heads of the second through 12th ribs articulate with the bodies of the corresponding vertebrae and the one above, as well as with the corresponding intervertebral disk. However, the first rib articulates only with the superior aspect of T1. The costovertebral articulation is a synovial joint, with a joint capsule that is strengthened by the radiate ligament (see below, Costovertebral Ligaments).

COSTOTRANSVERSE ARTICULATIONS
The costotransverse articulation is a joint representing the articulation of the tubercle of a rib with the transverse process of the corresponding vertebra. The joint is surrounded by a weak capsule that is greatly strengthened by the costotransverse ligaments.

ANTERIOR ARTICULATIONS
The anterior end of the rib is joined to its costal cartilage by the costochondral joint. The costal cartilage articulates anteriorly in a number of ways:

1. The first rib is joined to the manubrium by a cartilaginous joint.
2. The cartilage of the second rib articulates with demifacets on both the manubrium and the body of the sternum by way of synovial joints.
3. The cartilages of the third through seventh ribs create small synovial joints with the body of the sternum.
4. The eighth through tenth costal cartilages do not join the sternum but are continuous with the costal cartilage immediately above.
5. The 11th and 12th costal cartilages are free. These ribs are known as the floating ribs.

Ligamentous Attachments
Seven ligaments connect adjacent vertebrae in the thoracic spine.

1. The anterior longitudinal ligament is attached to the anterior surface of all vertebral bodies.

2. The posterior longitudinal ligament runs down the posterior surface of all vertebral bodies.
3. Intertransverse ligaments pass between the transverse processes in the thoracic spine.
4. Capsular ligaments are attached just beyond the margins of the adjacent articular processes.
5. Ligamenta flava (arcuate, flaval, or yellow ligaments) extend from the anterior inferior border of the laminae above to the posterior superior borders of the laminae below.
6. Interspinous ligaments connect adjacent spinous processes; they extend from the root to the apex of each spinous process.
7. The supraspinous ligament originates in the ligamentum nuchae and continues along the tips of the spinous processes.

COSTOVERTEBRAL LIGAMENTS

There are two kinds of costovertebral ligaments, interosseous ligaments and radiate ligaments, the latter consisting of three bands. Interosseous ligaments are attached to the head of the rib between the two articular demifacets and to the corresponding intervertebral disk. In the radiate ligaments, the superior band of tissue runs from the head of the rib to the vertebral body above. The inferior band runs from the head of the rib to the corresponding vertebral body, and the intermediate band runs from the head of the rib to the corresponding intervertebral disk.

COSTOTRANSVERSE LIGAMENTS

There are three kinds of costotransverse ligaments, determined by anatomic location with respect to the ribs and vertebrae—interosseous, posterior, and superior. The interosseous costotransverse ligament runs from the transverse process to the posterior surface of the neck of the corresponding rib. The posterior costotransverse ligament runs from the tip of the transverse process to the lateral border of the corresponding costal tubercle. The superior costotransverse ligament runs from the inferior border of the transverse process to the superior border of the neck of the underlying rib.

Thoracic Spinal Motion

INTERVERTEBRAL MOTION, EXCLUDING RIBS

Extension (least motion). In extension, the vertebrae approximate posteriorly. The inferior articular process of the superior vertebra glides posteriorly and inferiorly on the inferior vertebra. Motion is limited by approximation of the articular processes and spinous processes. These structures are sharply inclined posteriorly and inferiorly, and in normal anatomic relation are almost touching. The anterior longitudinal ligament is stretched, while the posterior longitudinal ligament, the ligamenta flava, and the interspinous ligaments are relaxed.

Flexion (second least motion). During flexion, the interspace between vertebrae increases posteriorly. The inferior articular process of the superior vertebra glides anteriorly and superiorly. Motion in the flexed spine is limited by the tension developed in the interspinous ligaments, the ligamenta flava, and the posterior longitudinal ligament.

Lateral flexion (second greatest motion). In lateral flexion, the articular surfaces on each side of a vertebra glide in opposite directions: on the contralateral side they glide upward, as in flexion; on the ipsilateral side they glide downward, as in extension. Lateral flexion to one side is accompanied by axial rotation to the opposite side, for three reasons: (1) One articular surface glides anteriorly while the other glides posteriorly. (2) Compression developed in the intervertebral disk, the anterior aspect of the unit, causes the vertebral body to move in the direction opposite to that of side bending. (3) Lateral flexion tends to stretch the contralateral ligaments, located at the posterior aspect of the unit, which causes these ligaments to move toward the midline posteriorly to minimize their lengths.

Motion in the laterally flexed thoracic spine is limited by the impact of the articular processes on the ipsilateral side and by the tension developed in the contralateral ligamenta flava and intertransverse ligaments.

Rotation (greatest motion). In rotation, the orientation of the thoracic articular facets allows them to glide relative to each other with an axis of rotation near the center of the vertebral body. Thus, one vertebra can rotate around an axis, producing a simple twisting of the thoracic intervertebral disk. In contrast, the facets of the lumbar vertebrae are aligned such that the axis of rotation is at the spinous process. For rotation to occur one vertebral body must glide laterally with respect to its adjacent vertebrae. This results in shearing forces at the intervertebral disk. The articulation at T12–L1 is identical to the articulations found in the lumbar spine, so that the degree of rotation is greatly reduced. For the thoracic spine, motion in rotation is limited by multiple ligamentous tensions.

STABILITY AFFORDED BY THE COSTAL CAGE
There are two mechanisms by which the ribs tend to increase the stability (and decrease the motion) of the thoracic spine. The first mechanism involves the articulation of the head of the ribs with the body and transverse processes of the vertebrae. The second mechanism increases the spine's moment of inertia via an increase in the transverse and anteroposterior dimensions of the spine structure. This results in increased resistance to motion in all directions

Although no studies have compared the motion of the thoracic spine with and without intact costovertebral joints, Panjabi et al have determined that the costovertebral joint plays a critical role in stabilizing the thoracic spine during flexion and extension.

The rib cage as a whole greatly enhances the stiffness of the spine, despite the flexibility of the individual components of the rib cage—the ribs, sternum, and their joints. Using a mathematical model of the thoracic and lumbar spine and the rib cage, Andriacchi et al performed computer simulations to determine the effect of the rib cage on the stiffness of the normal spine during flexion, extension, side bending, and axial rotation. They also studied the effect of removing one or two ribs or the entire sternum from an intact thorax. The stiffness properties of the spine were found to be greatly enhanced by the presence of an intact rib cage for all four motions, especially extension. The percentage increase in the stiffness of the spine with an intact rib cage, as compared with the spine and ligaments alone, was 27% for flexion, 132% for extension, 45% for lateral bending, and 31% for axial rotation. Removal of the sternum virtually nullified the stiffening effect of the costal cage. Removal of one or two ribs had minimal effect.

Thus, the intact thoracic cage, rather than individual elements or articulations, is a major factor contributing to the increased stability of the thoracic spine.

OVERALL MOTION OF THE THORACIC SPINE
The thoracic spine is a transitional region be-

tween the relatively more mobile cervical and lumbar regions. It is designed for rigidity and support of vital structures. The extent of each of the four physiologic motions varies throughout the region, owing to variable effects of the costal cage and to changes in vertebral osteology from a cervical-like osteology to a lumbar-like osteology.

Flexion/extension. Flexion and extension are the least of the motions of the thoracic spine and occur to the smallest extent in the upper thoracic spine, gradually increasing in amplitude in the lower thoracic spine. This transition is largely due to the stiffening effect of the costal cage in the upper thoracic spine, which is most evident during extension. The first seven ribs are attached directly to the sternum, promoting greatest stability. The next three ribs are only indirectly attached via costal cartilage. The last two ribs are not attached at all anteriorly and therefore resemble the cylinder with a strip cut out, providing considerably less stability than the ribs higher in the costal cage.

The motions of flexion and extension in the thoracic spine are further limited by costovertebral articulations. This stabilization is lost at T11–T12 and T12–L1, as the 12th rib articulates only with the body of T12, thus losing the support found when a rib articulates with two adjacent vertebrae.

Lateral bending. Lateral bending is the second greatest motion in the thoracic spine. The amplitude of motion remains fairly constant throughout the region but is restricted by articular impingement, by ligamentous attachments (including costovertebral and costotransverse ligaments), and by the resistance afforded by the intact costal cage.

Rotation. Rotation is the greatest motion in the larger part of the thoracic spine (T1–T10). The amplitude of rotation is markedly decreased in the lower part of the region. The articular orientation of the thoracic vertebrae allows them to rotate about a point in the center of the vertebral body. The articular orientation of the lower thoracic vertebrae, however, is similar to that of the lumbar vertebrae and permits rotation only about a point near the spinous process. This rotation is greatly resisted by shearing forces in the intervertebral disk. The extent of rotation is further diminished by the resistance afforded by the intact costal cage.

MOTION TESTING
Donald E. Phykitt

Gross Motion Testing
LATERAL FLEXION, T1–T12
1. Patient position: seated.
2. Physician position: standing behind patient.
3. **Technique:**
   a. The physician places his hands on the patient's shoulders with the web of the thumb and first finger over the acromion. The thumb rests posteriorly, pointing to T12, and the fingers rest anteriorly.
   b. To evaluate *right* lateral flexion:
      i. The physician exerts *downward* pressure accompanied by *left* translatory force on the *right* shoulder (Fig. 8-1A). The resulting force is transmitted downward through the body of T12.
      ii. Note the ease and degree of lateral flexion (normal = approximately 20 degrees) and the smoothness of the right lateral curve created in the thoracic spine.
   c. To evaluate *left* lateral flexion:
      i. The physician exerts *downward* pressure accompanied by a *right* translatory force on the left shoulder. The resulting force will be directed downward through the body of T12.
      ii. Note the ease and degree of lateral flexion (normal = approximately 20 degrees) and the smoothness of the left lateral curve created in the thoracic spine.
   d. Compare the degree of lateral flexion in each direction.
   e. Note the presence and location of any pain experienced by the patient during these maneuvers.

Figure 8-1. Localization of force induced on thoracic side bending. (**A**) T1 through T12. (**B**) T1 through T8. (**C**) T1 through T4.

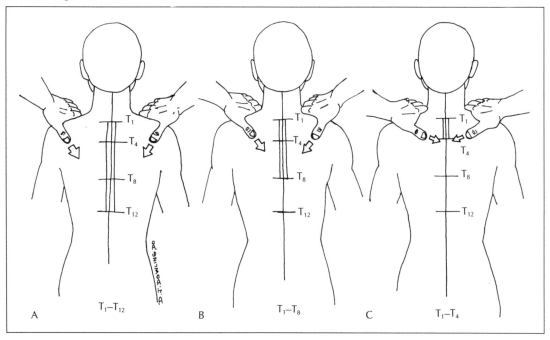

LATERAL FLEXION, T1–T8
1. Patient position: seated.
2. Physician position: standing behind the patient.
3. **Technique:**
   a. The technique is similar to that described for lateral flexion of T1–T12, with the following modifications. The physician's hands are placed with the web of the thumb and first finger halfway between the base the patient's neck and the acromion process. The thumbs point toward T8. Greater force is required to induce lateral flexion in the T1–T8 region. The resulting force exerted by the physician is directed downward and through the body of T8 (Fig. 8-1B).
   b. Compare the angle of lateral flexion (left vs right), and note any difference (normal = approximately 10 degrees).
   c. Observe the smoothness of the lateral curve created.

LATERAL FLEXION, T1–T4
1. Patient position: sitting.
2. Physician position: standing behind patient.
3. **Technique:**
   a. The technique is similar to that described for testing lateral flexion of T1–T12 and T1–T4, with the following modifications. The physician's hands are placed with web of the thumb and first finger as close as possible to the patient's shoulders at the base of the neck. The thumbs point toward T4. Greater force is required to induce lateral flexion than in the previous two tests. The force induced by the physician is directed downward and through the body of T4 (Fig. 8-1C).
   b. Compare the degree of lateral flexion (right vs left) and note any differences (normal = approximately 5 degrees).
   c. Note: Asymmetry in lateral flexion (right vs left) can be caused by single dysfunctions, group curves, or myofascial tension in the area being examined.

Discrepancies in findings between areas of the thoracic spine (T1–T12, T1–T8 or T1–T4) may indicate an area of dysfunction and should prompt the physician to examine this area more closely with the techniques of rotoscoliosis testing and intersegmental motion testing, described below.

ROTATION IN THE THORACIC SPINE
1. Patient position: seated, straddling the table, with his back near the end of the table.
2. Physician position: standing behind patient.
3. **Technique:**
   a. The physician places a hand on each of the patient's acromion processes.
   b. Rotation is induced by the physician drawing one shoulder toward himself while simultaneously pushing away the opposite shoulder (Fig. 8-2).
      i. *Right rotation:* The physician draws the right shoulder toward himself while pushing away the left shoulder.
      ii. *Left rotation:* The physician draws the left shoulder toward himself while pushing away the right shoulder.
   c. *Note:*
      i. The degree of rotation in each direction. This is best measured by noting the deviation of the shoulder line from the frontal plane. Normal rotation is approximately 40 degrees in each direction.
      ii. The symmetry of right rotation versus left rotation.
      iii. The presence and location of pain during this maneuver.

FORWARD BENDING/BACKWARD BENDING
It is quite difficult to separate the motions of forward and backward bending in the thoracic spine from the same motions in the lumbar spine. Therefore, these motions are considered for the combined thoracolumbar region, and the technique is described in Chapter 10.

Rotoscoliosis Testing
Rotoscoliosis testing and intersegmental motion testing are two diagnostic modalities for evaluating somatic dysfunction at a vertebral level. They can be used alone or in conjunction with each other, according to physician preference.

Rotoscoliosis testing evaluates the rotational position of the vertebrae with respect to the position of the transverse processes. This position is

Figure 8-2. Positions for thoracic left rotation.

Figure 8-3. Rotoscoliosis testing for type II dysfunction in the upper thorax.

evaluated with the spine in neutral position, in flexion, and in extension.

Vertebrae involved in a group curve will exhibit the greatest positional rotation in neutral position. From Fryette's first law, side bending and rotation should occur in opposite directions. Single somatic dysfunctions exhibit the greatest positional rotation in either flexion or extension. From Fryette's second law, side bending and rotation should occur in the same direction. Furthermore, in single somatic dysfunctions the freedom of motion (the direction for which the dysfunction is named) in flexion or extension will be opposite to the position in which the rotation is exaggerated.

The positions described in the following sections are the positions in which the patient is examined. Examples of examination findings and the corresponding diagnoses are given at the end of the chapter.

THE DOMINANT EYE

The dominant eye is the eye through which most information about the outside world is conveyed. A dominant eye develops in every person shortly after birth and does not change for the duration of life. It has no relationship to handedness.

Technique for Determining Dominant Eye
1. Make a circle by apposing your thumb and index finger.

2. Fully extend the arm in front of you.
3. With both eyes open, locate an object at least 10 feet away so that it is enclosed in the circle formed by your two fingers.
4. Maintaining this position, close each eye alternately, so that you are looking through the circle with each eye alternately.
5. The dominant eye is the one that "sees" the object as within the circle. The nondominant eye "sees" the object as outside the circle.

ROTOSCOLIOSIS TESTING FOR TYPE II DYSFUNCTIONS, T1–T3

1. Patient position: seated.
2. Physician position: standing behind the patient.
3. **Technique:**
   a. The physician uses his thumbs to palpate the tips of the transverse processes, located one-half inch lateral to and at the same level of the corresponding spinous process (Fig. 8-3).
   b. Evaluate for the presence of pain, increased myofascial tension, and one transverse process (right or left) more posterior than the other. The latter can be detected either by palpating a more posterior transverse process or by sensing a decreased tissue depth on the side of the posterior transverse process.
   c. At each level, have the patient begin with

Figure 8-4. Rotoscoliosis testing for type II dysfunction in extension in midthoracic region, patient prone.

Figure 8-5. Rotoscoliosis testing for type II dysfunction in flexion in midthoracic region, patient seated.

the neck fully flexed. Instruct the patient to slowly bring his head back into neutral position and then into full extension.
  d. Observe the changes under your palpating fingers. *Note* the position (flexion, extension) in which the maximum positional rotation occurs, and the direction of positional rotation (side of the posterior transverse process).
  e. Repeat these steps for T2 and T3.

ROTOSCOLIOSIS TESTING FOR
TYPE II DYSFUNCTIONS, T4–T12
Rotoscoliosis testing in the region of T4–T12 is identical to testing in the upper thoracic region, with the exception of differences in patient position for the different physiologic motions.

Extension
1. Patient position: prone, resting on his elbows. The upper thoracic musculature should be relaxed to allow full extension and to facilitate palpation (Fig. 8-4).
2. Physician position: seated or standing at the side of the patient, facing the patient's head. The physician's dominant eye is closest to the patient.
3. **Technique:** described under Flexion, which follows.

Flexion
1. Patient position: seated, with the feet supported on the floor or a stool. The hands are locked behind the neck and the patient is instructed to bend forward as far as he can (Fig. 8-5).
2. Physician position: standing in front of or behind patient.
3. **Technique** (for all lower thoracic rotoscoliosis diagnoses):
  a. The physician uses the thumbs or index fingers to palpate the tips of the transverse processes, located one-half to one inch lateral to the spinous processes. (The caudad-cephalad relationship between a vertebra's spinous process and its transverse processes is governed by the rule of 3's, described earlier in this chapter.)
  b. Evaluate:
    i. Pain on palpation.
    ii. Increased myofascial tension.
    iii. Posterior transverse process. Increased musculature in this region makes direct palpation of transverse processes difficult. Posterior rotation will most likely be detected from a decreased tissue depth.
  c. The physician positions himself so that he can visualize the midline of the patient's back parallel to the spine. *Note* the relative

heights of the palpating fingers. Are they even? Is one finger more posterior?

d. Begin by examining the entire lower thoracic region in neutral position and noting findings. Then instruct the patient move up into extension, and note findings in this position. Finally, instruct the patient to move into flexion, and note findings in this position.

e. After evaluating the lower thoracic region in all three positions, note in which position positional rotation was greatest at each vertebral level. It may be necessary to reevaluate one or more levels to determine the position in which the transverse process was most posterior.

ROTOSCOLIOSIS TESTING FOR TYPE I DYSFUNCTIONS

Evaluation of the thoracic spine for the detection of type I dysfunctions entails three different kinds of examinations:

1. Static symmetry scan (see Chap. 3). Observation from behind the patient may reveal side bending of a group of vertebrae, asymmetry in the *height* of paired landmarks (e.g., shoulders), or asymmetry in the *prominence* of paired landmarks (e.g., scapulae).

2. Regional motion testing. The physician observes for asymmetric lateral flexion. Restricted motion to the side of the convexity is common.

3. Rotoscoliosis testing. The diagnosis of type I dysfunctions is based on detecting three or more adjacent vertebrae whose positional rotation is greatest in neutral. Testing is done separately for the upper and lower thoracic regions.

Upper thoracic region (T1–T3)
1. Patient position: seated.
2. Physician position: standing behind patient.
3. **Technique:**
   a. The patient is instructed to sit up straight, thus placing the vertebrae in neutral position.
   b. Using the thumbs, the physician palpates the transverse processes of T1 bilaterally.
   c. The physician determines which transverse process is more posterior.
   d. Repeat these steps at T2 and T3.

Lower thoracic region (T4–T12)
1. Patient position: prone, head resting on chin and facing forward, arms either at the side or hanging down from table (Fig. 8-6).
2. Physician position: standing at the side of the patient, facing the patient's head. The physician's dominant eye is closest to the patient.
3. **Technique:** Repeat test as described for rotoscoliosis testing for Type II dysfunctions, T4–T12.

Alternative Methods of Rotoscoliosis Testing, T4–T12
The methods described here are alternatives to conventional rotoscoliosis testing. Their advantages include ease and speed of diagnosis. The patient remains in a single position in all three methods. Furthermore, the physician can more readily compare findings in neutral, flexion, and extension. These techniques require greater palpatory skill, and should be used only by an experienced physician.

Alternate technique 1
1. Patient position: seated on a stool with the feet resting firmly on the ground, shoulder width apart.
2. Physician position: standing behind the patient.
3. **Technique:**
   a. The physician's thumbs are used to palpate the tips of the transverse processes bilaterally (Fig. 8-7).
   b. At each vertebral level, evaluation begins with the patient in neutral position (sitting straight up). *Note* pain, tissue changes, and vertebral rotation, as in conventional rotoscoliosis testing of T4–T12.
   c. With the physician's thumbs at the same vertebral level, the patient is asked to bend over as far as possible. *Note* changes in vertebral positional rotation.
   d. With the physician's thumbs at the same level, the patient is asked to sit up and position himself in extension.
      i. To evaluate T4–T8, ask the patient to thrust his chest out as far as possible.
      ii. To evaluate T9–T12, ask the patient to thrust his abdomen out as far as possible.
      iii. Note changes in vertebral positional rotation.

Figure 8-6. Rotoscoliosis testing for type I dysfunction, lower thorax, neutral position.

Figure 8-7. Rotoscoliosis testing, T4–T12, hand position.

e. Note in which position (neutral, flexion, or extension) vertebral positional rotation is greatest.

f. Repeat these steps for all levels, T4 through T12.

Alternate technique 2

1. Patient position: prone, head resting on chin, arms at sides.
2. Physician position: standing at the patient's side, with the dominant eye closest to patient.
3. **Technique:**
   a. The physician's thumbs or index fingers are used to palpate the tips of the transverse processes bilaterally.
   b. At each level, the physician begins by palpating the vertebra in the neutral position by pressing straight down on the transverse processes.
      i. Note tissue tension and vertebral positional rotation, as described for the conventional method.
      ii. Visualize the relative heights of thumbs, as described for the conventional method.
   c. With the thumbs at the same level, the physician evaluates the vertebrae in flexion.
      i. Roll the thumbs superiorly and press down on the superior aspect of the transverse processes, thus placing the vertebrae into flexion (Fig. 8-8).
      ii. Evaluate as above.

d. With the thumbs at the same level, the physician evaluates the vertebrae in extension.
   i. Roll the thumbs inferiorly and press down on the inferior aspect of the transverse processes, thus placing the vertebrae into extension (Fig. 8-9).
   ii. Evaluate as above.

e. Determine in which position (neutral, flexion, extension) the greatest positional rotation is found.

f. Repeat these steps at all levels, T4 through T12.

Alternate technique 3

1. Patient position: prone, head resting on chin, arms at sides.
2. Physician position: standing at the patient's side.
3. **Technique:**
   a. The physician places his hand on the patient's back with his fingers perpendicular to the patient's spine. One finger is placed in the interspinous space above and one finger in the interspinous space below the vertebra being evaluated.
   b. *Note:*
      i. Symmetry of interspinous spaces above and below vertebra in question.
      ii. Lateral deviation of spinous process of vertebra in question.

Figure 8-8. Rotoscoliosis testing, T4–T12, alternate technique 2, flexion testing.

Figure 8-9. Rotoscoliosis testing, T4–T12, alternate technique 2, extension testing.

iii. Anteroposterior deviation of spinous process of vertebra in question.
c. **Interpretation:**
  i. Flexion (freedom of motion) dysfunction:
    a. Superior interspinous space narrower
    b. Inferior interspinous space wider
    c. Spinous process less prominent
  ii. Extension dysfunction:
    a. Superior interspinous space wider
    b. Inferior interspinous space narrower
    c. Spinous process more prominent
  iii. Neutral dysfunction (group curve):
    a. Superior and inferior interspinous spaces equal
  iv. Rotation:
    a. Spinous process deviated to the side opposite that of vertebral rotation
  v. **Example:** The spinous process of T6 is less prominent and rotated to the left; the space between the spinous processes of T5 and T6 is narrower than the space between the spinous processes of T6 and T7. The diagnosis is T6 flexion, rotation, and lateral bending to the right.
d. Repeat these steps at each level, T4 through T12.

EXAMPLES OF ROTOSCOLIOSIS FINDINGS AND CORRESPONDING DIAGNOSES

Example 1. Transverse process of T8 is posterior on the right and most prominent in flexion. Diagnosis: T8 E Rr Sr.

Example 2. Transverse processes of T4–T10 are posterior on the right and most prominent in neutral position. Diagnosis: T4–10 N Rr Sl.

Example 3. The same finding as in example 2, except that the transverse process of T7 is posterior on the left and most prominent in extension. Diagnosis: group curve (T4–T10 N Rr Sl) with a single somatic dysfunction (T7 F Rl Sl) at the apex. *Note:* Single somatic dysfunctions can occur within a group curve. They are most common at the apex (center) and the ends of a curve.

Intersegmental Motion Testing

TISSUE TEXTURE CHANGES AND SYMMETRY
1. Patient position: seated comfortably, with the hands on the thighs and the cervical spine in neutral position.
2. Physician position: standing behind the patient.
3. **Technique:**
   a. The physician slides one finger along the spinous processes from T1 to T12. *Note:*
     i. Deviation from midline.
     ii. Any change in the size of the space between spinous processes.
     iii. Displacement of the spinous processes in the sagittal plane.
     iv. Point tenderness along the spinous processes.
   b. Place the pads of the second and third

Figure 8-10. Intersegmental motion testing, flexion/extension, T1–T4.

Figure 8-11. Intersegmental motion testing, rotation, T1–T4.

fingers on each side of the spinous process of T1, over the transverse processes. Slide them down from T1 to T12. *Note:*

   i. Tissue texture changes (firmness, bogginess).

   ii. Posterior prominence of transverse processes.

   iii. Change in size of space between transverse processes.

   iv. Deviation of spinous process from the midline.

   v. Point tenderness.

    Interpretation: For a detailed interpretation of deviations found on static evaluation of the spinous processes, see preceding, Alternate Method 3.

INTERSEGMENTAL MOTION TESTING, T1–T4

1. Patient position: seated comfortably, with the hands on the thighs and the cervical spine in neutral position.
2. Physician position: behind and to one side of the patient. The hand farthest from the patient (the motion-inducing hand) is placed on top of the patient's head. The position of the other hand (the palpating hand) varies with the motion being tested and is described below for the individual cases.
3. **Technique:**
   a. In evaluating **flexion/extension,** the physician's palpating hand is placed so that the fingers are oriented horizontally and pointing away from the physician. The pad of the third finger lies in the interspinous space of the level being tested (i.e., for testing T1, it lies in the interspinous space between T1 and T2). The pads of the second and fourth digits lie in the interspinous spaces one level above and one level below, respectively. The patient's head is passively bent forward and backward until motion is palpated at the level in question, but not at the level below (Fig. 8-10). *Note* symmetry of flexion versus extension at the vertebral level.

      Interpretation: The dysfunction is named for the direction (flexion or extension) where greater motion is detected.

   b. To evaluate **rotation,** the physician places one or two fingers on either side of the spinous process, over the transverse processes of the vertebrae being tested. The patient's head is bent forward or backward (the direction in which least motion was detected on flexion/extension testing) down to the level in question. The patient's head is then rotated to the left until full motion is palpated at the transverse process in question (Fig. 8-11). This process is repeated to the right. *Note* symmetry of rotation right versus rotation left.

      Interpretation: The dysfunction is named for the direction of greater rotation.

Figure 8-12. Intersegmental motion testing, lateral flexion, T1–T4.

Figure 8-13. Intersegmental motion testing, rotation, T5–T12.

c. To evaluate **lateral flexion**, the physician places one or two fingers on both sides of the spinous process, between the transverse processes of the level being tested and the level below. The patient's head is bent forward or backward (in the direction of least motion) down to the level being tested, then is bent laterally to both sides (Fig. 8-12). Lateral flexion is detected as separation or approximation of the transverse processes under the palpating fingers. Note symmetry of right lateral flexion versus left lateral flexion.

 Interpretation: The dysfunction is named for the direction of greater lateral flexion.

Note that lateral flexion on intersegmental motion testing is greatly restricted by the ribs and may be difficult to evaluate. In normal spines or in group curves, lateral flexion is in the direction opposite the direction of rotation. In type II single-segment somatic dysfunctions, lateral flexion occurs in the same direction as rotation. The diagnosis of lateral flexion limitation relies primarily on the finding of asymmetric motion in flexion/extension and in rotation.

INTERSEGMENTAL MOTION
TESTING, T5–T12
The methods of diagnosing intersegmental dysfunction in the lower thoracic spine are quite similar to the techniques used in the upper thoracic

spine. The patient position is the same except that the patient must sit up straight. The positions of the palpating hand are the same. However, the physician is positioned differently with respect to the patient, and different techniques are used to induce motion in the lower thoracic spine. Only these differences are described.

1. Patient position: as for intersegmental motion testing of the upper thoracic spine (see p. 136).
2. Physician position: behind and to one side of patient. The hand closer to patient serves as the palpating hand. The other arm is positioned so that axilla rests on the patient's near shoulder. The arm reaches across the patient's sternum and the hand grasps the patient's far shoulder.
3. **Technique:**
   a. **Flexion** is induced by applying a downward and slightly anterior force to both of the patient's shoulders.
   b. **Extension** is induced by applying a caudal and slightly posterior force to both of the patient's shoulders.
   c. **Rotation** is induced by rotating the shoulders in the desired direction (Fig. 8-13).
   d. **Lateral flexion** is induced by exerting a caudal force to one shoulder (the side ipsilateral to the desired lateral flexion), accompanied by a translatory force to the opposite side.

Palpation and interpretation are identical to those described for intersegmental motion testing of the upper thoracic spine.

References

Andriacchi TP, Schultz AB, Belytscko TB, Galante JO. 1974. A model for studies of mechanical interaction between the human spine and ribcage. J Biomech 7:497.

Fryette H. 1954. Principles of Osteopathic Technique. Colorado Springs: Academy of Applied Osteopathy.

Kapandji IA. 1974. The Physiology of the Joints. Vol 3. The Trunk and the Vertebral Column. Edinburgh: Churchill Livingstone.

Schiowitz S, DiGiovanna E. 1981. An Osteopathic Approach to Diagnosis and Treatment. Old Westbury, New York: New York College of Osteopathic Medicine.

Warwick R, Williams P. 1973. Gray's Anatomy, 35th British ed. Philadelphia: W.B. Saunders Co.

White A, Panjabi MM. 1978. Biomechanics of the Spine. Philadelphia: J.B. Lippincott Co.

9   Treatment of the Thoracic Spine

MYOFASCIAL TECHNIQUES
Toni Murphy

The principles of myofascial treatment were discussed in Chapter 5. Several of the techniques described in this section are good general techniques for relaxing and stretching the muscles of the thoracic and shoulder girdle.

Passive Techniques
PERPENDICULAR STRETCH
Perpendicular stretch techniques can be used to treat any muscles of the thoracolumbar region that run parallel to the spinous processes, including the erector spinae and its subdivisions.

1. Patient position: prone, with the head turned to the side of most comfort.
2. Physician position: standing at the side of the table and opposite the side being treated.
3. **Technique:**
   a. The physician places the thumb and thenar eminence of one hand at the medial edge of the muscle to be treated and lateral to the spinous processes. The thumb is parallel to the spinous processes (Fig. 9-1).
   b. He then places the thenar eminence of the other hand over the thumb of the first hand (Fig. 9-2).

c. The physician applies a slow, gentle pressure downward (toward the table) and laterally. The pressure is held for 3 seconds and gently released.

   Note: The direction of the force is lateral and parallel to the table. Do not press down into the muscle belly when using this technique.
   d. The physician may shift his hands up or down the spine to treat different areas of the thoracolumbar region.
   e. The technique may be repeated.

Treatment of Muscles Running Along Suprascapular Area from Cervical Region to Shoulder (e.g., Superior Trapezius)
1. Patient position: prone, with the head turned toward the physician.
2. Physician position: standing at the side of the table and opposite the side of the patient being treated, near shoulder level.
3. **Technique:**
   a. The physician places the thumb and thenar eminence of one hand perpendicular and slightly caudad to the fibers being treated.
   b. The other hand may reinforce the first or may be placed beside it to extend the area of treatment.

Figure 9-1. Myofascial perpendicular stretch technique: thumb position.

Figure 9-2. Myofascial perpendicular stretch technique: both hands in place.

Figure 9-3. Myofascial perpendicular stretch of trapezius muscle.

c. The physician applies a slow gentle force downward and perpendicular to the muscle fibers (Fig. 9-3). This force is maintained for 3 seconds and gently released.

   Note: Always push the muscle perpendicular to the fibers.

d. The technique may be repeated.

Treatment of Superior Border of Trapezius

1. Patient position: prone, with the head turned to the side of most comfort.
2. Physician position: standing at the side of the table and opposite the side being treated, near shoulder level.
3. **Technique:**
   a. The physician places his caudal (with respect to the patient) hand over the patient's shoulder (the side to be treated).
   b. The fingers of the other hand are wrapped around the superior border of the trapezius.
   c. The physician applies gentle traction on the trapezius while applying a downward counterpressure on the shoulder. The direction of traction should be upward and perpendicular to the muscle fibers (Fig. 9-4).
   d. The traction is held for 3 seconds and gently released.
   e. The physician may slide his cephalad hand

closer to the patient's neck or shoulder in order to treat other parts of the muscle.
Modification: The same technique can be performed with the patient supine (Fig. 9-5).

TREATMENT OF SUBSCAPULAR MUSCLES (E.G., SERRATUS ANTERIOR)

1. Patient position: prone, with the head turned away from physician.
2. Physician position: standing at the side to be treated, slightly cephalad to the scapula.
3. **Technique:**
   a. The patient places his hand (on the side to be treated) behind his back until the scapula abducts away from the rib cage.
   b. The physician wraps his fingers around the medial border of the scapula (Fig. 9-6).
   c. A gentle upward and lateral traction is applied, pulling the scapula away from the rib cage. This force is maintained for 3 seconds and gently released.
   d. The technique may be repeated.

PARALLEL STRETCH

1. Patient position: prone, with the head turned to the side of most comfort.

Figure 9-4. Myofascial stretch of trapezius muscle, patient prone.

Figure 9-5. Myofascial stretch of trapezius muscle, patient supine.

Figure 9-6. Subscapular muscle myofascial stretch.

2. Physician position: standing at the side of the table and opposite the side of the patient being treated.
3. **Technique:**
   a. The physician's forearms are crossed and heels of his hands are placed on the body of the muscle with the fingers of each hand parallel to each other. One hand is directed cephalad, the other is directed caudad (Fig. 9-7).
   b. A gentle downward pressure is applied as the hands are separated.
      Note: To avoid excessive stretching of the skin, the hands are placed approximately one inch apart, then moved together to create slack in the skin. This will bring the hands to the position shown in Figure 9-7.

PERPENDICULAR TRACTION
Upper Thoracic Region
1. Patient position: lying on his side, the side to be treated facing up. The hips and knees are flexed 90 degrees.
2. Physician position: standing at the side of the table and facing the patient.
3. **Technique:**
   a. The physician places her hands around the patient's scapula, allowing the patient's arm to hang over hers.

b. The physician gently grasps the muscle to be treated (erector spinae, trapezius), separating it from the spine.
c. The physician rocks her body backward while simultaneously applying a lateral and anterior (with respect to the patient) traction on the muscle (Fig. 9-8). The traction is held for 3 seconds and released.
   Note: The physician's hands should not slide over the patient's skin, as this will cause friction and irritation. To avoid fatigue, the physician should use leverage and rock her body rather than apply the traction force with her arms.
d. The physician can move her hands (and body) caudad and cephalad to treat other muscle groups.

Thoracolumbar Area
1. Patient position: lying on his side, the side to be treated facing up. The knees and hips are flexed 90 degrees.
2. Physician position: standing at the side of the table, facing the patient. Her thighs rest against patient's knees.
3. **Technique:**
   a. The physician wraps the fingers of both hands around the paravertebral muscles to be treated.

Figure 9-7. Parallel stretch of muscle.

Figure 9-8. Perpendicular traction applied to muscle.

Figure 9-9. Perpendicular stretch of thoracolumbar paravertebral muscles, patient in lateral recumbent position.

Figure 9-10. Thoracolumbar bidirectional stretch.

 i. The fingers are directed perpendicular to the muscle fibers being treated.
 ii. The tips of the fingers are between the spinous processes and the muscle being treated.
 b. The physician rocks her body backward while simultaneously applying a gentle lateral and anterior traction to the muscle (Fig. 9-9).
  i. The physician exerts a counterforce with her thighs against the patient's knees.
 c. The traction is held for 3 seconds and gently released.
 d. The physician can move her hands caudad or cephalad to treat other parts of the paravertebral musculature.

Modification of Thoracolumbar Technique
1. Patient position: same as above.
2. Physician position: same as above, except the physician need not place her thighs against the patient's knees.
3. **Technique:**
 a. The physician grasps the muscle to be treated, as above.
 b. The physician braces her cephalic (with respect to the patient) elbow against patient's axilla and the other elbow against patient's hip. The elbows should not dig into the patient's body.
 c. The physician applies a gentle traction to the muscle while simultaneously pressing downward and cephalad on the axilla and downward and caudad on the hip (Fig. 9-

10). This induces both a parallel stretch and perpendicular traction on the muscle.

Medial Scapular Area (Levator Scapulae, Rhomboids, Superior Trapezius)
1. Patient position: lying on his side, the side to be treated facing up.
2. Physician position: standing at the side of the table, facing the patient.
3. **Technique:**
   a. The physician grasps the medial scapular muscles with her cephalic (with respect to the patient) hand and places the patient's arm over hers, toward the patient's head.
   b. The physician's other hand is placed over the inferior portion of the scapula and is used to stabilize the patient.
   c. Gentle traction is applied in a direction perpendicular to the muscle fibers (Fig. 9-11).
   d. The traction is held for 3 seconds and gently released.

Subscapular Area
1. Patient position: lying on his side, the side to be treated facing up.
2. Physician position: standing at the side of the table, facing the patient.

Figure 9-11. Medial scapular stretch, patient in lateral recumbent position.

Figure 9-12. Subscapular stretch.

3. **Technique:**
   a. The physician places her cephalic (with respect to the patient) hand over the patient's suprascapular area and grasps the upper medial border of the scapula with her fingers.
   b. With her other hand, the physician reaches under the patient's arm and grasps the inferior angle and border of the scapula (Fig. 9-12).
   c. The physician applies gentle traction laterally and caudally (relative to the patient), lifting the scapula into abduction and away from the rib cage.
      i. The physician may also try to insert her fingers under the scapula and pull the scapula away from the rib cage (as previously described and illustrated in Fig. 9-6).
      ii. This technique must be done gently so as not to cause the patient discomfort.
   d. The traction is held for 3 seconds and gently released.

Active Direct Techniques: I
In the active direct techniques described below, the patient pushes his hand toward the floor. The first two techniques can be used to treat the paravertebral muscles, the rhomboids, the levator scapulae, and the trapezius muscle.

1. Patient position: lying on his side, the side to be treated facing up.

Figure 9-13. Active direct myofascial technique for thoracolumbar muscles. The patient pushes his fingers toward the floor while the physician applies an isometric counterforce.

Figure 9-14. Active direct myofascial technique. The patient pushes his elbow toward the ceiling.

Figure 9-15. Active direct myofascial technique with patient's arm supported.

2. Physician position: standing at the side of the table, facing the patient.
3. **Technique:**
   a. With her caudal hand, the physician palpates (monitors) the muscles to be treated.
   b. The other hand grasps the patient's upper arm at the elbow such that the arm is fully supported. The patient's arm is flexed at the elbow and the fingers point toward the floor.
   c. Once the area to be treated has been localized (see below), the physician instructs the patient to push his fingers toward the floor (Fig. 9-13).
   d. The physician provides an isometric resistive counterforce to the patient's arm with her cephalic hand.
   e. To localize the muscle fibers to be treated she monitors the muscles with her caudal hand during the isometric contraction. The localization is controlled by the position (caudad or cephalad) of the patient's arm during isometric contraction.
      i. The further cephalad the physician positions the patient's elbow during contraction, the further cephalad are the fibers that will contract (i.e., be treated).
      ii. The further caudad the physician positions the elbow, the further caudad are the fibers being treated.
      iii. The caudal hand monitors for muscle contraction localized to the fibers being treated.
   f. The isometric contraction is held for 3 seconds, then the patient is instructed to relax.
   g. This technique can be repeated at the same location, or the elbow can be repositioned to treat a different area.

Active Direct Techniques: II

In the technique described below, the patient pushes his elbow toward the ceiling while the physician applies an isometric counterforce.

1. Patient position: same as for previous technique.
2. Physician position: same as for previous technique.
3. **Technique:**
   a. The physician's caudal hand monitors the muscle being treated, as in the previous technique.

The patient reaches toward the floor against isometric resistance.

The patient pushes his elbow toward the ceiling against an isometric resistance.

D. J. DOWLING, DO

Figure 9-16. Localization of active myofascial treatment of the thoracic region.

b. The patient's arm is positioned as in the previous technique (elbow flexed, fingers pointing toward the floor). The physician grasps the dorsal aspect of the patient's elbow, the part closest to the ceiling (Figs. 9-14, 9-15).

c. The physician instructs the patient to push his elbow to the ceiling while she provides an isometric resistive force with her cephalic (with respect to the patient) hand.

d. With this technique the area being treated is in a direct line with the long axis of the patient's upper arm (Fig. 9-16).

   i. If the patient's elbow is placed more cephalad the fibers being treated are located more caudad.

   ii. If the elbow is placed more caudad, the fibers being treated are located more cephalad.

e. The isometric force is maintained for 3 seconds, then the patient is instructed to relax.

f. The technique can be repeated at the same location, or the elbow can be repositioned to treat another area.

Active Direct Techniques: III. Scapula

This technique is good as an initial treatment to facilitate general relaxation of the entire scapular area.

1. Patient position: lying on his side, the side to be treated facing up.
2. Physician position: standing at side of table, facing the patient.
3. **Technique:**

   a. The physician grasps the superior border of the scapula with her cephalic (with respect to the patient) hand and the inferior angle with her other hand. The patient's arm rests on her caudal arm.

   b. The physician gently presses her sternum against the patient's shoulder.

c. Using the weight of her upper torso against the patient's shoulder, the physician gently pushes the scapula medially and either superiorly or inferiorly (whichever motion is more free). The scapula is held in this position.

d. The patient pushes his shoulder straight up against physician's chest while she applies an isometric resistive force.

e. The contraction is maintained for 3 seconds, then the patient relaxes.

f. The physician moves the scapula further medially and either superiorly or inferiorly.

g. The technique is repeated three times.

Active Indirect Technique

The active indirect technique described below is a generalized technique for all the muscles in the upper and middle thoracic region.

Figure 9-17. Active indirect myofascial technique for thoracic spine. The physician provides a resistive counterforce to the patient's rotation of the torso.

1. Patient position: supine.
2. Physician position: standing at the side of the table near the patient's head, on the side opposite that being treated.
3. **Technique:**
   a. The patient grasps the wrist on the side being treated with his other hand. He is then instructed to rotate his upper torso away from the physician while keeping his lower body flat on the table.
   b. The physician reaches across the table and holds the patient's opposite wrist.
   c. The patient pulls the arm he is holding (the one opposite the physician) across his body toward the physician, thus rotating his torso toward the physician.
   d. The physician provides an isokinetic counterforce to this motion (Fig. 9-17).
   e. The patient's active motion will end when his upper torso is fully rotated to the side of the physician.
   f. The patient is instructed to relax.
   g. The physician applies a passive stretch to increase the rotation while stabilizing the lower body at the opposite anterior superior iliac spine.
   h. The technique is repeated three times, with the physician providing increasingly greater counterforce each time.

MUSCLE ENERGY TECHNIQUES

Lillian Somner
Eileen L. DiGiovanna

This section describes muscle energy techniques for somatic dysfunctions, types I and II, of the thoracic spine. All of the techniques begin with the patient sitting erect and his feet adequately supported on the floor.

Type I Group Curve

1. Patient position: seated, feet on the floor, weight equally distributed on the buttocks.
2. Physician position: standing behind the patient and slightly to the side of the convexity.

Figure 9-18. Muscle energy treatment for a type I group curve, convex right.

Figure 9-19. Muscle energy treatment for an upper thoracic type II somatic dysfunction.

Figure 9-20. Muscle energy treatment for an upper thoracic type II somatic dysfunction. The barriers to flexion have been engaged, with left rotation and side bending of the patient's head.

3. **Technique:**
   a. The physician monitors at the apex of the curve being treated.
   b. The physician induces side bending toward the convexity and rotation away from the convexity by applying a caudal and anterior force to the ipsilateral shoulder. Motion is induced down to the monitoring finger at the apex of the curve (Fig. 9-18).
   c. If the patient becomes unbalanced by the above movement, a translatory force should be applied toward the concavity. *Note* that the spine is kept in neutral position (i.e., no flexion or extension).
   d. The patient then side bends toward the concavity (the freedom of motion) while the physician maintains a resistance on the shoulder closest to him (i.e., the side of the convexity).
   e. The force is held for 2 or 3 seconds, then the patient relaxes.
   f. After 2 seconds of rest, the new motion barriers to side bending and rotation are engaged.
   g. The procedure is repeated twice more.

Type II Single-Segment Somatic Dysfunction

UPPER THORACIC REGION (T1–T4)

1. Patient position: seated, with feet on the floor.
2. Physician position: standing behind the patient and to the side of the motion barriers.
3. **Technique:**
   a. One hand monitors the involved vertebra to detect motion.
   b. The other hand holds the patient's head, or the arm is wrapped around it turban-style to control its motion and to provide a resistance to the patient's motion.
   c. The patient's neck is either flexed or extended to its motion barrier, while the physician monitors at the vertebra being treated. The patient's head is then side bent and rotated into the barriers to motion (Fig. 9-19).
   d. The patient is instructed to side bend or rotate his head toward the freedom of motion against the physician's resistive force (Fig. 9-20).

Figure 9-21. Muscle energy treatment for a flexion type II somatic dysfunction of the middle and lower thoracic region. The barriers to extension have been engaged, with right rotation and side bending of the patient.

Figure 9-22. Muscle energy treatment for an extension type II somatic dysfunction of the middle and lower thoracic region. The barriers to flexion have been engaged, with right rotation and side bending of the patient.

    e. This is held 3 to 4 seconds, then the patient relaxes.
    f. New motion barriers are engaged.
    g. The process is repeated twice more.

MIDDLE AND LOWER THORACIC REGION
1. Patient position: seated, with the feet on the floor.
2. Physician position: Standing behind the patient and to the side of the motion barriers.
3. **Technique:**
    a. The physician places one arm over the patient's shoulder on the side of the motion barriers. He may use either his axilla or forearm.
    b. The patient is flexed or extended to the motion barrier. Extension may be achieved by asking the patient to sit up straight or to stick his belly out (Fig. 9-21). Flexion is achieved by having the patient slump forward (Fig. 9-22). Motion should be to the involved segment.
    c. Using his axilla or arm, the physician side bends the patient and rotates him into the motion barriers at the involved segment.
    d. If the dysfunction is low enough that side bending unbalances the patient, a translatory force in the opposite direction will aid in keeping both buttocks on the table.
    e. The patient then side bends or rotates toward the freedom of motion. The physician provides a resistance with his arm. This is held for 3 to 4 seconds.
    f. The patient relaxes, and the new motion barriers are engaged.
    g. The process is repeated twice more.

COUNTERSTRAIN TECHNIQUES
Eileen L. DiGiovanna
Lillian Somner

As in other areas of the body, when counterstrain treatment is used in the thoracic spine, the positions for treating tender points, corresponding to vertebral segment dysfunctions, are held for 90 seconds. The patient is returned to neutral position slowly and without active engagement of his muscles.

Anterior Tender Points

Figure 9-23 shows the locations of the anterior tender points for the thoracic spine. All anterior tender points are treated in flexion.

UPPER THORACIC SPINE (T1–T4)
1. Patient position: supine. The head and upper torso rest on the physician's knee so that the upper thoracic spine is flexed to the desired level.
2. Physician position: standing at the head of the table and resting his knee on the table. One

Figure 9-23. Locations of anterior tender points, thoracic spine.

hand monitors the tender point.
3. **Technique:** Pure flexion is usually all that is necessary. However, some slight side bending and rotation modification may help localize and reduce the point tenderness (Fig. 9-24).

MIDTHORACIC SPINE (T5–T8)
Midthoracic dysfunctions may require such marked flexion that flexion of the upper body alone may not be sufficient. Flexion may be increased if the patient's hips are bent and the spine is allowed to flex from the lumbar area into the lower thoracic area.

1. Patient position: supine, upper body supported by pillows, hips bent to 90 degrees, with lower legs resting on the physician's knee.
2. Physician position: side of table, one foot on the table with the knee bent, supporting the patient's lower legs.
3. **Technique:** Patient is flexed up by bringing the knees toward the abdomen while monitoring the tender point. When tenderness is relieved, the position is held for 90 seconds (Fig. 9-25).
4. **Modifications:**
   a. The technique may be performed with the patient in a lateral recumbent position with hips and knees flexed; the physician flexes the patient's torso until the tender point is relieved.
   b. Another alternative is similar to that used for the upper thoracics, with the upper back supported by the physician's knee.

LOWER THORACIC SPINE (T9–L1)
1. Patient position: supine, with knees and hips flexed and supported by the physician's knee. A pillow may be placed under the hips to aid flexion if necessary.
2. Physician position: standing at the side of the table next to the side of the tender point, one foot on the table and supporting the patient's legs.

Figure 9-24. Counterstrain treatment of anterior tender points, upper thoracic spine.

Figure 9-25. Counterstrain treatment of anterior tender points, midthoracic spine.

Figure 9-26. Counterstrain treatment of anterior T10 tender point, knees rotated to side of dysfunction.

3. **Technique:** The patient's knees and hips are flexed and the physician supports the patient's thighs on her thigh. Pressure is applied cephalad as the knees are rotated toward the side of dysfunction (Fig. 9-26).

Posterior Tender Points

Figure 9-27 shows the locations of the posterior tender points. All posterior tender points are treated in extension with the patient prone. The patient's position varies only so that motion may be localized to a given point.

UPPER THORACIC SPINE (T1–T2)
1. Patient position: prone, with arms at his side.
2. Physician position: standing on the side of the patient opposite the tender point.
3. **Technique:** One hand supports the patient's chin, the other hand monitors the tender point on the opposite side of the spinous process. The head and neck are extended to the involved segment (Fig. 9-28). Rotation and side bending will be away from the point.

MIDTHORACIC SPINE (T3–T5)
1. Patient position: same as above, except the arms are extended over the head.

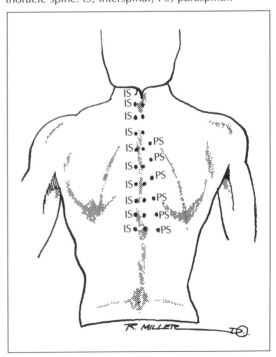

Figure 9-27. Location of posterior tender points, thoracic spine. *IS,* interspinal; *PS,* paraspinal.

Figure 9-28. Counterstrain treatment of posterior tender points, upper thoracic spine.

Figure 9-29. Counterstrain treatment of posterior tender points, midthoracic spine. Tender point is right; slight rotation is induced to the left.

Figure 9-30. Counterstrain treatment of posterior tender points, lower thoracic spine.

2. Physician position: same as above.
3. **Technique:** same as above (Fig. 9-29) with slight rotation.

LOWER THORACIC SPINE (T6–L2)
1. Patient position: prone, arms extended above head.
2. Physician position: as above. The cephalic (with respect to the patient) hand supports the patient's axilla on the side of the tender point.
3. **Technique:** Rotation and side bending are induced through pull on the axilla to the opposite side and cephalad, with care not to irritate the skin and other tissue. Extension may be facilitated by placing pillows under the patient's chest (Fig. 9-30).
4. **Variation:** The physician may use the pelvis to increase the rotation of a spinous process that is already rotated to one side. This relieves a tender point directly on the spinous process.

HIGH VELOCITY, LOW AMPLITUDE THRUSTING TECHNIQUES

Barry Erner
Paula D. Scariati

This section describes high velocity, low amplitude thrusting techniques for treating somatic dysfunctions of the thoracic spine by region—upper, middle, and lower spine. For most of the techniques the patient is supine; a variation is illustrated in which the patient is seated.

Upper Thoracic Somatic Dysfunction (T1–T3)
1. Patient position: supine.
2. Physician position: standing at the side of the table opposite the side of the posteriorly rotated transverse process.

Figure 9-31. High velocity, low amplitude thrusting technique for upper thoracic somatic dysfunction.

Figure 9-32. Hand placement for midthoracic high velocity, low amplitude thrusting technique.

Figure 9-33. Downward thrust on midthoracic segment.

3. **Technique:**
   a. The patient places his clasped hands behind her neck and approximates his elbows.
   b. The physician palpates the restricted segment and rests its posterior transverse process on the thenar eminence of his thrusting hand.
   c. With his other hand, the physician grasps the patient's elbows and rolls the patient's body over his thenar eminence.
   d. The physician exerts a rapid antero-posterior thrust through the patient's arms onto the transverse process resting on his thenar eminence (Fig. 9-31).

Midthoracic Somatic Dysfunction

1. Patient position: supine.
2. Physician position: standing at the side of the table opposite to the side of dysfunction.
3. **Technique:**
   a. The patient crosses his arms over his chest. The upper arm is the arm on the side of the posterior transverse process.
   b. The physician palpates the restricted

segment and rests its posterior transverse process on the thenar eminence of his thrusting hand (Fig. 9-32).
   c. With his other hand, the physician grasps the patient's elbows and rolls the patient's body onto his thenar eminence.
   d. The physician exerts a rapid downward thrust through the patient's arms into the transverse process resting on his thenar eminence (Fig. 9-33).

Lower Thoracic Somatic Dysfunction

1. Patient position: supine.
2. Physician position: standing at the side of the table opposite to the side of the posteriorly rotated transverse process.
3. **Technique:**
   a. The patient crosses his arms over his chest. The upper arm is the arm on the side of the posterior transverse process.
   b. The physician palpates the restricted segment and rests its posterior transverse process on the thenar eminence of his thrusting hand.
   c. With his other hand, the physician grasps

Figure 9-34. High velocity, low amplitude thrusting technique for somatic dysfunction of a lower thoracic segment.

Figure 9-35. Alternative high velocity, low amplitude thrusting technique for somatic dysfunction of the thoracic spine, patient supine.

Figure 9-36. Alternative high velocity, low amplitude thrusting technique for somatic dysfunction of the thoracic spine, patient seated.

the patient behind the shoulders and "hugs" him, creating and localizing flexion down to the restricted segment.

d. The physician rolls the patient over his thenar eminence and exerts a rapid thrust, creating a vector force through the posterior transverse process (Fig. 9-34).

Alternative Techniques for Thoracic Somatic Dysfunction

ALTERNATIVE 1

1. Patient position: on table reclined with back supported by physician's knee.
2. Physician position: standing at the head of the table, with one knee on table.
3. **Technique:**
   a. The physician places his knee under the posterior transverse process of the restricted segment.
   b. The patient is instructed to reach back and grasp his hands together around the physician's waist.
   c. The physician grasps the patient beneath the scapulae bilaterally and exerts an

upward cephalad traction force. Simultaneously, the physician rolls the patient over his knee (Fig. 9-35).

ALTERNATIVE 2

1. Patient position: seated on a stool, feet flat on the floor.
2. Physician position: standing behind the patient.
3. **Technique:**
   a. A pillow is placed between the patient's spine and the physician's knee for comfort.
   b. The patient is instructed to interlock her fingers behind his neck.
   c. The physician localizes the rotated transverse process with his knee (with the right knee for a right-sided lesion).
   d. The physician grasps the patient's forearms by sliding his arms underneath the patient's armpits and resting on the dorsal surface of the patient's wrists.
   e. The physician exerts an upward cephalad force while simultaneously rolling the patient's spine over his knee (Fig. 9-36).

EXERCISE THERAPY
Stanley Schiowitz
Albert DeRubertis

The thoracic region is much more complex than the cervical region. It consists of the thoracic spine, rib cage, shoulder girdle, and the intricate musculature that accompanies the functioning of each of the above. Prescribing exercise treatment for dysfunctions of any of these areas should include recognition of their interdependence. Pain and limited motion in one segment can be secondary to dysfunction of another.

Regional motions and functions can be divided as follows:

1. Thoracic spine: forward bending, backward bending, rotation, side bending.
2. Scapula: elevation, protraction, retraction, rotation.
3. Ribs: individual ribs have rotary elevating or depressing motions. The entire thorax, however, expands in the anteroposterior plane (pump handle motion) and in the frontal plane (bucket handle motion).

Regional Stretch
FORWARD BENDING
1. Patient position: seated, with back upright.

2. **Instructions:**
   a. Drop your head forward, allowing its weight to create forward bending.
   b. Allow the forward bending to continue gradually into the thoracic region, from the first thoracic vertebra down. Do not create pain.
   c. To increase stretch, maintain your body in its position of forward bending, drop both hands between your legs, and reach for the floor (Fig. 9-37). Do not change or increase your forward bending position.
   d. Hold for 5 to 15 seconds, then slowly return to upright position.
   e. Relax, rest, and repeat.

BACKWARD BENDING
1. Patient position: seated, with back upright and hands at sides.
2. **Instructions:**
   a. Drop your head backward, allowing its weight to create backward bending.
   b. Allow the backward bending to continue into the thoracic region.
   c. To increase stretch, push out your chest and abdomen and point your hands downward

Figure 9-37. Thoracic stretch, forward bending.

Figure 9-38. Thoracic stretch, backward bending.

Figure 9-39. Thoracic stretch, side bending.

Figure 9-40. Thoracic stretch, rotation.

Figure 9-41. Passive upper back stretch, patient seated.

and backward toward the floor (Fig. 9-38). Do not change or increase your backward bending position.

  d. Hold for 5 to 15 seconds. Slowly return to the upright position.
  e. Relax, rest, and repeat.

SIDE BENDING

1. Patient position: standing, back upright, hands at sides.
2. **Instructions:**
   a. Tilt your head, neck, and thoracic region to the right as you walk your right hand down your right leg toward the floor (Fig. 9-39).
   b. To increase stretch, raise your left arm over your head and try to touch the top of your right shoulder.
   c. Hold for 5 to 15 seconds. Slowly return to the upright position.
   d. Relax, rest, and repeat.
   e. To stretch the left side laterally reverse the instructions.

ROTATION

1. Patient position: seated, facing backward, on an armless chair, with legs straddling the seat.
2. **Instructions:**
   a. Fold your arms in front of your chest, each hand holding the opposite elbow.

   b. Slowly turn your head, then your neck, and then your back to the right, as far as possible without pain. Do not change your seated position.
   c. To increase stretch, with your right hand pull your left elbow toward the right, increasing the rotary motion (Fig. 9-40).
   d. Hold for 5 to 15 seconds. Slowly return to the starting position.
   e. Relax, rest, and repeat.
   f. To stretch in left rotation, reverse the instructions.

Upper Back Stretch

PASSIVE STRETCH

1. Patient position: standing.
2. **Instructions:**
   a. Raise your left elbow to shoulder level and place that hand over your right shoulder.
   b. Place your right hand on your left elbow and gently push it toward your back (Fig. 9-41). This will create a passive left upper back stretch.
   c. Maintain at maximum painless stretch for 5 to 15 seconds. Return to starting position.
   d. Relax, rest, and repeat.
   e. To stretch the right side, reverse the instructions.

ACTIVE STRETCH

Exercise 1

1. Patient position: prone, forehead touching the table.
2. **Instructions:**
   a. Abduct shoulders to 90 degrees and bend elbows to 90 degrees. Hands, elbows, and arms rest on the table (or floor).
   b. Simultaneously raise both upper extremities off the table, including the hands, elbows, and arms (Fig. 9-42).
   c. Hold for 5 to 15 seconds.
   d. Return arms to table, relax, rest, and repeat.
      Note: Modifying the degree of shoulder abduction will change the area of the back that is stretched.

Exercise 2

1. Patient position: prone, forehead touching the table.
2. **Instructions:**
   a. Place both arms, elbow straight and palms down, raised over your head.
   b. Simultaneously raise both upper extremities off the floor, including the hands, elbows, and arms (Fig. 9-43).
   c. Hold for 5 to 15 seconds.
   d. Return arms to table, relax, rest, and repeat.

Exercise 3

1. Patient position: sitting, with back upright.
2. **Instructions:**

Figure 9-42. Active upper back stretch, patient prone.

   a. Stretch both arms over your head, with fingers interlocked.
   b. Press both arms backward.
   c. Tilt your upper body to one side (Fig. 9-44). Hold for 5 seconds, then tilt upper body to other side.
   d. Return to starting position. Relax, rest, and repeat.

KYPHOSIS

Exercise 1

1. Patient position: supine, knees flexed, with a small pillow under the midthoracic region.
2. **Instructions:**
   a. Clasp your hands behind your neck.

Figure 9-43. Active upper back stretch, patient prone.

Figure 9-44. Active upper back stretch, patient seated.

Figure 9-45. Stretch for kyphosis.

Figure 9-46. Stretch for kyphosis.

Figure 9-47. Stretch for kyphosis, with pole.

b. Try to touch the shoulder blades together at the midline (Fig. 9-45).
c. Hold for 5 to 15 seconds.
d. Relax, rest, and repeat.

Exercise 2
1. Patient position: same as in previous exercise.
2. **Instructions:**
   a. Bring both arms fully extended over your head.
   b. Press your forearms and elbows down toward table (Fig. 9-46).
   c. Hold for 5 to 15 seconds.
   d. Relax, rest, and repeat.

Exercise 3
1. Patient position: seated, back upright.
2. **Instructions:**
   a. Hold broomstick or pole at each end, your hands facing forward.
   b. Raise the pole over your head.
   c. Tuck in your chin and, holding your neck in a fixed position, bring the pole down between your shoulder blades (Fig. 9-47).
   d. Hold for 5 to 15 seconds. Return to starting position.
   e. Relax, rest, and repeat.

Scapular Motions

ELEVATION STRETCH (SHRUG)
1. Patient position: standing, back upright, arms extended down at sides.
2. **Instructions:**
   a. Raise your shoulders straight up trying to touch them to your ears (Fig. 9-48).
   b. Hold for 5 to 15 seconds.
   c. Slowly return to starting position.
   d. Relax, rest, and repeat.

PROTRACTION STRETCH
1. Patient position: standing, back upright, arms extended at sides.
2. **Instructions:**
   a. Raise your shoulders straight up, trying to touch your ears.
   b. Roll your shoulders forward, separating the shoulder blades (Fig. 9-49).
   c. Hold for 5 to 15 seconds.
   d. Slowly relax, rest, and repeat.

RETRACTION STRETCH
1. Patient position: standing, back upright, arms extended at sides.
2. **Instructions:**
   a. Raise your shoulder straight up, try to touch your ears.

Figure 9-48. Scapula elevation
stretch (shrug).

Figure 9-49. Scapula protraction.

Figure 9-50. Scapula retraction.

Figure 9-51. Scapula rotation.

Figure 9-52. Pectoral muscle stretch.

b. Roll your shoulders backward, trying to
   bring the shoulder blades together (Fig. 9-50).
c. Hold for 5 to 15 seconds.
d. Slowly relax, rest, and repeat.

The previous two exercises can be modified to
create increased strength and stretch. Perform the
shrug maneuver, then with your shoulders elevated, proceed into the anterior and posterior
shoulder roll.

ROTATION
1. Patient position: standing, back upright.
2. **Instructions:**
   a. Place both hands on your shoulders and
      raise your arms away from the body
      (abduct) to 135 degrees (Fig. 9-51).
   b. Maintain this raised position.
   c. Hold for 5 to 15 seconds.
   d. Relax, rest, and repeat.

Figure 9-53. Inspiration rib stretch.

Figure 9-54. Inspiration rib isometric stretch.

Thorax

PECTORAL MUSCLE STRETCH

1. Patient position: standing, facing a corner, with hands on adjacent walls and feet away from the wall.
2. **Instructions:**
   a. Drop your body forward, supported by your hands. This will bring the shoulder blades together and create pectoral muscle stretch (Fig. 9-52).
   b. Hold this position for 5 to 15 seconds.
   c. Return to starting position, relax, rest, and repeat.

Figure 9-55. Passive abdominal expiration stretch.

INSPIRATION RIB STRETCH

1. Patient position: supine, both knees bent, feet on table, entire spine flattened.
2. **Instructions:**
   a. Raise both fully extended arms off the floor, while breathing in deeply (Fig. 9-53).
   b. Hold this position for 4 to 5 seconds.
   c. Lower both arms to floor as you slowly breathe out.
   d. Relax, rest, and repeat.

INSPIRATION RIB ISOMETRICS

1. Patient position: supine, both knees bent, feet on table, hands on sides of the rib cage.
2. **Instructions:**
   a. Inhale deeply while pressing firmly against your rib cage (Fig. 9-54). Try to prevent lateral chest expansion.
   b. Hold this position for 4 or 5 seconds.

   c. Exhale while you maintain your hand pressure.
   d. Relax, rest, and repeat.

EXPIRATION ABDOMINAL STRETCH

1. Patient position: supine, hips and knees flexed to 90 degrees, feet supported by chair.
2. **Instructions:**
   a. Place both hands on your upper abdomen and breathe out slowly while contracting the abdominal muscles.
   b. Press both hands firmly down on abdomen to create forced exhalation (Fig. 9-55).
   c. Maintain firm hand pressure on abdomen as you slowly inhale, resisting abdominal stretch.
   d. Hold full inhalation 4 to 5 seconds.
   e. Relax, rest, and repeat.

A

B

Figure 9-56. Abdominothoracic stretch. (**A**) Abdominal inspiration with expansion of the abdominal cavity. (**B**) As air is transferred to the thoracic cage, the abdominal muscles are contracted and the chest cavity is expanded.

ABDOMINOTHORACIC STRETCH

1. Patient position: supine, knees bent, feet on floor, both hands over head, elbows bent to 90 degrees.
2. **Instructions:**
    a. Inhale deeply. Try to use the abdomen only, with maximum abdominal muscle stretch (Fig. 9-56A).
    b. Close your throat to prevent the escape of air.
    c. Transfer the air to your upper chest by contracting your abdominal muscles. Your rib cage should rise (Fig. 9-56B).
    d. Hold this position for 4 or 5 seconds. Release the air.
    e. Relax, rest, and repeat.

10

Evaluation of the Lumbar Spine

FUNCTIONAL ANATOMY AND BIOMECHANICS
Stanley Schiowitz

The five lumbar vertebrae are separated from one another by intervertebral disks. The combined unit of the vertebrae and disks, in the upright position, forms the anteroposterior lordotic lumbar spinal curve.

Osteology

The lumbar vertebral bodies are larger than the thoracic vertebral bodies. They are wider transversely than in the anteroposterior dimension and are higher in front than in back, creating a posterior body wedge. In conjunction with a similar intervertebral disk shape, the wedge shape of the lumbar vertebral bodies helps maintain lumbar lordosis.

The spinous processes of the lumbar vertebrae are large, quadrangular, and directed dorsally in a horizontal plane. The transverse processes are long, thin, and directed laterally in a horizontal plane. In contrast to the different planar relationships of the thoracic vertebral structures, in the lumbar spine the spinous process, transverse processes, and vertebral body all lie at the same spinal level.

The fifth lumbar vertebra differs from those above it in having a larger body, thicker and shorter transverse processes, a smaller spinous process, and is markedly higher in its anterior aspect. The largest number of congenital defects occur at the level of the fifth lumbar vertebra.

The superior articular facets of the lumbar vertebrae are concave and face primarily medially and backward. They are rotated 45 degrees from the sagittal plane toward the frontal plane. The inferior articular facets are convex and face laterally and forward. The superior and inferior articular facets of the contiguous lumbar vertebrae fit into each other, forming zygophyseal joints.

Many variations of articular facets occur in the lumbar region, notably at the lumbosacral articulation. These variations include sagittal plane rotations of 0 to 90 degrees, a horizontal planar orientation, and facet asymmetries. These variants contribute to low back instability, disk disease, and somatic dysfunction.

Intervertebral Motion

All individual vertebral motions follow the rules of coupled motions:

1. Flexion and extension are coupled with a ventrad-dorsad translatory slide in the sagittal plane.

2. Lateral flexion is coupled with a contralateral translatory slide in the frontal plane.
3. Rotation is coupled with disk compression in the horizontal plane.

The motions of flexion and extension are greatest at all levels, as influenced by the vertical sagittal orientation of the facets. There is a small degree of lateral flexion present which is always accompanied by very limited rotation. The convex-concave articular shapes mandate the combined roll and slide motion.

Somatic Dysfunction

Group curves are common in the lumbar region and are usually secondary to thoracic scoliosis or to sacral base unleveling. Single-segment intervertebral somatic dysfunctions involve restricted motion in all three planes; however, rotation is the primary motion most commonly restricted. This rotation restriction is accompanied by ipsilateral lateral flexion.

Somatic dysfunctions are commonly diagnosed by monitoring the rotary motions of the lumbar transverse processes.

Intervertebral Disks

A healthy disk consists of a jelly-like substance, the *nucleus pulposus*, surrounded by a fibrotic ring, the *annulus fibrosis*. The annulus comprises a series of collagen fibers that are firmly attached to their superior and inferior vertebral end-plates. The fibroelastic mesh is formed by concentric circumferential lamellae. The collagen fibers of the lamellae lie at a 65-degree angle from the vertical, and their vertical orientation alternates in successive lamellae. This anatomical arrangement allows the disk to undergo rotary motions and shearing forces while still maintaining a restrictive stability. The nucleus moves in a direction opposite to vertebral motion, creating pressure on the annulus and a normalizing feedback mechanism.

The lumbar intervertebral disks sustain the most degenerative changes and dysfunctions of all the spinal disks, with the possible exception of the C5–C6 disk. It is thought that sitting postures in which the lumbar spine is flexed cause more fluid to be expressed from the lumbar disks than do erect postures. Restriction of this motion by extensive standing, fusion, degenerative arthritis, or spinal motion restriction of any cause is postulated to reduce nutrient flow to the disks and hasten lumbar disk degeneration. Degenerative changes result in loss of tissue elasticity, loss of restrictive stability, depressed feedback mechanisms, and loss of disk height. The relationships of the superior to inferior articular facets become abnormal. The ligaments connecting the vertebrae and disks become lax, and there is a greater tendency toward dysfunction.

Neurology

The lumbar plexus lies within the posterior part of the psoas major muscle and in front of the transverse processes of the lumbar vertebrae. It consists of the ventral rami of the first, second, third, and part of the fourth lumbar nerves.

The spinal cord ends at about the level of the second lumbar vertebra. Lower nerve roots run caudally and laterally to exit from the intervertebral foramina. Diskogenic herniation disturbs the nerve root of the lower vertebra involved. Therefore, an L5–S1 herniated disk will cause dysfunction of the first sacral nerve root.

Herniated disks are most common in the lower lumbar region, owing to narrowing of the posterior longitudinal ligament, the increased incidence of degenerative disk disease, ligament laxity, and excessive stress placed on the disks in this location. At a minimum, the clinician should be able to recognize the symptoms of L4, L5, and S1 nerve root dysfunctions. Dysfunction of the L4 nerve causes diminution in the patellar reflex, reduction of strength in the quadriceps and anterior tibialis muscles, and cutaneous sensation changes on the medial aspect of the leg and foot. Dysfunction of the L5 nerve does not affect a reflex but does impose a loss of strength of the first toe in dorsiflexion, loss of strength of the extensor hallucis muscle, and cutaneous sensation changes on the side of the leg and top of the foot. Dysfunction of the S1 nerve causes diminution in the Achilles reflex, a reduction of strength in the peroneus longus and brevis muscles, and sensation changes on the lateral aspect of the foot.

Myology

The erector spinae is a large muscle group lying at each side of the vertebral column. It originates at the sacrum and continues through to the cervical region. At the lumbar region it is divided, medially to laterally, into the spinalis, longissimus, and iliocostalis muscles. Bilateral muscle contraction causes extension of the vertebral column. Unilateral contraction causes ipsilateral extension and side bending.

The multifidus and rotatores muscles are small muscles of the back lying deep to the erector spinae. They function primarily as postural muscles, with control of individual vertebral motions. Bilateral contraction creates local extension, unilateral contraction causes lateral flexion with contralateral rotation.

The quadratus lumborum is a lateral muscle attached to the 12th rib, iliac crest, and vertebral column. Its rib attachment allows it to function with respiration by fixing the last rib and assisting in stabilizing the origin of the diaphragm. Bilateral contraction creates extension; unilateral contraction causes extension with ipsilateral sidebending.

The synergistic action of the abdominal muscles creates forward bending. External oblique contraction creates rotation to the opposite side; internal oblique contraction creates rotation to the same side. The combined actions of the abdominal muscles provide a coordinated mechanism for controlling dangerous torque, bending, and shear stresses in the lumbar spine. Their normal functioning is essential to the maintenance of the spinal mechanism.

The iliopsoas muscle plays an important role in the function and stability of the lumbar region. It is composed of two muscles. The psoas major originates from the anterior surfaces and lower borders of the transverse processes of all the lumbar vertebrae by five digitations, each extending from the body of the two vertebrae and their intersegmental disks, starting from the 12th thoracic vertebra and ending at the fifth lumbar vertebra. The muscle descends along the pelvic brim, passes behind the inguinal ligament and in front of the capsule of the hip joint, and ends in a tendon that receives, on its lateral side, nearly the whole of the fibers of the iliacus. The psoas major inserts into the lesser trochanter of the femur. The iliacus muscle originates from the superior two thirds of the concavity of the iliac fossa, from the inner lip of the iliac crest, from the ventral sacroiliac and iliolumbar ligaments, and from the upper, lateral surface of the sacrum. In front, it reaches as far as the anterior superior and anterior inferior iliac spines, and receives some fibers from the upper part of the capsule of the hip joint. It inserts into the lateral side of the tendon of the psoas major, which inserts into the lesser trochanter of the femur.

From above, the iliopsoas flexes the thigh on the pelvis; from below, it flexes the trunk forward by bilateral contraction. Unilateral contraction creates lateral trunk flexion with a pelvic shift to that side.

The iliopsoas remains in constant activity in the erect posture and prevents hyperextension of the hip joint in a standing subject. An increase in lumbar lordosis while standing erect causes increased activity of the psoas and low back instability and dysfunction.

The cardinal signs of iliopsoatic dysfunction in the standing and supine positions are as follows:

1. Standing: hip and knee flexion and pelvic tilt on the side of the dysfunction, a positive Trendelenburg sign, and a typical psoatic stance and gait.
2. Supine: exaggerated lumber lordosis and a positive Thomas test.

Somatic dysfunction of the lumbar region that is related to iliopsoas contracture usually occurs at the upper lumbar vertebral levels.

In the pelvis, these muscles create a supportive mechanism for the abdominal viscera, the psoas shelf, as they traverse the pubic bones in their descent to the lesser trochanters. Any somatic dysfunction that changes this structural relationship can cause visceral symptoms and pathology. Anterior sacral or pelvic tilt, psoas contracture, abdominal muscle weakness, pregnancy, wearing of high heels, poor posture, and somatosomatic reflexes can all increase the stress of the viscera onto the abdominal wall, which in turn can lead to diaphragmatic hernia, inguinal and femoral hernias, retroverted uterus, renal and visceral ptosis, and syndromes such as dysmenorrhea, menorrhagia, polyuria, constipation, and colitis.

The iliopsoas muscle also plays an important role in the synergistic activities of the muscles of the low back in maintaining a normal lumbosacral angle and proper postural balance.

LUMBOSACRAL ANGLE
(FERGUSON'S ANGLE)

The lumbosacral angle is the angle formed, in the lateral upright position, by extending the line of inclination of the sacrum as it meets a line parallel to the ground. This angle is normally between 25 and 35 degrees. A major portion of low back pain is attributable to an increased lumbosacral angle. The greater the angle, the greater is the inclination and the higher the shear stress placed on the lumbosacral joint and its attachments. In addition, the increased angle increases lumbar lordosis.

Factors that can influence the lumbosacral angle are obesity, pregnancy, abdominal muscle weakness, wearing of high heels, foot pronation, Achilles valgus, atypical lumbosacral facets, spondylolisthesis, diminished disk height, ligamentous weakness, organic kyphoscoliosis, poor posture, occupation, somatotype, heredity, psoatic dysfunction, anterior sacral/pelvic tilt, and somatic dysfunction.

An increased lumbosacral angle changes the articular relationships, as the inferior lumbar facets slide caudally on their matched superior sacral facets.

SYNERGISTIC ACTION OF THE MUSCLES
IN MAINTAINING LUMBAR CURVATURES

The abdominal muscles support and assist in the flattening of the lumbar lordosis. The psoas muscles pull on the vertebrae and anterior pelvis, increasing the lumbar lordosis. The gluteus maximus and hamstrings pull on the posterior pelvis, decreasing the lumbar lordosis. The erector spinae muscles and the abdominal muscles assist in flattening the lumbar lordosis.

Lumbar-Pelvic Rhythm

When a subject bends forward to touch the floor, combined motions of the lumbar vertebrae, pelvis, and hip joints are put into play. The individual vertebrae flex on each other, straightening the lumbar lordosis and sometimes causing a mild reversal of that curve. Simultaneously, a secondary pelvic rotation motion occurs around the axis of the hip joints as the hip joints move posteriorly in the horizontal plane. These are smooth, interrelated motions, both in total forward bending and in its reversal, straightening up.

In evaluating gross body movement, the physician must examine all three aspects of lumbosacral rhythm. It is common to relate all forward bending restrictions to lumbar dysfunction. This assumption is not correct. Hip joint or pelvic dysfunctions are often at fault.

MOTION TESTING
Lisa R. Chun

Thoracolumbar Regional
Motion Testing

1. Patient position: standing with his weight evenly distributed and feet placed four to six inches apart and parallel.
2. Physician position: kneeling directly behind the patient, his eyes level with the lumbar region.
3. Hand position: on the iliac crests and monitoring the anterior superior iliac spines.
4. Evaluation:
   a. The physician notes the limitation of

motion, the progression from thoracic through the lumbar spine, the fluidity with which the motion is achieved, and the symmetry or asymmetry created.
   b. Rotation of the lumbar spine is usually no more than 5 degrees in each direction. The test is more for thoracic than for lumbar rotation.
   c. Pelvic rotation will occur with this technique; however, it can be minimized by having the patient lock his knees.
5. Techniques:

Figure 10-1. Thoracolumbar region testing: forward bending.

Figure 10-2. Thoracolumbar region testing: backward bending.

Figure 10-3. Thoracolumbar region testing: side bending.

Forward bending:
a. The patient is instructed to slowly bend forward as if to touch his toes; the knees remain locked (Fig. 10-1).
b. Forward bending is continued until movement is felt at the anterior superior iliac spines, at which time the patient is instructed to stop.
c. The physician determines the angle created by the anterior displacement in a sagittal plane of the spinous process of the first thoracic vertebra from a position of neutral to one of flexion. The angle of flexion normally approximates 105 degrees.
d. The patient is instructed to return to a neutral standing position.

Backward bending:
a. The patient is instructed to slowly bend backward toward the physician (Fig. 10-2). The movement should be mainly from the waist up.
b. Once motion is felt at the anterior superior iliac spines, the patient is instructed to stop bending backward.
c. The physician determines the angle created by the posterior displacement of the first thoracic spinous process from a position of

neutral to one of extension. The normal angle of extension is approximately 60 degrees.
d. The patient is instructed to return to a neutral standing position.

Side bending:
a. The patient is instructed to slowly slide one hand down the lateral aspect of the ipsilateral leg without deviating into lumbar flexion or extension and without flexing or hyperextending the knee (Fig. 10-3).
b. The side bending motion is continued until movement of the contralateral iliac crest is felt by the physician, at which time the patient is instructed to stop side bending.
c. The physician determines the angle created by the lateral displacement in the frontal plane of the first thoracic spinous process from a position of neutral to one of side bending. The normal angle of side bending is approximately 40 degrees.
d. The patient is instructed to return to a neutral standing position.
e. Repeat procedure for the other side of the body.
f. The physician compares right side bending with left side bending.

Figure 10-4. Thoracolumbar regional motion testing: rotation.

Figure 10-5. Lateral lumbar flexion: hip drop test.

Rotation:
a. The patient is instructed to turn his body, from the waist up, to one side, while keeping his feet firmly on the ground with the knees straight (Fig. 10-4).
b. This motion is continued until movement is felt at the contralateral anterior superior iliac spine, at which time the patient is instructed to stop rotation.
c. The physician determines the angle created by the posterior displacement of the lateral tip of the posteriormost acromion process from a position of neutral to one of rotation. The normal angle of rotation is approximately 40 degrees.
d. The patient is instructed to return to a neutral standing position.
e. The procedure is repeated for the other side of the body.
f. The physician compares right rotation to left rotation.

Lateral Lumbar Flexion: Hip Drop Test
1. Patient position: standing relaxed, facing forward, with weight evenly distributed over feet, feet placed four to six inches apart.
2. Physician position: facing the patient's back, his eyes level with the lumbar region.
3. **Technique:**
   a. The patient is instructed to bend one knee, keeping the corresponding foot on the ground and keeping the other knee straight (Fig. 10-5).
   b. The patient should allow the compensatory shift in body weight distribution.
   c. The physician notes the degree of lumbar lateral flexion and the degree of curve created, as measured by the drop in the iliac crest.
   d. The patient is instructed to return to a neutral standing position.
   e. The procedure is repeated with the patient bending the other knee.
   f. The physician compares right lateral flexion with left lateral flexion. Lateral flexion is most restricted to the side of greatest iliac crest lowering.

Intersegmental Motion Testing
See intersegmental motion testing for the thoracic spine. Similarities in patient position, physician position, and technique exist. Modify the hand position to palpate the lumbar vertebrae.

INTERSEGMENTAL MOTION TESTING: ALTERNATIVE TECHNIQUE
1. Patient position: varies according to motion being tested. *Rotation:* prone, with arms on the table. *Flexion, extension, and lateral*

flexion: lateral recumbent, with both hips and knees flexed and on the table, head supported.

2. Physician position: standing at the side of the table facing the patient.

3. Hand position: varies according to motion being tested. *Rotation:* monitoring fingers are placed on the transverse processes of the lumbar vertebra to be examined. *Lateral flexion:* monitoring fingers are placed on the transverse processes of the lumbar vertebra to be examined and of the vertebra above it. *Flexion and extension:* monitoring finger between the spinous processes of the vertebra to be tested, as well as the one above it.

4. **Technique:**

Rotation:

a. The physician assesses the symmetry or asymmetry of both soft tissue and bone at the transverse processes of the vertebra being examined.

b. The physician applies a firm, equal pressure in a ventral direction on the transverse processes of the vertebra being assessed.

c. The ease of ventral motion of one transverse process indicates a rotation to the contralateral side. For example, if the right transverse process moves more freely ventrally than the left, the left transverse process is rotated posteriorly. The vertebra is rotated left.

d. The procedure is repeated at each lumbar level.

e. The physician compares rotation between levels.

Rotation, patient laterally recumbent

a. The physician flexes the patient's hips and knees until motion is felt at the spinous processes.

b. The physician leans into the patient's knees once this flexion position is attained.

c. Using the patient's knees as a fulcrum, the physician laterally flexes the lumbar spine by raising the patient's ankles to the ceiling (Fig. 10-6).

d. Lateral flexion is created until motion is felt at the monitoring finger.

e. The physician assesses the relationship created between the vertebra being monitored and the one above it. The physician should also note if there is a

Figure 10-6. Intersegmental motion testing: rotation, patient recumbent, alternative technique.

change in position of the monitored vertebra between the neutral position and lateral flexion.

f. Posterior protrusion (rotation) of the upper process indicates a type II somatic dysfunction, according to Fryette's second principle of physiologic motion of the spine. Ventral rotation of the upper transverse process indicates a type I somatic dysfunction, according to Fryette's first principle of physiologic motion of the spine.

g. The procedure is repeated for each lumbar vertebra.

h. The physician compares the motions at various levels.

Flexion/extension, patient laterally recumbent

a. The physician creates flexion by moving the patient's legs and knees towards the patient's abdomen.

b. Motion is created only until it is felt at the monitoring finger.

c. The physician induces extension by moving the patient's legs and knees away from the patient's abdomen and applying axial compression through the patient's femurs.

d. Motion is created only until it is felt at the monitoring finger.

e. Each vertebra is assessed in both flexion and extension before continuing to the next vertebral level.

f. Ease of flexion with a barrier to extension indicates a flexion dysfunction.

g. The procedure is repeated for all lumbar vertebrae.

Note: In applying these techniques for intersegmental motion testing, the physician is no longer testing motion of a vertebra on the one immediately below it but on the one above it. Asymmetry of position and motion of the spinous process in the sagittal plane should raise suspicion of a flexion or extension dysfunction.

Rotoscoliosis Motion Testing

1. Patient position: prone.
2. Physician position: standing at the side of the table with his dominant eye over the midline of the patient's body. The physician's eyes should be as horizontal to the examining surface as is possible.
3. Hand position: monitoring fingers are placed on the transverse processes of the vertebra being examined.
4. **Technique:**
   a. Each vertebra is assessed in all three positions before the next vertebra is evaluated.
   b. The monitoring fingers remain in contact with the patient's skin until all positions have been assessed for one vertebra.
   c. After the motions of one vertebra have been compared in all three positions, the

physician compares the anteroposterior symmetry or asymmetry of that vertebra with the symmetry or asymmetry of the other lumbar vertebrae.

d. **Neutral**
   i. With the patient prone, the physician determines the anteroposterior symmetry or asymmetry of a vertebra by comparing the corresponding right and left transverse processes (Fig. 10-7).
   ii. The physician then continues to the next positional motion testing.

e. **Flexion**
   i. The patient is seated with his feet firmly and equally supported.
   ii. The patient is instructed to bend forward, allowing the arms to fall between the knees.
   iii. This flexion motion is discontinued when motion is felt at the monitored transverse processes.
   iv. The physician determines the anteroposterior symmetry or asymmetry of the corresponding transverse processes (Fig. 10-8).

f. **Hyperextension**
   i. The patient is prone.
   ii. The patient hyperextends the lumbar spine by placing either his elbows on the table or his hands on the table with his elbows extended (Fig. 10-9).

Figure 10-7. Lumbar rotoscoliosis testing in neutral position.

Figure 10-8. Lumbar rotoscoliosis testing in flexion.

Figure 10-9. Lumbar rotoscoliosis testing in extension.

   iii. Extension is created until motion is felt at the transverse processes of the monitored vertebra.

   iv. The physician determines the anteroposterior symmetry or asymmetry of the corresponding transverse processes.

References

Adams MA, Hutton HC. 1983. The effect of posture on the fluid content of lumbar intervertebral discs. Spine 8(6):665–671.

Bogduk N, Twomey T. 1987. Clinical Anatomy of the Lumbar Spine. Edinburgh: Churchill Livingstone.

Cailliet R. 1968. Low Back Syndrome, 2nd ed. Philadelphia: F.A. Davis Co.

Farfan HF. 1975. Muscular mechanism of the lumbar spine and the position of power and efficiency. Orthop Clin North Am 6(1):135–144.

Farfan JF, Sullivan JD. 1967. The relation of facet orientation to intervertebral disc failure. Can J Surg 10:179.

Jayson IV. 1976. The Lumbar Spine and Back Pain, 3rd ed. Edinburgh: Churchill Livingstone.

Jones L. 1955. The Postural Complex. St. Louis: Charles C Thomas, Publisher.

Kapanji IA. 1974. The Physiology of the Joints. Vol 3. The Trunk and the Vertebral Column. Edinburgh: Churchill Livingstone.

Michele AA. Iliopsoas. St. Louis: Charles C Thomas, Publisher.

Schiowitz S, DiGiovanna E, Ausman P. 1983. An Osteopathic Approach to Diagnosis and Treatment. Old Westbury: New York College of Osteopathic Medicine of the New York Institute of Technology.

Warwick R, Williams PL. 1973. Grays Anatomy, 35th British ed. Philadelphia: W.B. Saunders Co.

Weisel SW, Bernini P, Rothman RH. 1982. The Aging Lumbar Spine. Philadelphia: W.B. Saunders Co.

White AA, Panjabi MM. 1978. Biomechanics of the Spine. Philadelphia: J.B. Lippincott Co.

11

Treatment of the Lumbar Spine

MYOFASCIAL TECHNIQUES
Toni Murphy

The principles of myofascial therapy were discussed in Chapter 5. This section describes the application of passive, active direct, and active indirect techniques to the lumbar region. In all of the techniques the patient lies recumbent on his side. The affected side is down or up, according to the technique used.

Passive Techniques
1. Patient position: recumbent on his side, with the affected side up. The patient's head is supported and the hips and knees are flexed to 90 degrees.
2. Physician position: standing at the side of the table facing the patient's front.
3. Hand position: Grasping the paravertebral muscle body to be treated and gently separating it from the spine.
4. **Technique:**
   a. The physician stabilizes the patient and herself by leaning into the patient's knees.
   b. The physician pulls the muscle body toward herself and simultaneously pushes the patient's knees backward to gain more stretch on the muscle (Fig. 11-1).
   c. Rest; repeat.

Many of the passive techniques used to treat thoracolumbar disorders (Chap. 9) may also be applied to the lumber region. Because the lumbar region has greater muscle mass, the pelvis and lower extremities can be used for leverage and stabilization. Do not be afraid to be creative.

Active Direct Techniques
1. Patient position: recumbent on his side, with the affected side down. The patient's head is supported and his hips and knees are flexed to 90 degrees.
2. Physician position: standing at the side at the table facing the patient's front.
3. Hand position: grasping the patient's ankles with one hand.
4. **Technique:**
   a. The physician leans into the patient's knees with her body to keep the knees in place on the table. She then raises the patient's ankles off the table. (Fig. 11-2). The knees therefore become the fulcrum of the side bending motion off the table, thus creating passive lateral flexion (side bending) of the lumbar spine.
   b. The patient is instructed to push his ankles down toward the table and to hold this

Figure 11-1. Passive myofascial technique applied to the lumbar spine, patient recumbent.

Figure 11-2. Active direct myofascial lumbar technique, patient recumbent.

position for approximately 6 seconds.

c. The physician applies an isometric resistive force to the motion of the patient's ankles.

d. The patient relaxes. The physician then induces further sidebending by lifting the patient's ankles more than before, further stretching the paravertebral muscles.

e. The physician may localize the treatment by flexing the patient's hips. Approximately 90 degrees of hip flexion localizes the treatment to the lower lumbar spine. With greater hip flexion the treatment is effective higher in the lumbar spine. The patient's muscles closest to the table are being treated.

Modification

1. Patient position: recumbent on his side, with the affected side up. The patient's head is supported and his hips and knees are flexed to 90 degrees.

2. Physician position: standing at the side of the table facing the patient's front.

3. Hand position: grasping the patient's ankles with one hand.

4. **Technique:**

a. The physician leans into the patient's knees.

b. As the patient attempts to push his ankles toward the ceiling, the physician applies an isometric counterforce. The patient's upper muscles are being treated (Fig. 11-3).

Active Indirect Techniques

1. Patient position: recumbent on his side with the affected side down. The patient's head and neck are supported; his hips and knees are flexed to 90 degrees and are close enough to the edge of the table to allow his feet and legs to fall off the table when not supported by the physician.

2. Physician position: standing at the side of the table facing the patient's front.

3. Hand position: one hand grasps the patient's ankles, the other hand monitors the patient's lower paravertebral muscle.

Figure 11-3. Modified active direct myofascial lumbar technique.

4. **Technique:**
   a. The physician gently leans into the patient's knees to maintain knee and hip flexion and to keep the knees in place on the table.
   b. The physician raises the patient's ankles off the table cephalad, causing side bending of the spine (convexity down). The knees act as the fulcrum for the side bending motion.
   c. The patient is instructed to push his feet downward toward the floor while the physician applies an isokinetic counterforce at the patient's ankles. This allows the patient to move his feet toward the floor slowly against a resistive force. The muscles being treated are on the side the patient is lying on.
   d. At the end of a session, the lumbar convexity should be sidebent up. At this point the physician applies a gentle passive stretch at the patient's ankles, inducing further stretch of the muscle.

MUSCLE ENERGY TECHNIQUES
Sandra D. Yale
Nancy Brous

The principles of muscle energy therapy were discussed in Chapter 5. This section describes the application of techniques to group curves and single-segment dysfunctions in the lumbar spine. In all of these techniques the patient lies on his side on the table or in a modified Sims's position; the transverse processes of the segment being treated face up or down, according to the precise technique.

Type I Neutral (Group) Curves
1. Patient position: lateral recumbent with concavity toward the table; therefore, the posteriorly rotated transverse processes are up.
2. Physician position: standing at the side of the table facing the patient.
3. **Technique:**
   a. The physician monitors the apex of the curve with one hand.
   b. The physician flexes the patient's hips to 90 degrees.
   c. The physician side bends the lumbar spine to the apex by elevating the patient's ankles with the nonmonitoring hand (Fig. 11-4).
   d. The patient is then instructed to push his feet toward the floor for 3 seconds.
   e. The physician provides resistance, producing a static contraction.
   f. The patient is asked to relax.
   g. The physician further elevates the patient's legs until motion is felt at the new apex of the curve.
   h. The procedure is repeated three times.

Type II Somatic Dysfunction (Single-Segment Dysfunction)
FLEXED SOMATIC DYSFUNCTION
1. Patient position: lying on the table in a lateral recumbent position. The posteriorly rotated transverse process to be treated faces down, toward the table.
2. Physician position: standing at the side of the table facing the patient.

Figure 11-4. Muscle energy treatment for a type I curve, convex right.

3. **Technique:**

   a. The physician instructs the patient to lie on his side with the posterior transverse process down.

   b. The physician stands facing the patient and monitors the somatic dysfunction with one hand at the interspinous region.

   c. With the other hand the physician flexes the patient's hips and knees until motion is felt at the level below the dysfunction (i.e., at L2 on L3).

   d. The patient straightens his lower leg and the physician extends it until motion is felt at the same level. The flexed upper leg is "locked" in place with the dorsum of the foot of the top leg placed in the popliteal space of the lower leg by the physician.

   e. The physician changes hands so that the caudal (with respect to the patient) hand is now monitoring the involved segment.

   f. With his other hand the physician grasps the patient's lower arm and pulls it upward, causing rotation of the torso, until motion is felt at the level of the restriction.

   g. Further rotation and localization are achieved by directing the patient to use his top hand to grasp the table edge behind his back.

   h. The physician places his cephalic hand on the patient's shoulder.

   i. The patient is instructed to take a deep breath, then exhale. Thereafter the patient is directed to reach farther down the table edge. The physician places light pressure against the patient's shoulder and more precisely localizes the somatic dysfunction.

   j. The physician again switches hands and uses his cephalic hand to monitor the level of the restriction.

   k. The physician grasps the ankle of the patient's upper leg and elevates it until the lumbar spine side bends to the motion barrier.

   l. The patient pushes his elevated foot down toward the table while the physician maintains resistance, producing a static contraction (Fig. 11-5).

   m. After 3 seconds, the patient is asked to relax.

   n. The physician then increases extension, side bending, and rotation into the new

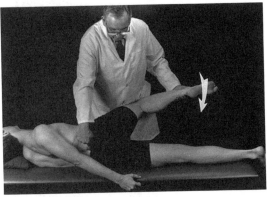

Figure 11-5. Muscle energy treatment for a flexed somatic dysfunction.

   motion barriers by again elevating the patient's upper ankle.

   o. The procedure is repeated three or four times.

Variation: The patient is instructed to push the upper knee upward rather than the foot down.

EXTENDED SOMATIC

1. Patient position: lying on the table in a lateral recumbent position. The posteriorly rotated transverse process to be treated faces up. The patient is then placed in the modified Sims's position.

2. Physician position: standing at the side of the table facing the patient.

3. **Technique:**

   a. The patient is instructed to lie on his side with the posterior transverse process up.

   b. The physician faces the patient and monitors the somatic dysfunction with his cephalic hand.

   c. The physician flexes the patient's knees and hips until motion is felt at the area of somatic dysfunction.

   d. The physician switches monitoring hands so that the caudal (with respect to the patient) hand is on the somatic dysfunction.

   e. Rotation is achieved by placing the patient in the lateral Sims's position.

   f. Additional rotation is induced by having the patient inhale, then exhale and simultaneously reach toward the floor.

   g. The physician pushes down on the shoulder with his cephalic hand until the

A

B

Figure 11-6. Muscle energy treatment for an extended somatic dysfunction. (**A**) Physician standing. (**B**) Physician seated.

torso is rotated down to the monitored segment, exaggerating the Sims's position.

h. The patient's legs are lowered off the side of the table to create lumbar side bending up to the restricted area (Fig. 11-6A).

i. Since this position is uncomfortable for the patient, the physician may either place a pillow under the patient's lower knee or sit behind the patient and put his thigh between the patient's legs and the table (Fig. 11-6B). (This position requires the physician to change the hand monitoring.)

j. The patient pushes his feet toward the ceiling while the physician resists, creating an isometric contraction, which is held for 3 seconds.

k. The patient relaxes. The physician engages a new motion barrier by further lowering the patient's legs.

l. The procedure is repeated three times.

Summary of Muscle Energy Techniques for Lumbar Somatic Dysfunction

Extension somatic dysfunctions: S.U.E.
S: Lateral Sims's position.
U: Posterior process is up.
E: Extension somatic dysfunction.

Flexion somatic dysfunctions: F.D.R.
F: Flexion somatic dysfunction.
D: Posterior process is down.
R: Lateral recumbent position.

COUNTERSTRAIN TECHNIQUES
Eileen L. DiGiovanna

Many of the counterstrain techniques for lumbar somatic dysfunctions are facilitated by slight rotation of the patient's thighs or hips, and by resting some part of the patient's leg on the physician's thigh or knee. Anterior tender points are treated with the patient supine, posterior tender points with the patient prone.

Anterior Tender Points

Figure 11-7 shows the locations of the anterior lumbar tender points.

L1 TENDER POINT (MEDIAL TO ANTERIOR SUPERIOR ILIAC SPINES)
1. Patient position: supine.
2. Physician position: standing next to the table on the side of the tender point.

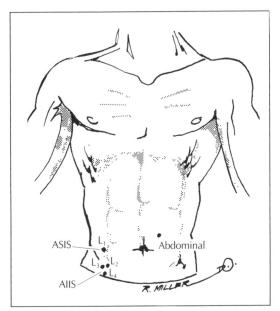

Figure 11-7. Anterior lumbar tender point locations.

Figure 11-8. Treatment for L1 lumbar tender point, L1.

3. **Technique:**
   a. The patient's upper body is propped up on pillows.
   b. Both knees are flexed and rotated toward the tender point. Because the lower body is rotated, this position is equivalent to upper body rotation away from the tender point (Fig. 11-8).
   c. The hips are side bent toward the tender point.
   d. The patient's legs may be supported on the physician's thigh if desired.

Note: The L1 tender point is treated in the same manner as the tender points corresponding to vertebrae T9–T12.

L2 TENDER POINT
1. Patient position: supine.
2. Physician position: standing at the side of the table opposite the tender point, which is located on the inferior medial surface of the anterior inferior iliac spine.
3. Both thighs are rotated 60 degrees away from the tender point, with side bending away (Fig. 11-9).

Figure 11-9. Treatment for L2 lumbar tender point, L2.

ABDOMINAL L2 TENDER POINT
The abdominal L2 tender point is found 2 inches lateral to the umbilicus. The treatment is the same as for the anterior inferior iliac spine tender point except that the thighs are rotated toward the tender point (the equivalent of rotation away from the tender point at the vertebral level) (Fig. 11-10).

L3, L4 TENDER POINTS
1. Patient position: supine.
2. Physician position: standing at the side of the table on the side of the tender point, with one foot on the table.

Figure 11-10. Treatment for abdominal lumbar tender point.

Figure 11-11. Treatment for anterior L5 tender point.

3. **Technique:**
   a. The patient's hips and knees are flexed. His legs rest on the physician's thighs.
   b. The spine is side bent away from the tender point with slight rotation toward the tender point.

L5 TENDER POINT
1. Patient position: supine.
2. Physician position: standing at the side of the table next to the tender point, which is on the pubic ramus. Her foot is on the table.
3. **Technique:**
   a. The patient's hips and knees are flexed. His legs rest on the physician's thighs.
   b. The far ankle is crossed over the one closer to the physician. The knees are dropped slightly apart (Fig. 11-11).
   c. There is side bending away from the tender point and slight rotation toward it.

Posterior Tender Points
Figure 11-12 shows the locations of the posterior tender points.

L1–L5 TENDER POINTS (SPINOUS OR TRANSVERSE PROCESS)
1. Patient position: prone.
2. Physician position: standing at the side of the table.

Figure 11-12. Posterior lumbar tender point locations.

Figure 11-13. Counterstrain treatment for posterior lumbar tender points, spinous process.

Figure 11-14. Counterstrain treatment for posterior transverse process lumbar tender points with rotation introduced.

Figure 11-15. Counterstrain treatment for lower pole L5 tender point.

3. **Technique:**
   a. The extended leg is elevated, extending the lumber spine. Both legs may be used.
   b. If the tender point is near the midline, this position may be sufficient. It is best if the physician stands on the same side as the leg being elevated (Fig. 11-13).
   c. If the tender point is over the transverse process, some rotation may be necessary. This is best done with the physician standing at the side opposite the tender point. The leg is elevated and adducted over the other leg enough to cause rotation at the vertebral level being treated. External rotation of the thigh assists this process (Fig. 11-14).

L3, L4, L5 UPPER POLE TENDER POINTS
The L3 to L5 vertebrae also have tender points on the lateral buttocks. The L5 tender point is superior to the posterior inferior iliac spines. These tender points are treated in a manner similar to that described for tender points on the transverse processes. The leg is elevated and adducted. It may rest on the operator's knee, which is placed on the table.

L5 LOWER POLE TENDER POINT
1. Patient position: prone.
2. Physician position: seated on a stool at the side of the table next to the tender point.

3. **Technique:**
   a. The patient's leg is dropped off the table with the knee and hip flexed. The hip is slightly rotated internally.
   b. While supporting the patient's leg, the physician pushes the knee toward the table, adducting the thigh (Fig. 11-15).
   c. Treatment is monitored at the tender point just medial to the posterior inferior iliac spine and just inferior to it.

HIGH VELOCITY, LOW AMPLITUDE THRUSTING TECHNIQUES

Barry Erner
Paula D. Scariati

This section describes high velocity, low amplitude thrusting techniques for treating somatic dysfunctions of the lumbar spine.

Lumbar Somatic Dysfunction

1. Patient position: lateral recumbent, with the posteriorly rotated transverse process up.
2. Physician position: standing facing the front of the patient.
3. **Technique:**
   a. The physician uses one hand to monitor the posteriorly rotated transverse process at all times while positioning and treating the patient.
   b. The physician flexes the hip and knee of the patient's superior leg until he feels motion in his monitoring hand. He then hooks the patient's foot in the popliteal fossa of the inferior leg, which is resting on the table in an extended position.
   c. The physician rotates the patient's torso in the same direction as the posteriorly rotated transverse process by pulling on the patient's underneath arm. Rotation is induced down to but not including the vertebral segment of the somatic dysfunction.
   d. The physician places the forearm of his thrusting arm over the patient's superior iliac crest and maintains finger monitoring of the dysfunction.
   e. The physician places his other arm beneath the patient's upper arm and stabilizes the patient's lateral torso and rib cage.
   f. The patient inhales deeply and exhales.
   g. The physician exerts a rapid rotary thrust at the end of exhalation. This is achieved by rotating the patient's pelvis forward and toward the table (Fig. 11-16).

Figure 11-16. High velocity, low amplitude treatment of the lumbar region.

Alternative Technique

a. Patient position: lateral recumbent position with the posteriorly rotated transverse process up.
b. Physician position: standing facing the front of the patient.
c. **Technique:**
   i. The method is the same as in the technique just described, except that the patient's superior leg is dropped off the table into full hip flexion. This leg is then locked between the physician's legs and maintained in full hip flexion.
   ii. Localization and thrust are the same as in the first technique.

EXERCISE THERAPY
Stanley Schiowitz
Albert R. DeRubertis

Low back pain is the single most common cause of work absenteeism in the United States. Some 70% to 80% of adults suffer from low back pain at some time in their lives. It is important that primary care physicians understand low back structural biomechanics as they will regularly encounter patients with low back pain.

A comprehensive therapeutic approach includes exercises designed to establish and maintain musculoskeletal structural integrity. A simple approach is to evaluate the lumbar lordosis, the structures involved in its formation, and the muscles that act synergistically to maintain it.

The three questions to be answered are:

1. Is the anteroposterior lumbar curve flattened or exaggerated?
2. Do the individual vertebrae move freely?
3. Do the muscles involved require stretching (extensibility) or strengthening (contractility)?

The muscles involved in creating low back pain are usually the erector spinae, the gluteus maximus, the hamstrings, the iliopsoas, and the abdominals. With the exception of the abdominals and occasionally the back extensors, these muscles require stretching. Regional motion testing may demonstrate restriction caused by muscle contraction. Specific testing for motion, stretch, and strength should be employed.

The exercises described in this chapter are based on the above approach. Many serve more than one function.

Abdominal Muscles
UPPER ABDOMINAL
STRENGTHENING EXERCISE
1. Patient position: supine, hips and knees flexed, feet on floor, arms extended.
2. **Instructions:**
   a. Roll your head, neck, and upper back off the floor.
   b. Try to touch your knees with your hands (Fig. 11-17).

Figure 11-17. Upper abdominal strengthening exercise.

Figure 11-18. Rotary abdominal strengthening exercise.

   c. Hold this position for 5 to 15 seconds. Slowly lower your body to the floor.
   d. Relax, rest, and repeat.

ROTARY ABDOMINAL
STRENGTHENING EXERCISE
1. Patient position: supine, hips and knees flexed, feet on floor, arms extended.
2. **Instructions:**
   a. Roll your head, neck, and upper back off the floor.
   b. Try to touch your left knee only with both hands, creating a body twist (Fig. 11-18).
   c. Hold this position for 5 to 15 seconds. Slowly lower your body back to floor.

Figure 11-19. Lower abdominal strengthening exercise, one leg raised.

Figure 11-20. Lower abdominal strengthening exercise, both legs raised.

Figure 11-21. Lower back muscle stretch, seated on chair.

Exercise 2
1. Patient position: supine on floor, both hands over head and firmly holding onto a solid structure.
2. **Instructions:**
    a. Tighten your abdominal muscles, keeping your back flat against the floor.
    b. Flex both knees to 45 degrees. Now raise both feet six to eight inches off the floor (Fig. 11-20).
    c. Hold this position for 5 to 15 seconds.
    d. Slowly lower both feet to the floor.
    e. Relax, rest, and repeat.

Lower Back Muscles
STRETCH
Exercise 1
1. Patient position: seated on edge of chair, both feet flat on floor.
2. **Instructions:**
    a. Cross both arms in front of your chest.
    b. Let your body bend forward between your legs. Let the body weight create low back stretch (Fig. 11-21).
    c. Hold for 5 to 15 seconds.
    d. Return slowly to the upright position. Relax, rest, and repeat.
        Caution: This can create vertigo and hypotension.

    d. Relax and rest.
    e. Repeat by trying to touch your right knee.

LOWER ABDOMINAL
STRENGTHENING EXERCISES
Exercise 1
1. Patient position: supine on floor, both knees slightly bent, heels on floor.
2. **Instructions:**
    a. Tighten your abdominal muscles and maintain your back flat against the floor.
    b. Raise your left leg off the floor six to eight inches. Maintain both knees in their slightly flexed position (Fig. 11-19).
    c. Hold this position for 5 to 15 seconds.
    d. Slowly lower the left leg to the floor.
    e. Relax, rest, and repeat by raising your right leg.

Figure 11-22. Lower back muscle stretch, seated on floor.

Figure 11-23. Lower back muscle rotary stretch, legs extended.

Exercise 2

1. Patient position: seated on the floor or a table with both legs extended.
2. **Instructions:**
   a. Lean forward and grasp your shins with each hand.
   b. Pull your trunk into further forward bending by bringing your hands down your legs (Fig. 11-22).
   c. Feel stretch in the lower back. Hold for 5 to 15 seconds. Slowly return to the starting position.
   d. Relax, rest, and repeat.

ROTARY STRETCH

Exercise 1

1. Patient position: supine, arms and legs extended.
2. **Instructions:**
   a. Bend your right knee up, cross it over your left leg, and place the right foot flat on the floor, close to the left knee.
   b. Grasp your right knee with your left hand and slowly pull it toward the left side of the floor. Keep your shoulders flat on floor (Fig. 11-23).
   c. This will create a right low back rotary stretch. Hold for 5 to 15 seconds.
   d. Release right knee, relax, and repeat.
   e. For left low back rotary stretch, reverse the knee and hand instructions.

Figure 11-24. Lower back muscle rotary stretch, hips and knees bent.

Exercise 2

1. Patient position: supine, both hips and knees bent, feet together and flat on the floor.
2. **Instructions:**
   a. Using your left foot as a fulcrum, pivot both knees to the left. Allow the weight of the legs to create a right low back rotary stretch (Fig. 11-24).
   b. Keep your shoulders flat on the floor. Do not use muscular contraction to increase stretch.
   c. Hold at maximum relaxed stretch for 5 to 15 seconds. Return knees to starting position.
   d. Relax, rest, and repeat.
   e. For left rotary stretch, reverse the instructions.

Figure 11-25. Gluteus maximus active muscle stretch.

Figure 11-26. Gluteus maximus passive muscle stretch.

Figure 11-27. Pelvic tilt.

Gluteus Maximus Muscles

ACTIVE STRETCH

1. Patient position: supine, both knees bent, feet on floor.
2. **Instructions:**
   a. Bring your right knee up to your chest as far as possible and grasp with both hands. At the same time fully extend your left leg (Fig. 11-25).
   b. Hold for 5 to 15 seconds.
   c. Reverse procedure by bringing your left knee up to your chest and fully extend your right leg.
   d. Hold this position for 5 to 15 seconds. Return to starting position.
   e. Relax, rest, and repeat.

PASSIVE STRETCH

1. Patient position: supine, arms at sides, knees bent, feet on floor.
2. **Instructions:**
   a. Bring your right knee to your chest. Clasp both your hands over that knee.
   b. Passively and slowly, pull your right knee to your chest (Fig. 11-26). Hold this position for 5 to 15 seconds.
   c. Return to starting position, repeat with other knee.
   d. Repeat, flexing both hip and knees to chest at one time.
      Note: If you have knee dysfunction, clasp both hands on the posterior thigh near the popliteal region.

Lumbar Spine

LUMBAR FLATTENING (PELVIC TILT TO DECREASE LORDOSIS)

1. Patient position: supine, arms above head, both knees bent, feet on floor.
2. **Instructions:**
   a. Tighten your abdominal muscles and your buttocks at the same time.
   b. Flatten your back firmly against the floor. Roll your pelvis backward if necessary to achieve full flattening (Fig. 11-27).
   c. Hold this position for 5 to 15 seconds.
   d. Relax, rest, and repeat.

Figure 11-28. Lumbar flexibility—flexion (cat back).

Figure 11-29. Lumbar flexibility—extension (cat back).

CAT BACK—LUMBAR FLEXIBILITY

1. Patient position: hands and knees on the floor, back up, fully lengthened and straight.
2. **Instructions:**
   a. **Flexion**
      i. Drop your head down between your arms, looking toward your thighs.
      ii. Arch your back upward and try to bring your pelvis toward your head (Fig. 11-28).
      iii. Try to achieve full back flexion with reversal of lumbar lordosis.
      iv. Hold this position for 5 to 15 seconds, return to starting position.
      v. Relax, rest, and then do the following extension exercise.
   b. **Extension**
      i. Bring your head back into full head and neck extension.
      ii. Arch your back down toward the floor. Try to bring your buttocks toward your head.
      iii. Try to achieve full back extension, exaggerating the lumbar lordosis (Fig. 11-29).
      iv. Hold this position for 5 to 15 seconds. Return to starting position.
      v. Relax, rest, and repeat the entire exercise.
         Note: Try to maintain your abdominal muscles in a flattened, mildly contracted position throughout the exercise.

LUMBAR FLATTENING

1. Patient position: kneeling, buttocks resting on heels.

Figure 11-30. Lumbar flattening stretch.

2. **Instructions:**
   a. Bring both fully extended arms forward. Touch both palms to floor, bringing your chest parallel to floor.
   b. Contract your abdominal muscles while pushing both arms forward. This should bring your chest against your knees (Fig. 11-30).
   c. Maintain maximum stretch for 5 to 15 seconds. Return to starting position.
   d. Relax, rest, and repeat.

FULL BODY STRETCH (FLATTEN ALL CURVES)

1. Patient position: supine, arms fully extended overhead, legs fully extended downward.
2. **Instructions:**
   a. Stretch your arms overhead and your legs

Figure 11-31. Full body stretch.

downward. Point your toes into plantar
flexion.
b. Tighten your abdominal muscles and flatten
your lumbar spine.
c. Tuck in your chin and flatten your cervical
spine (Fig. 11-31).
d. Hold this position for 5 to 15 seconds.
e. Relax, rest, and repeat.

Anterior Pelvic Muscle Stretch

1. Patient position: prone, legs extended, arms at
sides.
2. **Instructions:**
   a. Place both hands, palms down, on the floor
   at shoulder level.
   b. Raise your upper body off the floor by fully
   extending your arms. Keep your upper
   thighs on the floor (Fig. 11-32).

Figure 11-32. Anterior pelvic muscle stretch.

c. Allow your abdomen and pelvis to sag
(stretch) toward the floor. Your body weight
will perform the necessary stretch.
d. Hold this position for 5 to 15 seconds.
Lower your body to the floor.
e. Relax, rest, and repeat.

Back Extensor Muscle Strengthening

1. Patient position: prone, arms fully extended
upward, legs fully extended downward. Two
pillows are placed under the abdomen.
2. **Instructions:**
   a. Raise your left arm and right leg up off the
   floor, fully extended (Fig. 11-33). Hold for 5
   seconds. Lower and repeat with your left
   arm and right leg.
   b. Raise your right arm and right leg off the
   floor, fully extended. (Fig. 11-34). Hold for

Figure 11-33. Back extensor muscle strengthening,
left arm and right leg raised.

Figure 11-34. Back extensor muscle strengthening,
right arm and right leg raised.

Figure 11-35. Back extensor muscle strengthening, both arms raised.

Figure 11-36. Back extensor muscle strengthening, both legs raised.

Figure 11-37. Back extensor muscle strengthening, all extremities raised.

5 seconds. Lower and repeat with your left arm and left leg.

c. Raise both arms, fully extended, off the floor (Fig. 11-35). Hold for 5 seconds. Lower. Now raise both legs fully extended off the floor (Fig. 11-36).

d. Raise all four fully extended extremities off the floor simultaneously (Fig. 11-37). Hold for 5 seconds. Lower.

e. Relax, rest, and repeat the entire exercise.

Hip Flexor Stretch

PSOAS—UNASSISTED

1. Patient position: supine on edge of table or bed, so that side to be stretched can drop off toward the floor (right side).

2. **Instructions:**

a. Bend your left hip and knee to chest and hold them with both hands. Keep your low back flat on the table.

b. Drop your right leg off the table toward floor.

c. The assistant holds the left hip and knee in full flexion, while gently pushing down on the right thigh, creating stretch (Fig. 11-38).

d. Hold maximum painless stretch for 5 to 15 seconds. Return both legs to the table in full extension.

e. Relax, rest, and repeat.

Figure 11-38. Psoas muscle stretch, assisted.

Figure 11-39. Psoas muscle stretch, unassisted.

Figure 11-40. Hamstring muscle stretch, seated.

Figure 11-41. Hamstring muscle stretch, supine.

PSOAS

1. Patient position: supine on edge of table or bed, so that side to be stretched can drop off toward the floor (right side).
2. **Instructions:**
   a. Bend your left hip and knee to chest. Hold them firmly against your chest. Keep your low back flat on the table.
   b. Drop your right leg off the table toward the floor. Allow its weight to create stretch.
   c. For additional stretch, a three- to five-pound weight can be added at the ankle (Fig. 11-39).
   d. Hold the maximum painless stretch for 5 to 15 seconds. Return both legs to the table in full extension.
   e. Relax, rest, and repeat.

Hamstring Stretch

SEATED STRETCH

1. Patient position: seated with the back upright and the left leg in full extension. The right leg is bent so that right foot is touching the left thigh.
2. **Instructions:**
   a. Bend forward from your hips. Place both hands on your left leg until you feel stretch (left-sided).
   b. Hold this position, then walk your hands farther down the left leg to increase the stretch to maximum (Fig. 11-40).
   c. Hold this position for 5 to 15 seconds. Return to the upright position.
   d. Relax, rest, and repeat.

   e. To stretch the right side, reverse instructions.

SUPINE STRETCH

1. Patient position: supine, hips and knees flexed, both feet flat on the floor.
2. **Instructions:**
   a. Flex the hip to be stretched toward your chest. Then extend that leg fully toward the ceiling. Bend your toes down toward your body. Hold in maximum painless stretch.
   b. Bring both hands or a towel around and behind the extended knee or thigh. Slowly pull your thigh toward your chest. Maintain full leg extension (Fig. 11-41).
   c. Hold this position for 5 to 15 seconds. Return to the original position.
   d. Relax, rest, and repeat.
   e. To stretch the other side, reverse instructions.

Figure 11-42. Hamstring muscle stretch, standing.

STANDING STRETCH
1. Patient position: standing near a table or other firm support. Support must be of sufficient height to allow stretch.
2. **Instructions:**
   a. Place the heel of the foot to be exercised on the support. Keep the knee fully extended.
   b. With both hands on your leg, slowly bend forward from your hips until you feel maximum painless stretch in the back of your raised leg (Fig. 11-42).
   c. Hold for 5 to 15 seconds, increasing the painless stretch as tolerated. Return leg to floor.
   d. Relax, rest, and repeat.
   e. To stretch the other side, reverse instructions.

Reference

Mitchell FL Jr, Moran PS, Pruzzo NT. 1979. An Evaluation and Treatment Manual of Osteopathic Muscle Energy Procedures. Valley Park, Mo: Mitchell, Moran, and Pruzzo.

12

Evaluation of the Pelvis and Sacrum

FUNCTIONAL ANATOMY AND BIOMECHANICS
Stanley Schiowitz

Anatomy

The pelvis consists of two innominate bones that meet at the midline anteriorly and end posteriorly in a wedge-shaped opening that is filled by the sacrum. This completes the overall ring shape of the pelvis.

Each innominate bone consists of three bones, the ilium, ischium, and pubes, which fuse in late adolescence to form one bone. On the lateral surface of the innominate is the acetabulum, which articulates with the head of the femur to create the hip joint.

The sacrum is a large bone in the shape of an inverted triangle that is formed by the fusion of the five sacral vertebrae. It is inserted between the two innominate bones in the upper, posterior aspect of the pelvic cavity. The upper aspect of the sacrum—the base of the triangle—articulates with the fifth lumbar vertebra, creating, with the L5 intervertebral disk, the lumbosacral articulation. The weight of the upper body is transmitted through the sacrum, innominate bones, and acetabulum to the femurs, then down to the feet and the supporting surface.

In the upright position the sacrum lies in an oblique plane, running from above downward in an anteroposterior direction. Its anterior surface is concave. Its posterior surface is convex and contains the palpable spinous tubercles. The sacrum contains the sacral canal, in which are located the cauda equina and four sacral foramina; these apertures provide passageway for the ventral and dorsal rami of the first four sacral spinal nerves. Bilaterally the sacrum has auricular surfaces that articulate with the innominate bones to form the sacroiliac joints.

The sacroiliac articulations are kidney-shaped and convex ventrally. The sacral and iliac articulations seem to match in a crescent-shaped, convex-concave arrangement, but this is not true for the joints' entire bony relationship. Horizontal sections from various levels of the sacroiliac articulation show that the convex-concave relationship exists only at the upper and middle portions. In the lower portion the relationship is variously described as a flattened, planar joint or a reverse, concave-convex relationship (Fig. 12-1); anatomists differ in their descriptions of the sacroiliac articulations.

Occasionally the right and left sacroiliac articulations do not mirror each other in the same body. It is generally agreed that the midarticulation has the greatest convex-concave relationship, promoting joint stability and flexion-extension

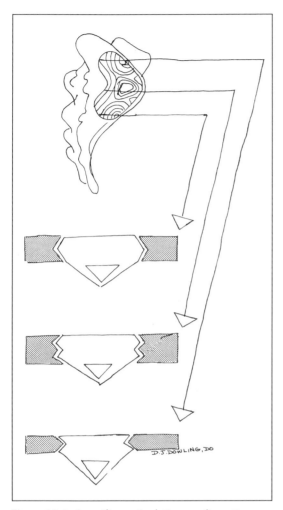

Figure 12-1. Sacroiliac articulation configurations as seen at different sacral levels.

Figure 12-2. An increase in the lumbosacral angle creates a greater anterior vector force, which increases the lumbosacral strain.

motions. This is usually found at the level of the second sacral vertebra.

The multiple forms and contours found at any sacroiliac articulation account for the diversity of motions of this joint. The joint is held together by its ligaments. There are no direct muscular attachments from the sacrum to the ilium.

Pelvic Motions

The pelvis moves as a single unit whose gross motions are initiated by the motions of other body segments. Rotation, side bending, and forward and backward bending are all related to the hip or trunk motions. In addition, there are patterns of movement between the sacrum and the ilium, and patterns of movement at the pubic articulation.

Review of some everyday activities will demonstrate their effect on the pelvic structures. In the standing position, body weight is transmitted through the fifth lumbar vertebra to the sacrum, where the force vector splits in two. One force vector drives the sacrum into its articulation, the other rotates the sacrum anteriorly. The greater the lumbosacral angle, the greater is the anterior vector force, which in turn increases the lumbosacral strain (Fig. 12-2).

During the act of walking, the ilium on the side of the stance leg is elevated, while the ilium on the swing side is tilted down and rotated toward the stance leg. This creates pubic shear and tor-

Figure 12-3. Pubic shear and torsion in walking (*top*), corresponding to the position of the weight-bearing ilium as the stance leg moves from heel strike to toe-off (*bottom*).

sion (Fig. 12-3, *top*). The stance leg, from heel strike to toe-off, is associated with a close-packed hip joint articulation and causes anterior rotation of the ilium (Fig. 12-3, *bottom*). The body weight shifts to the side of the stance leg, creating lateral flexion stress of the sacrum. The one-legged weight stress produces unilateral stance leg sacroiliac joint locking, allowing the creation of the oblique axis (Mitchell, 1965). This in turn permits sacral torsional motion.

Respiratory motions create sacral flexion/extension (Sutherland, 1936). Flexion and extension of the sacrum create pressure on the ilia that is transmitted to the pubic articulation.

The three principal kinds of motions that occur in the pelvis are sacral motions on the ilium, ilial motions on the sacrum, and pubic motions. Each is described below.

SACRAL MOTION ON THE ILIUM
The sacral motions on the ilium, and the axes on which they occur, are as follows:

1. Sacral flexion and extension are caused by respiratory motion and occur on a superior transverse axis, also known as the respiratory axis, that is located at the level of the articular processes of the second sacral segment.
2. Sacral flexion and extension are transmitted as force vectors through the lumbar spine to the middle transverse axis, located at the level of the second sacral body.
3. Rotation of the sacrum occurs on a vertical axis.
4. Lateral flexion of the sacrum occurs on an anteroposterior axis.
5. Torsional motions of the sacrum occur on a right or left oblique axis, located from the superior end of the articular surface of one side to the inferior end of the articular surface of the other side.

The axes of sacral motion on the ilium are shown in Figure 12-4.

The coupled motions of rotation and lateral bending of the sacrum are variable, depending

Figure 12-4. Axes of motion of the sacrum on the ilia. *1*, vertical axis; *2*, right oblique axis; *3*, sacroilial axis; *4*, respiratory axis; *5*, iliosacral axis; *6*, left oblique axis; *7*, anteroposterior axis.

somewhat on how those movements are initiated. According to Kappler, sacral rotation induced by lumbar spinal rotation occurs in the same direction as the lumbar spinal rotation, but lateral flexion of the sacrum occurs to the opposite side. When lateral sacral flexion is induced by lateral flexion of the lumbar spine, sacral rotation may occur to either side.

ILIAL MOTIONS ON THE SACRUM
The motions of the ilium on the sacrum, and the axes on which these movements occur, are as follows.

1. Anteroposterior rotation of the ilium on the sacrum occurs on the inferior transverse axis,

located at the inferior pole of the lower sacral articulation (Fig. 12-5).
2. Ilial translatory motions on the sacrum occur in a superoinferior direction (Fig. 12-6).
3. Ilial translatory motions on the sacrum occur in an anteroposterior direction (Fig. 12-7).

PUBIC MOTIONS
The pubic motions, shown in Figure 12-8, are as follows:

1. Caliper motion (flexion/extension of sacrum).
2. Torsional motion (swing/tilt of swing leg).
3. Superoinferior translatory motion (one-legged weight-bearing).

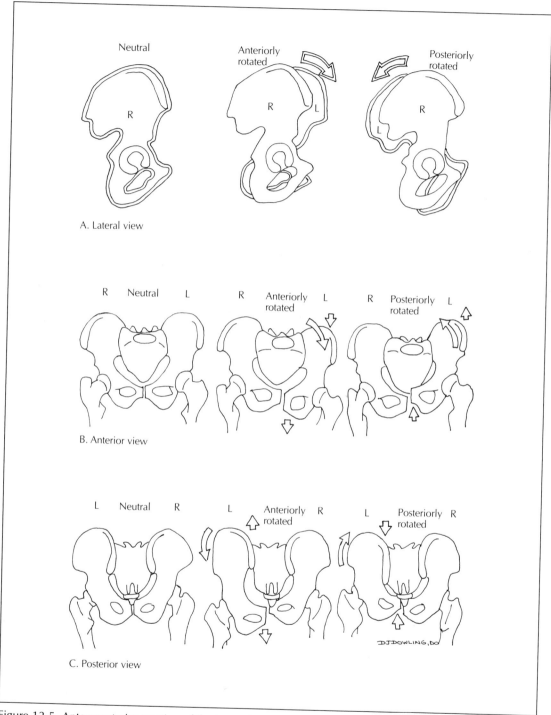

Figure 12-5. Anteroposterior rotation of the innominate on the sacrum. The directions are named for left-sided movement in this illustration.

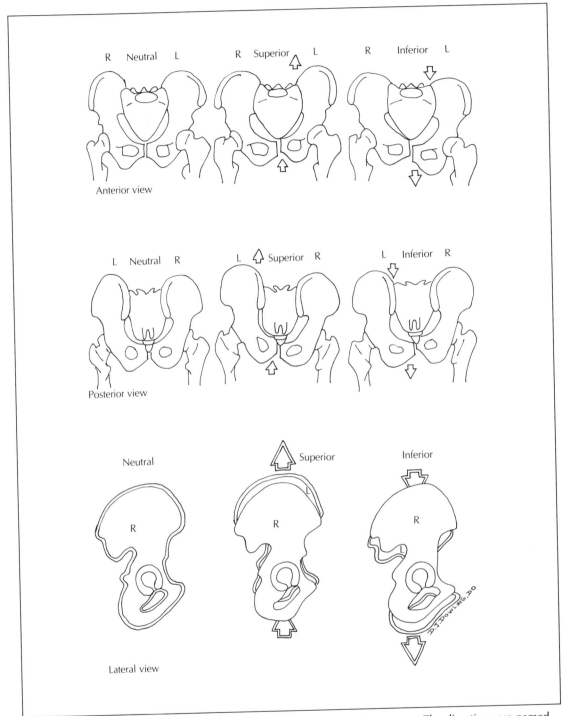

Figure 12-6. Superoinferior translatory motion of the innominate on the sacrum. The directions are named for left-sided movement.

Figure 12-7. Anteroposterior translatory motion of the innominate on the sacrum. The left side is illustrated.

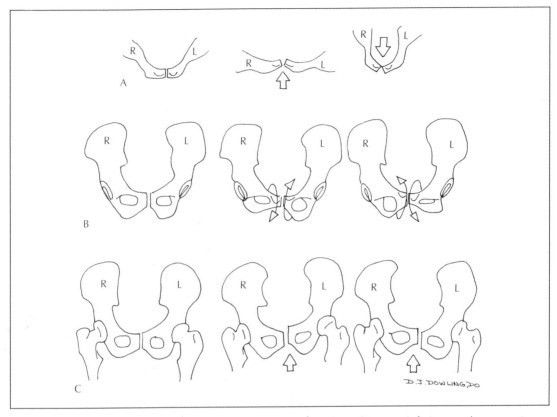

Figure 12-8. Pubic motions. (**A**) Caliper motion, (**B**) torsional motion, (**C**) superoinferior translatory motion.

The Pelvis During Pregnancy

During vaginal delivery, the sacrum undergoes a process called *nutation* (nodding) that facilitates delivery. In nutation the sacrum flexes at its middle transverse axis. This diminishes the anteroposterior diameter of the pelvic brim. At the same time the iliac bones approximate, narrowing the transverse diameter of the pelvic brim, and the ischial tuberosities separate, widening the pelvic outlet (Fig. 12-9).

The patient's position and the stress involved, when added to the laxity of the ligaments at delivery, can create sacroiliac dysfunctions. These dysfunctions worsen and are locked into malposition as the ligaments regain their normal rigidity post partum. Dysfunction can be prevented after delivery by holding the hip in internal rotation as each leg is removed from the lithotomy position and placed flat on the table.

Pelvic Somatic Dysfunctions

Pelvic somatic dysfunctions are of the following types:

1. Primary pubic dysfunctions are superior/inferior or abducted/adducted dysfunctions.
2. Dysfunctions of motion created by the sacrum moving on the ilium are commonly unilateral anterior sacral dysfunctions or oblique torsional sacral dysfunctions.
3. Dysfunction created by the ilium moving on the sacrum usually involves anteroposterior ilial rotation or superoinferior ilial shear.

These dysfunctions may be difficult to diagnose individually since many of the motion functions and diagnostic findings overlap. Specific treatment of a specific dysfunction is most effective. However, because of the firm ligamentous attachments of this articulation, nonspecific treatment may be equally as effective.

Figure 12-9. Sacral relations during vaginal delivery. (**A**) Counternutation, (**B**) nutation.

EXAMINATION AND MOTION TESTING
Dennis J. Dowling

Patient Standing
1. Patient position: standing, barefoot, with the feet parallel and six to eight inches apart.
2. Physician position: kneeling behind the patient with his eyes approximately at the level of the iliac crests and the posterior superior iliac spines (PSIS).

STATIC EXAMINATION (FIG. 12-10)
1. **Technique:**
   a. Iliac crests: The physician places his hands on the patient's iliac crests and evaluates the symmetry of heights of the two crests.
   b. Posterior Superior Iliac Spines: A landmark for the PSIS is usually visible as a skin

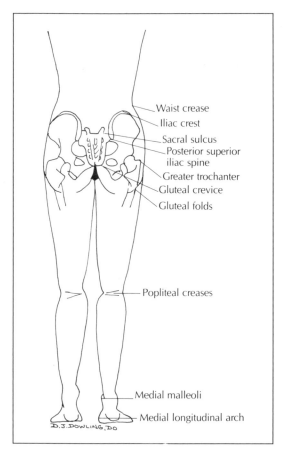

Figure 12-10. Relationship of pelvic structures on static examination, patient standing.

dimple indicating the location of attachment of the deep fascia. The physician places his thumbs at these locations, hooks his thumbs beneath the PSIS, and compares heights.

c. Gluteal folds: The physician observes directly these folds, which delineate the lower border of the gluteus maximus muscle, and compares heights. A variation in height may indicate the influence of habitual patterns, postural imbalances, leg length differences, neurologic dysfunction, or other factors.

2. **Other findings:** The physician may also examine asymmetry of the popliteal creases, greater trochanters of the femurs, medial malleoli, and the medial longitudinal arches of the feet.

MOTION TESTING (STANDING FLEXION TEST)

1. **Technique:**
   a. The physician places his thumbs at the inferior aspect of the PSIS.
   b. The patient is directed to bend forward from the waist and reach with his hands toward his toes, without bending his knees (Fig. 12-11).
   c. As the patient is flexing forward, the physician observes the movement of the PSIS as the ilium moves on the sacrum.
   d. Flexion of the spine carries the base of the sacrum anteriorly and motion is introduced into the sacroiliac joint. A certain amount of play occurs before the movement of the sacrum carries the ilium into anterior rotation, which in turn causes the PSIS to rise superiorly.
   e. Restriction on one side causes the iliosacral joint to lock prematurely on that side, causing the PSIS to elevate sooner and probably farther than the PSIS on the other side. This is considered a positive test result.
   f. A positive test indicates iliosacral somatic dysfunction on the ipsilateral side.

2. **Variations:**
   a. The PSIS may initially be at different heights. Asymmetry may indicate somatic dysfunction but does not determine which side is involved.
   b. Placement of a wooden shim under the foot on the same side as the lower PSIS, until

Figure 12-11. Static examination, standing flexion test.

Figure 12-12. Static examination, seated flexion test.

both PSIS are at the same level, facilitates diagnosis.

c. Proceed with test as outlined above.

Patient Seated—Seated Flexion Test

1. Patient position: seated on a stool, both feet flat on the floor and the arms resting comfortably on the thighs.
2. Physician position: kneeling behind the patient with his eyes at the level of the iliac crests.

MOTION TESTING (SEATED FLEXION TEST)

1. **Technique:**
   a. The physician places his thumbs at the inferior aspect of the PSIS.
   b. The patient is directed to bend forward from the waist and reach toward the floor (Fig. 12-12).
   c. As the patient bends forward, the physician observes the movement of the PSIS, indicating movement of the sacrum on the ilium.
   d. In the seated position the innominate is initially locked in place via the ischial tuberosity. The sacroilial portion of the joint becomes involved as the sacrum engages the ilium, which rotates anteriorly with sacral flexion, elevating the PSIS bilaterally.
   e. Restriction on one side causes the sacroiliac joint to lock prematurely. The ilium and PSIS begin and carry through excursion

sooner and probably farther than on the contralateral side. This is considered a positive test result.

   f. A positive test indicates sacroiliac somatic dysfunction on the ipsilateral side.
2. **Variations:** An uneven PSIS level may be related to such factors as wallets, clothing restriction, twisting of the torso, or other influences.

Patient Supine

1. Patient position: supine.
2. Physician position: varies according to the region examined.

STATIC EXAMINATION

1. Pubic tubercles
   a. The pubic tubercles are located on the anterior superior aspects of the pubic bones (Fig. 12-13). The pubic symphysis is located medially.
   b. The patient is more comfortable if he voids before the examination.
   c. The physician places the palm of one hand flat on the patient's lower abdomen.
   d. The physician gently slides this hand downward until the pubic bones are located.
   e. The tubercle positions are located by

Figure 12-13. Location of pubic tubercles.

Figure 12-14. Relationship of anterior superior iliac spines to other pelvic structures.

Anterior superior iliac spines

Pubic tubercles

Ischeal tuberosities

placing the pads of the index fingers gently on the cephalic aspect.

f. The physician brings his eyes directly over the pubic region and evaluates the position of his index fingers relative to each other.

g. Asymmetry of position indicates a pubic dysfunction. The diagnosis is named according to the side on which the standing flexion test is positive, and according to the relative position of the pubic tubercle involved.

2. Anterior superior iliac spines (ASIS)

a. The ASIS is a bony protuberance on the anterior portion of the ilium (Fig. 12-14).

b. The physician places the pads of his thumbs under the ASIS bilaterally.

c. With his eyes directly over the pelvic region, the physician evaluates the position of the ASIS (superior/inferior, ventral/dorsal) relative to each other.

d. Asymmetry of position may indicate ilial dysfunction. The diagnosis is named according to the side on which the standing flexion test is positive.

3. Medial malleoli

a. The physician stands at the foot of the table and places his thumbs under the distal ledge of the medial malleoli (Fig. 12-15).

b. The physician evaluates the relative positions of the malleoli (caudal/cephalad).

c. The side of the dysfunction is determined by the side of the positive standing flexion test.

MOTION TESTING

1. Innominate (ilial) rocking

a. The physician stands on the side of the table, facing toward the patient's head.

b. The physician places his thenar and hypothenar eminences against the ASIS.

c. A gentle but firm rocking motion against the ASIS is directed along planes that are roughly sagittal (Fig. 12-16). Each ASIS should be examined alternately.

d. The physician allows the ilia to recoil anteriorly against gentle pressure.

e. Ease of motion in anterior and posterior directions is noted as the innominates are rocked.

Figure 12-15. Medial malleoli.

Figure 12-16. Innominate rocking.

Figure 12-17. Hip flexion with external rotation and extension of the hip and knee.

Figure 12-18. Hip flexion with internal rotation and extension of the hip and knee.

f. The diagnosis is made by noting the resistance to motion.
2. Iliosacral dysfunction: Leg lengthening or shortening
  a. The physician stands at the foot of the table.
  b. The patient flexes his knees and places his feet flat on the table.
  c. The patient elevates his buttocks off the table, then lowers them onto the table.
  d. The physician extends the patient's legs to their full length and notes the relative position of the medial malleoli.
  e. The physician then:

    i. Fully flexes one of the patient's hips and knees.
    ii. Externally rotates and abducts the hip (Fig. 12-17).
    iii. Firmly extends the patient's leg.
    iv. Compares the change in position of the ipsilateral medial malleolus in relation to the contralateral medial malleolus.
    v. Fully flexes the ipsilateral hip and knee.
    vi. Internally rotates and adducts the hip (Fig. 12-18).
    vii. Firmly extends the patient's leg.
    viii. Compares the change in position of the

ipsilateral medial malleoli relative to each other.

  ix. Repeats the procedure for the other leg.

f. The physician notes the total excursion of each medial malleolus during the procedure.

g. A smaller amplitude of malleolar excursion on one side indicates dysfunction of the iliosacral joint on that side.

  Note: The physician should flex both sides equally. Inequality of motion testing may produce erroneous results.

i. The action of flexion, along with internal/external rotation, changes the orientation of the ilium relative to the sacrum if there is no restriction. Extension maintains this change in relationship. If the iliosacral joint is restricted, hip flexion induces posterior rotation of the ilium, which causes posterior movement of the sacral base. Little or no change occurs at the joint, as indicated by the small total excursion of the medial malleolus.

Patient Prone

1. Patient position: prone.
2. Physician position: varies according to the region examined.

STATIC EXAMINATION

1. Posterior superior iliac spines
   a. The physician stands at the side of the table and faces toward the patient's head.
   b. The physician places his thumbs on the inferior slope of each PSIS and, viewing them directly from above, notes their relative orientation (superior/inferior, ventral/dorsal).
   c. The dysfunction is named according to the side on which the standing flexion test is positive.
2. Sacral sulci
   a. The physician stands at the side of the table and faces toward the patient's head.
   b. The physician places his thumbs on each PSIS.
   c. The physician hooks his thumbs medially along the PSIS and into the sacral sulci (Fig. 12-19).
   d. The physician evaluates the relative depth of the sulci by two means:

Figure 12-19. Position for evaluating sacral sulci.

Figure 12-20. Position for evaluating inferior lateral angles.

  i. By palpating the depth of each sulcus by thumb position.

  ii. By lowering his eyes to the level of the sulci for visual evaluation of depth.

3. Inferior lateral angles
   a. The inferior lateral angles are bony protuberances located lateral to the sacral hiatus. They outline the inferior lateral aspect of the sacrum.
   b. The physician may locate the inferior lateral angles by palpating down the length of the sacral crest to the hiatus and then moving his thumbs laterally to the inferior lateral angles (Fig. 12-20).
   c. The position of the inferior lateral angles may be evaluated in two orientations:
     i. Posterior/anterior
       (a) The physician places his thumbs on the surface of the sacrum at the inferior lateral angles.

Figure 12-21. Evaluation of medial malleoli, patient prone.

Figure 12-22. Sacral motion testing, patient prone.

(b) He lowers his eyes to the level of the sacrum.

(c) The relative positions of inferior lateral angles are described as anterior or posterior.

   ii. Superior/inferior

     (a) The physician places his thumbs along the lower edges of the inferior lateral angles.

     (b) He views the sacrum from above.

     (c) The positions are described as superior or inferior.

       Note: Because of sacral structure and the types of movement available, the inferior lateral angles exhibit pairing in these positions: **posterior and inferior,** and **anterior and superior.**

4. Medial malleoli

  a. The physician places his thumbs on the underside of the medial malleoli and evaluates their relative position (Fig. 12-21).

  b. Asymmetry of the malleoli is named according to the side on which the standing flexion test is positive.

MOTION TESTING

1. Sacral mobility

  a. The physician stands at the side of the table and faces toward the patient's head.

  b. The physician places his palms on the patient's inferior lateral angles and the fingertips at the sacral sulci (Fig. 12-22).

  c. The physician directs a force cephalad from the inferior lateral angles into the sacroiliac joint on the same side. Force should not be directed obliquely as this may give erroneous findings.

  d. A positive test indicating dysfunction consists of a decrease in joint play on one or both sides and restriction of sacral motion.

2. Spring test

  a. The physician stands at the side of the table facing across the patient's body.

  b. The physician places his hands transversely across the patient's lumbar spine.

  c. Gentle pressure is exerted downward through the lumbar spine (Fig. 12-23).

Figure 12-23. Spring test, patient prone.

d. A positive test consists of a steel-like resistance to the exerted force. In a normal response some play is transmitted through the spine.

3. Sacral mobility, respiratory motion
   a. The physician stands at the side of the table facing across the table.
   b. The physician's cephalad hand is placed over the sacrum with the thenar and hypothenar eminences at the sacral base and the fingertips at the apex. The other hand is placed over the first hand. The physician should stand comfortably with elbows flexed (Fig. 12-24).
   c. The patient takes a deep breath. The sacral base moves posteriorly in response to inspiration.
   d. The physician monitors sacral motion during exhalation, with attention to asymmetric movement.

Figure 12-24. Test for sacral mobility during respiration.

ILIOSACRAL SOMATIC DYSFUNCTION DIAGNOSIS
Michael J. DiGiovanna

Somatic dysfunction at the sacroiliac joint can occur through one of two general mechanisms. A force can be exerted on the sacroiliac joint cephalad through a lower extremity, in which case the dysfunction is termed *iliosacral*. The dysfunctional force can also be exerted on the sacroiliac joint caudad through the spine, in which case the dysfunction is termed *sacroiliac*. The dysfunctions considered in this section are related to the iliosacral mechanism of injury and therefore are dysfunctions of the ilium moving on the sacrum, whereby the sacrum becomes a fixed point.

Primary iliosacral somatic dysfunctions are classified according to a system in which dysfunction is defined as unopposed freedom of motion in one of the planes of motion of the ilia moving on the sacrum. The ilium moving on the sacrum produces anterior and posterior rotation of the ilium about a slightly oblique axis (poste-

rior to anterior, medial to lateral) that passes approximately through the ipsilateral S2 vertebral foramen, a small amount of superior and inferior glide, and anterior and posterior glide along approximately sagittal planes. The dysfunctions that arise in ilial motion on the sacrum therefore are anterior and posterior rotation dysfunctions, and superior and inferior innominate shear dysfunctions.

One other problem that must be sought at the time of evaluation for iliosacral somatic dysfunction is the short leg syndrome. Although short leg syndrome may be of congenital, traumatic, or postoperative origin and thus not a true somatic dysfunction, it can cause a wide variety of iliosacral and sacroiliac somatic dysfunctions. The diagnostic tests used during the physical examination are similar to those used for iliosacral diagnosis, and may be employed here. These tests were described in the previous section.

Some iliosacral somatic dysfunctions are due to various injuries or chronic conditions. The shear phenomenon, specifically superior, has occasionally been related to falls in which the individual lands on one ischial tuberosity or leg. The upwardly directed force is sufficient to induce an iliosacral somatic dysfunction.

Determination of Iliosacral Somatic Dysfunction

The first step in the evaluation of iliosacral somatic dysfunction is to determine if such a dysfunction is present. The test used to determine the presence of iliosacral somatic dysfunction is the standing flexion test. This test was outlined earlier in this chapter (see Examination and Motion Testing). If positive, it should determine not only the presence of iliosacral somatic dysfunction but also the side of the dysfunction. Many of the tests described in this section can lead to one of two diagnoses; a positive standing flexion test will determine the side of the dysfunction.

If the iliac crests are of different height, the short leg syndrome should be considered, whether or not the standing flexion test is positive. If the anterior and posterior superior iliac spines (ASIS, PSIS) are more inferior on the same side as the inferior iliac crest, an even stronger suspicion of short leg syndrome should exist. Similar findings may be noted in cases of innominate shear.

A short leg can arise not only from differences in length between the femurs and tibias, but also from knee, ankle, and foot problems. Apparent differences in leg length may also be due to muscle imbalance, so a course of stretching and relaxation of the muscles likely to have an impact on leg length should be employed. In addition, ilial rotations may give rise to apparent leg length differences. These observations underscore the importance of correcting all somatic dysfunctions and musculoskeletal imbalances before diagnosing short leg syndrome. A more definitive diagnosis can be made with standing postural radiography. Treatment of short leg syndrome may be necessary to prevent further recurrence of existing iliosacral or sacroiliac somatic dysfunctions.

Criteria for Diagnosing Iliosacral Somatic Dysfunctions

1. Anterior ilial rotation
   a. PSIS: higher on involved side.
   b. ASIS: lower on involved side.
   c. Sacral sulcus: appears shallower on ipsilateral side.
   d. Standing flexion test: positive on ipsilateral side.
   e. Leg may appear longer on ipsilateral side.
   f. Sacral inferior lateral angles appear even.
2. Posterior ilial rotation
   a. PSIS: lower on involved side.
   b. ASIS: higher on involved side.
   c. Sacral sulcus: appears deeper on ipsilateral side.
   d. Standing flexion test: positive on ipsilateral side.
   e. Leg may appear shorter on ipsilateral side.
   f. Sacral inferior lateral angles appear even.
3. Superior innominate shear
   a. PSIS: higher on involved side.
   b. ASIS: higher on involved side.
   c. Sacral sulci: approximately equal depth.
   d. Standing flexion test: positive on ipsilateral side.
   e. Leg may appear shorter on ipsilateral side.
   f. Sacral inferior lateral angles appear even.
4. Inferior innominate shear
   a. PSIS: lower on involved side.
   b. ASIS: lower on involved side.
   c. Sacral sulci: approximately equal depth.
   d. Standing flexion test: positive on ipsilateral side.
   e. Leg may appear longer on ipsilateral side.
   f. Sacral inferior lateral angles appear even.

SACROILIAC SOMATIC DYSFUNCTION DIAGNOSIS
Michael J. DiGiovanna

The various methods of diagnosing sacroiliac somatic dysfunction can be categorized according to the physiologic motions of the sacroiliac articulation. These motions are the following:

1. **Flexion:** the sacral base moves anteriorly (Fig. 12-25A).
2. **Extension:** the sacral base moves posteriorly (Fig. 12-25C).
   Flexion and extension occur about an axis perpendicular to the sagittal plane.
3. **Rotation:** the sacrum rotates around a vertical axis perpendicular to the horizontal plane (Fig. 12-26).

4. **Lateral flexion:** the sacrum rotates around an anteroposterior axis perpendicular to the coronal plane (Fig. 12-27).
   Somatic dysfunction can occur in any one or a combination of these motions.
5. **Torsional motion** around diagonal axes, either forward or backward. By definition, a left diagonal axis runs from the superior end of the left articulation to the inferior end of the right articulation. A right diagonal axis runs from the superior end of the right articulation to the inferior end of the left articulation (Fig. 12-28).
   The sacrum may rotate forward on the left axis (left on left torsion) or backward (right on left torsion). It may rotate forward on the right axis (right on right torsion) or backward (left on right torsion) (Fig. 12-29).

Figure 12-25. Flexion and extension of the sacrum. (**A**) Flexion. (**B**) neutral, (**C**) extension.

Flexion

Extension

A   B   C

Figure 12-26. Rotation of the sacrum.

Figure 12-27. Lateral flexion of the sacrum.

Figure 12-28. Torsional axes.

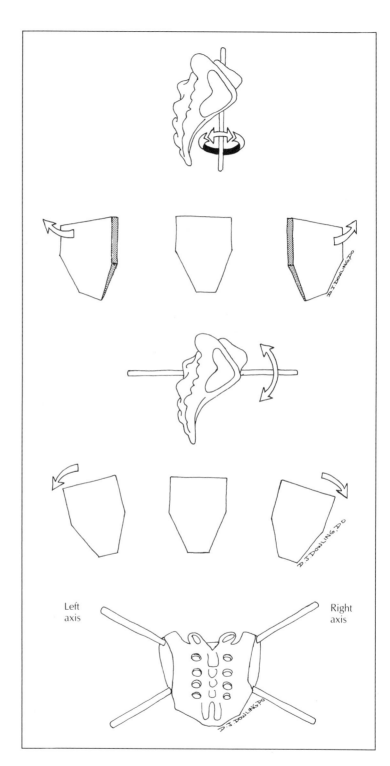

Diagnostic Test for Sacroiliac Somatic Dysfunctions

1. **Seated flexion test**
   a. **Interpretation:** The posterior superior iliac spine (PSIS) on the side of the dysfunction rises higher than the PSIS on the contralateral side. This test differentiates sacroiliac from iliosacral dysfunctions.
2. **Palpation of sacral sulci**
   b. **Interpretation:** The thumb that depresses further into the sacral sulcus indicates the side of the deep sacral sulcus.
3. **Palpation of inferior lateral angles (ILAs)**
   a. **Interpretation:** The side on which the physician's thumb is more posterior, according to palpation and visual observation, is the posterior inferior lateral angle. The more inferior ILA may be determined in similar fashion. Because of sacral biomechanics, the more posterior inferior lateral angle will also be the more inferior.
4. **Lumbar spring test:** Spring is defined as any amount of give in the forward direction, or as the lumbar vertebrae moving into extension. A positive test result is defined as no spring in the lumbar spine in the setting of a backward sacral torsion.

Findings on the above tests are written down in the order in which the tests were performed. The findings can then be more easily used to adduce the somatic dysfunction.

Types of Dysfunctions

1. Forward sacral torsions (see Fig. 12-29A & D)
   a. Left on left sacral torsion
   b. Right on right sacral torsion
2. Backward sacral torsions (see Fig. 12-29B & C)
   a. Left on right sacral torsion
   b. Right on left sacral torsion
3. Unilateral sacral flexions
   a. Left unilateral sacral flexion
   b. Right unilateral sacral flexion
4. Bilateral sacral flexion dysfunction
5. Bilateral sacral extension dysfunction

To diagnose a sacral somatic dysfunction on this list, the physician must adhere to a particular set of criteria. These criteria will be described below in terms of the anatomic nature of the dysfunction that leads to the diagnostic findings.

SACRAL TORSION

Sacral torsions occur around an oblique axis (see Fig. 12-29). In naming a sacral torsion, the direction of rotation of the side of the sacral base that undergoes motion is designated first, followed by the axis around which the torsional motion occurs.

The direction of rotation on axis torsions may be forward or backward. A forward sacral torsion is either a left on left or a right on right sacral torsion. These are considered forward torsions in that one side of the sacral base moves anteriorly. In a backward sacral torsion, one side of the sacral base moves posteriorly, producing either a left on right or a right on left sacral torsion. In sacral torsions, the direction of rotation will cause a slight amount of side bending in the same direction as rotation.

Forward Sacral Torsions

In forward sacral torsions, the sides of the deep sacral sulcus and the inferior/posterior inferior lateral angles are opposite and the lumbar spring test is negative (a good amount of spring is present in the lumbar spine). Since the base of the sacrum is moving forward (anteriorly), no locking of the lumbar vertebrae occurs; hence the negative lumbar spring test.

1. **Left on left sacral torsion**
   Deep sulcus: right.
   PSIS: even.
   Inferior/posterior ILA: left.
   Seated flexion test: positive right.
   Sacral restriction: right.
   Sacral mobility: right base anterior and to the left.
2. **Right on right sacral torsion**
   Deep sulcus: left.
   PSIS: even.
   Inferior/posterior inferior lateral angle: right.
   Seated flexion test: positive left.
   Sacral restriction: left.
   Sacral mobility: left base anterior and to the right.

Figure 12-29. Sacral torsion. (**A**) Left rotation of sacrum on left oblique axis, (**B**) Right rotation of sacrum on left oblique axis, (**C**) Left rotation of sacrum on right oblique axis, and (**D**) Right rotation of sacrum on right oblique axis.

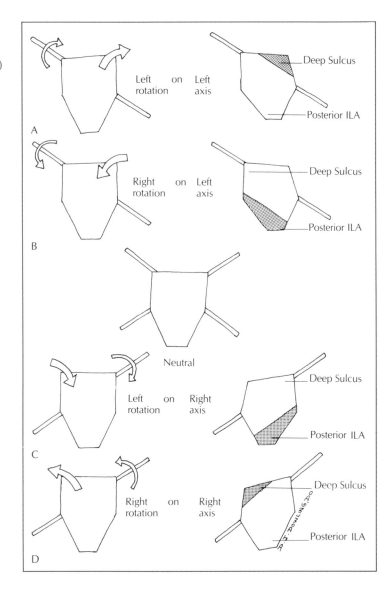

Backward Sacral Torsions

In backward sacral torsions the sides of the deep sacral sulcus and the inferior/posterior inferior lateral angles are opposite and the lumbar spring test is positive. There is little or no spring in the lumbar spine, owing to the locking that has occurred with the sacral base moving backward and engaging the lumbar verbebrae.

1. **Left on right sacral torsion**
   PSIS: even.
   Deep sulcus: right.
   Inferior/posterior ILA: left.
   Sacral restriction: left.
   Sacral mobility: left base posterior and to the left.

2. **Right on left sacral torsion**
   PSIS: even.
   Deep sulcus: left.
   Inferior/posterior ILA: right.
   Seated flexion test: positive right.
   Sacral restriction: left.
   Sacral mobility: right base posterior and to the right.

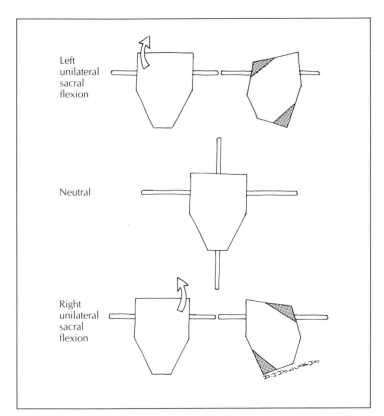

Figure 12-30. Unilateral sacral flexion.

UNILATERAL SACRAL FLEXIONS

In a unilateral sacral flexion the sacrum rotates around a midsagittal axis, with side bending occurring in the opposite direction. The side of the deep sacral sulcus is ordinarily the same side as the inferior/posterior inferior lateral angle. The lumbar spring test is negative (good motion) (Fig. 12-30).

1. **Left unilateral sacral flexion**
   Deep sulcus: left.
   Inferior/posterior ILA: left.
   Seated flexion test: positive left.
   Sacral restriction: left.
   Sacral mobility: left base anterior.
2. **Right unilateral sacral flexion**
   Deep sulcus: right.
   Inferior/posterior ILA: right.
   Seated flexion test: positive right.
   Sacral restriction: right.
   Sacral mobility: right base anterior.

BILATERAL SACRAL DYSFUNCTIONS

In bilateral sacral dysfunctions, the dysfunction occurs in one of the normal motions of the sacrum, flexion or extension. There is no difference in the depth of the sacral sulci or in the level of the inferior lateral angles. The amplitude of motion is decreased in the direction opposite to the dysfunction (Figs. 12-31, 12-32).

1. **Bilateral sacral flexion dysfunction**
   Sacral motion is decreased bilaterally on motion testing.
   The sacrum flexes but is restricted in extension.
   The lumbar spring test is normal, since flexion (anterior motion) of the sacrum does not lock the lumbar vertebrae.
   Seated flexion is symmetrically positive.
2. **Bilateral sacral extension dysfunction**
   Sacral motion is decreased bilaterally on motion testing.
   The lumbar spring test is positive, since extension (backward motion) of the sacrum does lock the lumbar vertebrae.

Figure 12-31. Bilateral sacral flexion dysfunction.

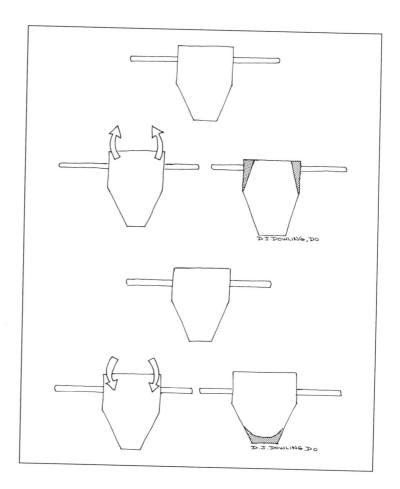

Figure 12-32. Bilateral sacral extension dysfunction.

PUBIC SOMATIC DYSFUNCTION DIAGNOSIS
Michael J. DiGiovanna

Somatic dysfunctions that occur at the pubic symphysis may be either primary pubic dysfunctions or secondary to ilial dysfunctions. Although pain is usually a poor indicator of dysfunction, the pubic symphysis is one area where pain is a fairly reliable indicator. Patients with primary or secondary pubic dysfunctions will present with midline groin pain. Other, nonmusculoskeletal causes of pain such as urinary tract infections and inguinal hernias must be ruled out.

Four dysfunctions are possible at the pubic symphysis: superior pubes, inferior pubes, abducted pubes, and adducted pubes. The last two dysfunctions are also known as an open pubic dysfunction and a closed pubic dysfunction, respectively. The distinction as to whether one pube is inferior or the other pube is superior is made on the standing flexion test. This test determines the side of the dysfunction, defined as the side on which the posterior superior iliac spine rides superiorly with trunk flexion.

Interpretation of Palpatory Findings

With the index finger in the midline over the pubic symphysis, the physician looks for the normal space between the pubic rami. If the space appears larger than normal, a pubic abduction (opened) dysfunction is present. If the space between the pubic rami appears narrower than normal, a pubic adduction (closed) dysfunction is present. Only through the experience of multiple palpations of pubic symphyses can appreciation of the normal width of the pubic symphysis be obtained.

With the index fingers on the pubic tubercles, the physician assesses the cephalic-caudal relationship of each to the other. The diagnosis is based on the results of the standing flexion test. If the standing flexion test is positive on one side and that same side appears to have a pubic ramus lower than the other, an inferior pubic dysfunction is present. Conversely, if a pubic ramus appears more cephalad on the same side as the standing flexion test, a superior pubic dysfunction is present.

References

Bourdillon JF. 1987. A torsion free approach to the pelvis. Manual Med 3(1):20–23.

Dowling DJ. 1985. An Illustrated Guide to OMT of the Neck and Trunk. Self-published.

Fryette HH. 1959. Principles of Osteopathic Technic. Carmel, CA: Academy of Applied Osteopathy.

Greenman PE. 1986. Innominate shear dysfunction in the sacroiliac syndrome. Manual Med 2:114–121.

Kapandji IA. 1974. The Physiology of the Joints. Vol III. The Trunk and Vertebral Column. New York: Churchill Livingstone.

Kappler, Robert. 1975. Lecture notes. Chicago: College of Osteopathic Medicine.

Kennedy, Hall. 1975. Unilateral sacroiliac dysfunction. 1975 Yearbook of Selected Osteopathic Papers. Ed: Ruth Hewitt. Colorado Springs: American Academy of Osteopathy.

Kidd R. 1988. Pain localization with the innominate up slip dysfunction. Manual Med 3(3):103–105.

Larson NJ. 1984. Physiologic movement of the Sacrum. Read before the Chicago College of Osteopathic Medicine, February 1984

Mitchell FL. 1965. Structural pelvic function. 1965 Year Book of Selected Osteopathic Papers, Vol II, pp. 178–199. M. Barnes, Ed. Carmel, CA: Academy of Applied Osteopathy.

Mitchell FL Jr, Moran PS, Pruzzo NT. 1979. An Evaluation and Treatment Manual of Osteopathic Muscle Energy Procedures. Valley Park, Mo: Mitchell, Moran, and Pruzzo Associates.

Moore KL. 1980. Clinically Oriented Anatomy. Baltimore: Williams & Wilkins.

Northup TL. 1943. Sacroiliac lesions primary & secondary. Academy of Applied Osteopathy Year Book, 1943–44. pp 53–54. Ann Arbor: Academy of Applied Osteopathy.

Schiowitz S, DiGiovanna EL, Ausman PJ. 1983. An Osteopathic Approach to Diagnosis and Treatment. Old Westbury, NY: New York College of Osteopathic Medicine.

Schwab WA. 1965. Principles of manipulative treatment: The low back problems. Academy of Applied Osteopathy 1965 Yearbook of Selected Osteopathic Papers, Vol II, pp. 65–69. M. Barnes, Ed. Carmel, CA: Academy of Applied Osteopathy.

Sutherland WG. 1936. The Cranial Bowl. Mankato, MN: Free Press Co.

Warwick R, Williams PL. 1973. Gray's Anatomy, 35th British Edition. Philadelphia: W.B. Saunders Co.

13

Treating Dysfunctions of the Innominate

MUSCLE ENERGY TECHNIQUES FOR ILIAC DYSFUNCTIONS
Lisa R. Chun

This section describes muscle energy techniques for anterior and posterior iliac dysfunctions and for superior and inferior innominate shear.

Anterior Iliac Dysfunction

1. Patient position: prone; the hip and knee on the ipsilateral side of the dysfunction are flexed and hanging off the edge of the table.
2. Physician position: standing on the same side of the table as the dysfunction, facing the patient. The physician supports the patient's flexed leg by placing the sole of the patient's foot against the physician's extended leg.
3. Hand position: one hand monitors the dysfunctional sacroiliac joint while also stabilizing the sacrum. The other hand grasps and supports the patient's flexed knee.
4. **Technique:**
   a. The physician flexes both the hip and the leg on the side of the dysfunction until motion is felt at the sacroiliac joint. This position is maintained by the physician.
   b. The patient is instructed to attempt to straighten the flexed leg by pushing the sole of the foot into the physician's extended leg, using five to ten pounds of force.

c. The physician resists this motion, causing a static contraction (Fig. 13-1).
d. After 3 to 5 seconds, the patient is instructed to stop the attempt and relax.
e. The physician allows the patient to relax, while supporting the lower extremity.
f. Once the tissue under the monitoring finger is relaxed, the physician engages the new motion barrier by flexing both the hip and the leg on the dysfunctional side until motion is felt at the involved sacroiliac joint.
g. Repeat steps b through f twice more.
h. The physician places the flexed lower extremity into a neutral midline position.
i. The physician reevaluates the dysfunction.
j. Treatment may be repeated if indicated.

Posterior Iliac Dysfunction

1. Patient position: prone, with extended lower extremities on the table.
2. Physician position: standing on the side of the table opposite the dysfunction, facing the patient.
3. Hand position: cephalic hand monitors the dysfunctional sacroiliac joint while stabilizing

Figure 13-1. Muscle energy technique for anterior iliac dysfunction, patient prone.

Figure 13-2. Muscle energy technique for posterior iliac dysfunction, patient prone.

the patient's ilium. The caudal hand grasps the patient's leg above the knee on the dysfunctional side.

4. **Technique:**
   a. The physician engages the restricted motion barrier by extending the lower extremity on the dysfunctional side until motion is felt at the sacroiliac joint.
   b. The physician maintains this position.
   c. The patient is instructed to attempt to bring the extended lower extremity down toward the table, using five to ten pounds of force.
   d. The physician resists this motion, causing a static contraction (Fig. 13-2).
   e. After 3 to 5 seconds, the patient is instructed to stop the attempt and to relax.
   f. The physician allows the patient to relax while maintaining the extension of the lower extremity.
   g. Once tissue of the sacroiliac joint is felt to loosen, the physician engages the new motion barrier by repositioning the involved lower extremity into extension until motion is felt at the dysfunctional sacroiliac joint.
   h. Steps b through g are repeated twice more.
   i. The physician places the extended lower extremity into a neutral midline position.
   j. The physician reevaluates the status of the dysfunction.
   k. Treatment may be repeated if indicated.

Superior Innominate Shear

1. Patient position: supine, with lower extremities extended and resting on the table.

2. Physician position: standing at the foot of the table, facing the patient.
3. Hand position: both hands grasping the distal portions of the tibia and fibula on the side of the dysfunction proximal to the ankle joint.
4. **Technique:**
   a. The physician abducts and extends the involved lower extremity until the loose-packed position of the sacroiliac joint is identified.
   b. The physician maintains this position.
   c. The physician internally rotates the involved lower limb until a close-packed position of the hip joint is felt by the physician.
   d. The physician applies a continuous long axis traction on the involved lower limb while maintaining the lower limb in extension, abduction, and internal rotation (Fig. 13-3).
   e. The patient is instructed to breathe deeply three or four times while the physician maintains traction on the lower limb position.
   f. After three or four complete respirations, the patient is instructed to cough forcibly, at which time the physician tugs sharply along the long axis of the involved limb.
   g. The physician places the involved limb into a neutral midline position.
   h. The physician reevaluates the status of the dysfunction.
   i. Treatment may be repeated if indicated.

Figure 13-3. Muscle energy technique for superior innominate shear.

Figure 13-4. Muscle energy technique for inferior innominate shear.

Inferior Innominate Shear

1. Patient position: lateral recumbent, with dysfunctional side up. The ipsilateral lower extremity, as the dysfunction, is flexed and placed on the physician's shoulder.
2. Physician position: sitting on the table behind the patient.
3. Hand position: one hand placed on both the pubic and ischial rami of the dysfunctional side, the other hand placed on both the ischial tuberosity and the posterior inferior iliac spine of the dysfunctional side.
4. **Technique:**
   a. With the patient relaxed, the physician laterally distracts the innominate bone.
   b. Maintaining this position, the physician then applies a cephalad force upon the pubic and ischial rami, ischial tuberosity, and posterior inferior iliac spine of the dysfunctional side (Fig. 13-4).
   c. The physician then instructs the patient to inhale deeply and exhale completely.
   d. The physician maintains the cephalad force, on the distracted innominate during the inspiratory phase of the patient's respiratory cycle.
   e. During the expiratory phase of the patient's respiratory cycle, the physician increases the cephalad force on the distracted innominate.
   f. Steps c through e are repeated twice more.
   g. The physician slowly releases the innominate and positions the patient's involved leg into a neutral midline position.
   h. The physician reevaluates the status of the dysfunction.
   i. Treatment may be repeated if indicated.

HIGH VELOCITY, LOW AMPLITUDE THRUSTING TECHNIQUES FOR ILIAC DYSFUNCTIONS
Barry Erner

This section describes high velocity, low amplitude thrusting techniques for dysfunctions of the posterior and anterior iliac. The patient assumes a lateral recumbent position with the side of dysfunction facing up or down.

Posterior Ilial Somatic Dysfunction

1. Patient position: lateral recumbent position with somatic dysfunctional side facing up.
2. Physician position: standing, facing the front of the patient.
3. **Technique:**
   a. The physician flexes the hip/knee of the patient's superior leg until motion is felt at the lumbosacral angle, then places the foot of this flexed leg in the popliteal fossa of the inferior leg.
   b. Using the patient's lower arm, the physician rotates the patient's torso away from the table until all spinal rotation up to the lumbosacral angle is removed.
   c. The physician places his other forearm over the patient's superior ilium.
   d. The physician exerts a rapid rotational

forward thrust through the dysfunctional ilium (Fig. 13-5).

Anterior Ilial Somatic Dysfunction

1. Patient position: lateral recumbent position with somatic dysfunction side up.
2. Physician position: standing, facing the front of the patient.
3. **Technique:**
   a. The physician flexes the hip of the patient's superior leg until motion is felt at the lumbosacral angle. This leg is then dropped off the table.
   b. The physician rotates the patient's torso by pulling on the lower arm until all spinal rotation up to the lumbosacral angle is removed, then maintains this position with his cephalad arm.
   c. The physician places the forearm of his caudal arm over the patient's superior ilium.
   d. The physician exerts a rapid, rotational, slightly downward thrust through the dysfunctional ilium following the long axis of the femur (Fig. 13-6).

Figure 13-5. High velocity, low amplitude thrusting technique for a posterior ilial somatic dysfunction.

Figure 13-6. High velocity, low amplitude thrusting technique for an anterior ilial somatic dysfunction.

MUSCLE ENERGY TECHNIQUES FOR PUBIC DYSFUNCTIONS
Lisa R. Chun

This section describes muscle energy techniques for treating somatic dysfunctions of the pubes (inferior and superior), and for open (abduction) and closed (adduction) pubic dysfunctions. The patient begins each treatment supine, often with the hips and knees flexed.

Inferior Pubic Dysfunction
1. Patient position: supine; hip and leg on the side of the dysfunction are flexed.
2. Physician position: sitting on or standing at the same side of the table as the dysfunction, facing the patient.
3. Hand position: monitoring finger on the anterior superior iliac spine of the dysfunctional side, other hand placed in a fist (palm up) on the ischial tuberosity of the dysfunctional side. The fist also rests on the table.
4. **Technique:**
   a. The physician places the patient's flexed knee onto the anterior aspect of her shoulder.
   b. The physician flexes the patient's involved hip until motion is felt at the monitoring finger.
   c. The patient is instructed to attempt to straighten the flexed hip using five to ten pounds of force.
   d. The physician resists this force, creating static contraction, while applying a cephalic force on the involved ischial tuberosity with the fist (Fig. 13-7).
   e. After 3 to 5 seconds, the patient is instructed to discontinue the attempt and to relax.
   f. The physician allows the patient to relax, while maintaining both hip flexion and the cephalic force at the ischial tuberosity.
   g. Once the tissue under the physician's monitoring finger is felt to relax, the physician engages the new restricted motion barrier by repositioning the

Figure 13-7. Muscle energy technique for inferior pubic dysfunction.

involved hip into flexion until motion is felt under the monitoring finger.
   h. Steps c through g are repeated twice more.
   i. The physician places the flexed lower extremity into a neutral, mid-line position.
   j. The physician re-evaluates the status of the dysfunction.
   k. Treatment may be repeated if indicated.

Superior Pubic Dysfunction
1. Patient position: supine, lower extremity on side of the dysfunctional side extended and hanging off the edge of the table.
2. Physician position: standing on the same side of the table as the dysfunction, facing the patient. The physician's legs are used to support the patient's hanging leg.
3. Hand position: monitoring finger on the anterior superior iliac spine contralateral to the dysfunctional side, other hand on the thigh of the patient's hanging leg.

Figure 13-8. Muscle energy technique for superior pubic dysfunction.

4. **Technique:**
   a. The physician extends the patient's involved side of the pelvis by pressing down on the patient's thigh.
   b. This extension is created only until motion is felt under the monitoring finger.
   c. The patient is instructed to attempt to raise the extended leg to the ceiling using five to ten pounds of forcè.
   d. The physician resists this force, creating static contraction (Fig. 13-8).
   e. After 3 to 5 seconds, the patient is instructed to stop the attempt and to relax.
   f. The physician allows the patient to relax, while maintaining the same degree of hip extension.
   g. Once the tissue under the monitoring finger is felt to loosen, the physician engages the new motion barrier by repositioning the involved hip into extension until motion is felt under the monitoring finger.
   h. Steps c through g are repeated twice more.
   i. The physician places the extended hip into a neutral position.
   j. The physician reevaluates the status of the dysfunction.
   k. Treatment may be repeated if indicated.

Abduction (Open) Pubic Dysfunction

1. Patient position: supine, hips flexed and knees flexed to 90 degrees; lying closer to one side of the table than the other.
2. Physician position: standing at the side of the table to which patient is closest and facing the patient.
3. **Technique:**
   a. The physician wraps her arms around the patient's flexed knees and draws them against herself.
   b. The patient is instructed to attempt to spread his knees apart with maximal force.
   c. The physician resists this force, creating static contraction.
   d. After 3 to 5 seconds, the patient is instructed to relax.
   e. The physician allows the patient to relax, while maintaining the position attained.
   f. Steps b through e are repeated twice more.
   g. The physician reevaluates the status of the dysfunction.
   h. Treatment may be repeated if indicated.

Adduction (Closed) Pubic Dysfunction

1. Patient position: supine, hips flexed and knees flexed to 90 degrees.
2. Physician position: standing at the side of the table facing the patient.
3. Hand position: the physician's forearm is placed between the patient's knees. One hand is on the medial aspect of one of the patient's knees, with the elbow joint on the medial aspect of the other knee.
4. **Technique:**
   a. The patient is instructed to attempt to bring his knees together with a maximal force.
   b. The physician's forearm resists this attempt by acting as a solid bar.
   c. After 3 to 5 seconds, the patient is instructed to relax.
   d. The physician allows the patient to relax while maintaining the position attained.
   e. Steps a through d are repeated twice more.
   f. The physician reevaluates the status of the dysfunction.
   g. Treatment may be repeated if indicated.

HIGH VELOCITY, LOW AMPLITUDE THRUSTING TECHNIQUES FOR PUBIC DYSFUNCTIONS
Barry Erner

This section describes high velocity, low amplitude thrusting techniques for treating a superior position of the pubic tubercle and pubic restriction.

Superior Pubes
1. Patient position: supine.
2. Physician position: standing at the side of the table, on the same side as the dysfunction.
3. **Technique:**
   a. The physician flexes the patient's knee/hip on the side of the dysfunction and rests the patient's ankle/calf on his shoulder.
   b. The physician makes a tight fist with his treating hand.
   c. The physician places his fist against the ischial tuberosity on the side of the pubic dysfunction.
   d. The physician exerts a rapid cephalad/clockwise thrust through the ischium (Fig. 13-9).

Figure 13-9. HVLA treatment for a superior pubic dysfunction.

Alternate Technique To Treat Pubic Restriction
1. Patient position: supine.
2. Physician position: standing at the side of the table.
3. **Technique:**
   a. The physician flexes, abducts, and externally rotates the patient's legs bilaterally.
   b. The patient's feet are placed with the soles approximated.
   c. The physician exerts a quick downward thrust through the patient's knees bilaterally, symmetrically, and simultaneously (Fig. 13-10).

Figure 13-10. An alternate HVLA treatment technique for pubic restriction.

References
Greenman PE. 1986. Innominate shear dysfunction in the sacroiliac syndrome. Manual Med 2:114–121.

Schiowitz S, DiGiovanna E, Ausman P. 1983. An Osteopathic Approach to Diagnosis and Treatment. Old Westbury, New York: New York College of Osteopathic Medicine of the New York Institute of Technology.

14

Treating Sacral Dysfunctions

MUSCLE ENERGY TECHNIQUES
Lisa R. Chun

This section describes muscle energy techniques for unilateral sacral flexion dysfunctions and dysfunctions of forward and backward sacral torsion.

Unilateral Sacral Flexion Dysfunction
1. Patient position: prone, arms hanging off the sides of the table.
2. Physician position: standing at the same side of the table as the dysfunction.
3. Hand position: the heel of the caudal hand is on the caudal edge of the inferior lateral angle of the sacrum on the side to be treated. The middle or index finger of that hand is placed in the sacral sulcus.
4. **Technique:**
   a. The physician abducts the lower extremity of the involved side until motion is felt at the sacral sulcus being monitored.
   b. The physician maintains the abduction while introducing internal rotation.
   c. Internal rotation is continued until motion is felt at the sacral sulcus being monitored. This position of abduction and internal rotation is maintained.
   d. Using the hand on the patient's sacrum and

an extended elbow, the physician applies a constant force at the posterior inferior lateral angle down toward the table and cephalad (Fig. 14-1). The force applied is more cephalad.
   e. The patient is instructed to inhale deeply and to hold his breath.
   f. The physician increases the pressure on the inferior lateral angle during the inspiratory phase.
   g. The patient is instructed to exhale completely.
   h. The physician maintains the cephalad force on the posterior inferior lateral angle during the expiratory phase.
   i. Steps e through h are repeated twice more.
   j. At the end of the last expiratory phase, an additional cephalad thrust is provided by the physician on the posterior inferior lateral angle.
   k. The physician places the abducted and internally rotated leg into a neutral midline position.
   l. The physician reevaluates the status of the dysfunction.
   m. Treatment may be repeated if indicated.

Figure 14-1. Muscle energy technique for treating unilateral sacral flexion dysfunction.

Figure 14-2. Muscle energy technique for treating forward sacral torsion dysfunction.

Forward Sacral Torsion Dysfunction

1. Patient position: Sims's position (lateral recumbent position with upper torso prone and hips and knees flexed), with the axis of the dysfunction down toward the table. The patient's arms hang off the sides of the table.
2. Physician position: standing at the side of the table facing the patient.
3. Hand position: monitoring finger(s) at the lumbosacral junction. The other hand is used to engage the motion barriers. To facilitate engagement of the restricted motion barriers, the hand monitoring the lumbosacral junction is switched.
4. **Technique:**
   a. The physician flexes the patient's hips until motion is felt at the lumbosacral junction.
   b. The physician maintains this position by leaning into the patient's knees.
   c. The patient is instructed to inhale deeply and exhale completely. During the exhalation, the patient is instructed to reach for the floor with the upper arm.
   d. The physician assists the patient in this rotational move by pressing the patient's shoulder toward the floor until motion is felt at the lumbosacral junction.
   e. To achieve rotation, steps c and d may have to be repeated.
   f. Once rotational motion is felt at the monitoring finger(s), the side bending component of the treatment is engaged by lowering the feet off the table.

   g. While maintaining flexion, the physician, using the patient's knees as a fulcrum, applies downward pressure on the patient's ankle (Fig. 14-2).
   h. The patient's lower legs may have to be side bent over the edge of the table.
   i. Once motion is felt at the lumbosacral junction, the position is maintained.
   j. The patient is instructed to attempt to raise his ankles to the ceiling using five to ten pounds of force.
   k. The physician isometrically resists this attempt.
   l. After 3 to 5 seconds, the patient is instructed to stop the attempt and to relax.
   m. Once the tissue of the lumbosacral junction is felt to loosen, the physician reengages the restricted motion barriers by repeating steps c through j.
   n. Repeat steps k through m twice more.
   o. The physician places the patient into a neutral position.
   p. The physician reevaluates the status of the dysfunction.
   q. Treatment may be repeated if indicated.

Backward Sacral Torsion Dysfunction

1. Patient position: lateral recumbent position with the axis of the dysfunction down toward the table; knees flexed.
2. Physician position: standing at the side of the table facing the patient's anterior.

Figure 14-3. Muscle energy technique for treating backward sacral torsion dysfunction.

3. Hand position: monitoring finger at the lumbosacral junction. The other hand is used to engage the restricted motion barriers. To facilitate engagement of the restricted motion barriers, the hand monitoring the lumbosacral junction is switched during the procedure.
4. **Technique:**
   a. The physician flexes the patient's hips and knees until motion is felt at the monitoring finger(s).
   b. The physician maintains this position by leaning into the patient's upper knee.
   c. The patient is instructed to straighten his lower leg.
   d. The physician hooks the foot of the patient's upper leg onto the straightened lower leg.
   e. While still leaning on the patient's upper knee, the physician moves the patient's lower thigh into extension.
   f. Hip extension is continued until motion is felt at the lumbosacral junction.
   g. The physician maintains this position by placing the forearm of her monitoring hand on the patient's hip.
   h. The physician grasps the lower arm, on which the patient is lying, and pulls directly up toward the ceiling, thereby rotating the patient's torso backward.
   i. The patient is then instructed to reach his top arm behind him and grasp the edge of the table.
   j. The patient is instructed to inhale deeply.

k. The patient is instructed to exhale completely and simultaneously to reach down the edge of the table. At the end of the exhalation, the patient grasps the edge of the table.
   l. The physician may facilitate this motion by pressing the patient's upper shoulder back toward the table and caudad while the patient is exhaling.
   m. For this rotation motion to be felt at the lumbosacral junction, steps k and l may have to be repeated. This is continued only until motion is felt at the monitoring fingers. Once motion is felt, the position is maintained.
   n. Using the patient's upper knee as a fulcrum, the physician lifts the ankle of the upper leg until motion is felt at the lumbosacral junction.
   o. Once motion is felt, this position is maintained.
   p. The patient is instructed to attempt to bring the elevated ankle to the floor using five to ten pounds of force (Fig. 14-3).
   q. The physician isometrically resists this attempt.
   r. After 3 to 5 seconds, the patient is instructed to stop the attempt and to relax.
   s. The physician allows the patient to relax while maintaining the above position.
   t. Once the tissue at the lumbosacral junction is felt to loosen, the physician reengages the restricted motion barriers by repeating steps j through o.
   u. Steps p through t are repeated twice more.
   v. The physician places the patient into a neutral position.
   w. The physician reevaluates the status of the dysfunction.
   x. Treatment may be repeated if indicated.

TECHNIQUE MODIFICATION: BACKWARD SACRAL TORSION DYSFUNCTION
1. Patient position: as above.
2. Physician position: as above.
3. **Technique:**
   a. Steps a through m in the above technique are performed.
   b. The patient is instructed to attempt to push his flexed knee up to the ceiling using five to ten pounds of force.

c. The physician isometrically resists this attempt with her hand on the side of the patient's flexed knee. The physician should feel a contraction under her monitoring fingers. If no contraction is felt, the physician repositions the involved hip and knee using flexion or extension. Once a contraction is felt by the monitoring fingers, the treatment has been localized to the lumbosacral junction.

d. After 3 to 5 seconds, the patient is instructed to stop the attempt and to relax

the involved lower extremity while maintaining the above position.

e. Once the tissue at the lumbosacral junction is felt to loosen, the physician reengages the restricted motion barriers by repeating steps j through m of the previous test.

f. Steps b through e of this section are repeated twice more.

g. The physician places the patient into neutral position.

h. The physician reevaluates the status of the dysfunction.

i. Treatment may be repeated if indicated.

COUNTERSTRAIN TECHNIQUES FOR THE SACRUM AND PELVIS
Eileen L. DiGiovanna

Anterior Tender Points

There are three significant tender points generally related to the pelvis or sacrum: the low ilial sacroiliac tender point, located on the superior surface of the ramus of the pubes; the iliacus tender point, located in the lower quadrant of the abdomen and deep in the fossa (often a tender point of concern in dysmenorrhagic women); and the inguinal ligament tender point, located on the inguinal ligament at its attachment to the pubes. Techniques for treating each of these tender points are described below.

LOW ILIUM SACROILIAC TENDER POINT
1. Patient position: supine.
2. Physician position: standing at either side of the table.
3. **Technique:**
   a. The thigh is flexed to about 40 degrees.
   b. Both thighs may be flexed with the legs resting on the physician's thigh, as in the treatment of the lumbar tender point (Fig. 14-4).

ILIACUS TENDER POINT
1. Patient position: supine.
2. Physician position: standing at the side of the table near the tender point, with one foot on the table.

3. **Technique:**
   a. Both of the patient's legs are flexed with the legs resting on the physician's thigh.
   b. The ankles are crossed and the knees are dropped apart, externally rotating the thighs (Fig. 14-5).

INGUINAL LIGAMENT TENDER POINT
1. Patient position: supine.
2. Physician position: standing at the side of the table opposite the tender point, with her foot on the table.
3. **Technique:**
   a. The patient's legs are flexed and rested on the physician's thigh.
   b. The leg nearest the physician is crossed at the knee over the further leg.
   c. The lower leg is internally rotated by the physician pushing laterally on the ankle (Fig. 14-6).

Posterior Tender Points

The locations of the posterior tender points are shown in Figure 14-7.

PIRIFORMIS TENDER POINT
This is the tender point most commonly associated with sacral dysfunctions and is frequently

Figure 14-4. Counterstrain treatment for a low ilium sacroiliac tender point.

Figure 14-5. Counterstrain treatment for an iliacus tender point.

Figure 14-6. Counterstrain treatment for an inguinal ligament tender point.

involved in sciatic radiation of pain, owing to its close association with the sciatic nerve.

1. Patient position: prone, with involved leg dropped off the side of the table.
2. Physician position: seated at the side of the dysfunction.
3. **Technique:**
   a. The patient's hip and knee are flexed.
   b. The leg is externally rotated and may be rested on the physician's lap (Fig. 14-8).
   c. The movement of flexion and external rotation may be modified to achieve maximal softening of the piriformis.

MIDPOLE SACRAL TENDER POINT

This tender point is palpated by pushing medially on the lateral side of the sacrum at the midpoint.

1. Patient position: prone.
2. Physician position: standing or sitting at the side of the table next to the tender point.
3. **Technique:**
   a. Leg is abducted straight laterally.
   b. Occasionally the thigh must be extended or flexed, although this is not usual (Fig. 14-9).

Figure 14-7. Tender point locations, posterior sacrum and pelvis. *Pir,* piriformis; *MpS,* midpole sacral; *HFOSI,* high flare-out sacroiliac; *LPL5,* lower pole L5; *UPL5,* upper pole L5.

Figure 14-8. Counterstrain treatment for a piriformis tender point.

Figure 14-9. Counterstrain treatment for a midpole sacral tender point.

Figure 14-10. Counterstrain treatment for a high flare-out sacroiliac tender point.

HIGH FLARE-OUT SACROILIAC TENDER POINT

This tender point, about 4 inches below and medial to the PSIS, is frequently associated with coccygodynia.

1. Patient position: prone.
2. Physician position: standing at the side of the table.
3. **Technique:**
   a. The leg nearest the tender point is extended.
   b. Some abduction may be needed, although occasionally adduction with external rotation of the thigh is needed (Fig. 14-10).

HIGH VELOCITY, LOW AMPLITUDE THRUSTING TECHNIQUES
Barry Erner

Anterior Sacral Flexion

1. Patient position: prone.
2. Physician position: standing at the same side of the table as the side of dysfunction.
3. **Technique:**
   a. The physician places the thenar eminence of his treating hand over the inferior lateral angle of the dysfunctional side of the sacrum.
   b. The physician extends and internally rotates the patient's leg on the side of the dysfunction. The leg is then abducted until motion is felt by the palpating hand.
   c. The patient is instructed to take a deep breath and hold it.
   d. The physician exerts a downward pressure over the sacrum at the inferior lateral angle, creating relative extension.
   e. At the end of inspiration, the physician exerts a quick downward thrust with his thenar eminence over the inferior lateral angle (Fig. 14-11).

Figure 14-11. High velocity, low amplitude thrusting technique for anterior sacral flexion dysfunction.

References

Greenman PE. 1986. Innominate shear dysfunction in the sacroiliac syndrome. Manual Med 2:114–121.

Jones L. 1981. *Strain and Counterstrain.* Colorado Springs: American Academy of Osteopathy.

Moran PS, Pruzzo NA, et al. 1973. An Evaluation and Treatment Manual of Osteopathic Manipulative Procedures. Vol I. The Postural Structural Model, and ed. Kansas City: Institute for Continuing Education in Osteopathic Principles.

Schiowitz S, DiGiovanna E, Ausmen P. 1983. An Osteopathic Approach to Diagnosis and Treatment. Old Westbury: New York College of Osteopathic Medicine of the New York Institute of Technology.

15

Locomotion
and Balance

THE FUNCTIONAL, BIOMECHANICAL, AND CLINICAL SIGNIFICANCE OF GAIT
Stanley Schiowitz

The first scientific observations of gait were probably made by Hippocrates and Aristotle. As clinicians, we continue that tradition by observing patients walking every day and by selecting certain characteristics for assessment.

The examiner focuses on asymmetric movement while viewing the patient from the front, side, or back. Asymmetric movements are characterized by reduced or excessive displacements or by a change in the speed of movement during parts of the gait cycle. Asynchronous movement in the sagittal plane is best observed from the side, while coronal plane dysfunction is best observed from the front or rear.

To use gait fully as a diagnostic tool, the clinician should be aware of the patient's normal gait parameters—his usual speed, step length, and step rate. A variation in any one of these parameters will affect the others.

Kinematics of Gait
Physiologic, efficient locomotion entails translation of the body's center of gravity through space along a path requiring the least expenditure of energy. The center of gravity is constantly being dis-

placed beyond the body's base of support. The resulting loss of balance is corrected by moving one lower extremity forward to change the base of support. Repetition of this pattern on alternating legs creates the walking cycle.

The normal walking cycle is divided into two phases—stance phase, when the foot is on the ground, and swing phase, when it is moving forward. Sixty percent of the normal cycle is spent in stance phase. Of this 60%, 25% is in double stance. The remaining 40% of the walking cycle is in swing phase.

Stance phase is divided into the following segments: heel strike, foot flat, midstance, and push-off or toe-off. Swing phase is divided into acceleration, midswing, and deceleration.

The average width of the base of gait, as measured from heel to heel, is between two and four inches. The average length of a step is 15 inches, with a cadence of 90 to 120 steps per minute. The feet are usually in slight abduction.

The forces acting in gait are gravity, muscle contraction, and momentum. Muscle contraction generally initiates motion; gravity and momentum then add their contributions. According to Winter and Robertson, during swing phase, gravity, muscle contraction, and knee acceleration cause the shank to rotate. In the first half of the swing, gravity and momentum contribute 80% of the force, while in the second half of the swing, muscles contribute 80% of the force.

The counterpressure of the ground against the feet is the force that propels the body. We are not usually aware of the earth's thrust. However, in soft snow, sand, or mud this thrust is reduced, necessitating increased muscular activity and energy used to maintain forward locomotion. Friction between the foot and the ground is essential for transmission of the ground's pressure. The friction must be sufficient to counterbalance the horizontal vector component of force. The greater the horizontal force, the greater is the dependence on friction. The corollary holds true: on icy streets, small, almost vertical steps are taken.

Walking is initiated through the complex interplay of neural mechanisms, muscular activity, and biomechanical forces. The triceps surae relaxes, permitting forward inclination of the body ahead of the center of gravity. The line of the center of gravity, which is midway between the feet and anterior to the ankle joint, moves toward the swing limb in a posterioanterior direction. As the swing limb prepares for toe-off, the center of gravity shifts to the stance side. The weight is balanced on the stance leg to allow forward propulsion of the swing limb.

Both phases of gait are in operation simultaneously, alternating sides at the completion of each cycle. The swing phase leg rotates the pelvis toward the stance side, with concomitant rotation of the spine to the swing side. The hip joint flexes with this swing action. The knee joint flexes during the first half and extends during the second half of swing, while the ankle and foot are dorsiflexed.

On the stance side, the hip joint extends, accompanied by muscular contraction that prevents dropping of the pelvis toward the swing side. The knee joint is in slight flexion at the moment of foot contact, heel strike, after which the knee is extended.

The foot and ankle in this segment, from heel strike to full weight-bearing, is in plantar flexion of the ankle. The foot then converts to a rigid lever for transferring the body weight to the forefoot for push-off. At this time the heel rises rapidly and the foot everts, causing increased external rotation of the leg with hyperextension of the meta-tarsophalangeal joints at the end of the propulsive phase. The clinical significance of the mechanics of the subtalar joint (as used in the stance phase) cannot be overemphasized. The slightest disturbance will cause noticeable dysfunction.

A definite sequence is observed in weight-bearing on the osseous tripod of the foot: the weight passes from the heel to the fifth metatarsal head and then across the metatarsal heads to the big toe. Any change in pressure on one of these points will be accompanied by a change in the normal sequence of motion and weight-bearing at other points. Calluses usually develop at these sites.

The normal walking cycle in the lower extremities is accompanied by regular motions of the shoulders, arms, and head. Their actions are part of any clinical evaluation. When the pelvis on the swing side moves forward, the shoulder on that side drops back. Therefore, the opposite arms and legs swing in tandem.

The action of the arm in the anteroposterior plane reduces rotation of the shoulders, which directly aids in keeping the head forward. Arm swing balances the rotation of the pelvis. These motions are in direct proportion to each other. If the arms do not swing, the upper trunk will rotate in the same direction as the pelvis.

Gait Efficiency

Efficiency of gait can be considered in terms of the translatory movement of the body's center of gravity through a smooth undulating pathway of low amplitude. The center of gravity in the erect, motionless human is just anterior to the second sacral vertebra. In walking it is displaced both vertically and horizontally, describing a sinusoidal curve.

Vertical displacement of the center of gravity occurs twice during the cycle from heel strike to heel strike of the same foot. The total amount of vertical displacement is about 1.8 inches. The summits occur at 25% and 75% of the cycle. At the midpoint of the gait cycle (double weight-bearing), the center of gravity is at its lowest point.

Saunders, Inman, and Eberhart have proposed six major determinants of gait for the maintenance of mechanical efficiency:

1. **Pelvic rotation.** The pelvis rotates on the swing side, approximately 4 degrees on either side of the central axis. Since the pelvis is a semi-rigid structure, this rotation occurs alternately at each hip joint as the hip passes from relative internal rotation to external rotation during stance phase.

2. **Downward pelvic tilt.** The pelvis tilts downward in the coronal plane on the swing side. The alternate angular displacement is 5 degrees at the stance hip joint, creating relative adduction of the extremity in stance and relative abduction in swing.

3. **Knee flexion of the swing leg.**

These three determinants of gait—pelvic rotation, pelvic tilt, and swing knee flexion—all act by flattening the vertical arc through which the center of gravity is moving. Pelvic rotation elevates the extremities of the arc, while pelvic tilt and knee flexion depress its summit.

4., 5. The combined actions of the foot, ankle, and knee of the stance leg constitute the fourth and fifth determinants of gait. These actions help maintain a smooth pathway for the translatory motion of the center of gravity. A first arc occurs at heel strike when the ankle rotates from dorsiflexion to plantar flexion, with the heel functioning as the fulcrum. A second arc occurs with rotation of the foot, with the forepart of the foot functioning as the fulcrum. This occurs with heel rise. Both arcs are accompanied by stance knee flexion, which maintains a level center of gravity.

6. **Displacement of center of gravity.** Displacement of the center of gravity over the weight-bearing extremity aids in maintaining body balance as the swing leg is lifted from the ground. The relative adduction of that hip, along with the tibiofemoral angle, reduces the amount of lateral displacement necessary for balance. The center of gravity deviates laterally about 1¾ inches. Thus, deviation of the center of gravity is almost equivalent in horizontal and vertical planes.

Pelvic Motion

The pelvis is not a rigid structure. It has an anterior articulation at the symphysis pubes and two articulations with the sacrum.

As the pelvis rotates and tilts, a torsional effect develops at the symphysis pubis. This is created because every part of the pelvis is moving at a different linear velocity. Measuring the displacement of rotation and tilt of the lateral edge of the right innominate from the fixed left hip will show that the angular velocity is constant from every part of the left and right innominates, but the linear velocity, and therefore the distance traveled, increases from left to right. Thus, the combined motions of rotation and tilt occur at different speeds of linear displacement for different parts of the pelvis and create a torsion at the symphysis pubis with every step taken.

The sacrum moves with the innominate and undergoes the same rotation, tilt, and lateral shift as does the innominate, but not at the same speed. When swing of the right leg initiates rotation of the right innominate toward the left, with right innominate tilt and left lateral shift, the sacrum will move on its vertical axis and rotate to the left, with right sacral flexion. Simultaneously the center of gravity in the horizontal plane shifts to the left, producing left sacral lateral flexion. The vertical center of gravity moves to the superior pole of the left sacroiliac, locking the articulation into a mechanical position that establishes movement of the sacrum on the left oblique axis. This sets the pattern so the sacrum can torsionally turn to the left (Mitchell, 1965). Walking creates the mechanics of oblique sacral motion without dysfunction, or, in the above example a left on left sacral torsional motion (Fig. 15-1).

During these motions, the lumbar spine rotates to the right and flexes laterally to the left, compensating for the right sacral flexion created by pelvic rotation toward the left with right pelvic tilt.

Asymmetric Motion

In the perfectly balanced, symmetric human, the joint motions of gait have little or no effect on the body's structural integrity. However, asymmetry develops in virtually everyone and causes constant small structural stress situations that can lead to somatic dysfunctions.

What happens to symmetry of gait in short leg syndrome? What happens to the comparative reversals of motions of lumbar rotation and lateral

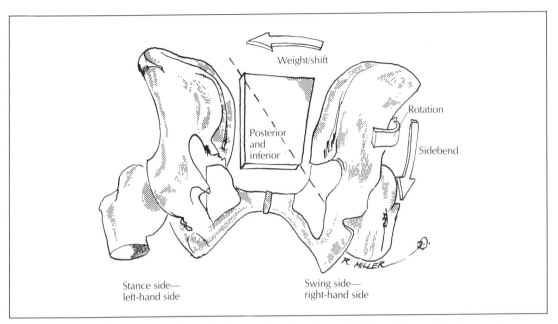

Figure 15-1. Pelvic determinants of normal gait, posterior view. Shown is left on left sacral torsional motion.

flexion if scoliosis is present? Radiographs of patients with low back problems often show lateral flexion, rotation deformity of one lumbar vertebra on the one below it. The intervertebral disk is wedged and spondylytic changes are present, yet the site has not sustained previous specific trauma. This condition is very likely produced by the constant stress of gait on a localized somatic dysfunction.

Structural deformities should be treated, even if asymptomatic, while the subject is young. This will prevent some of the constant microtrauma that occurs with daily locomotion, and will prevent symptomatic dysfunction in later life.

Neurologic Gait Patterns

Analysis of gait is the most important test in neurology and one of the least performed. The following points should be noted in this evaluation: the position of the body, movement of the legs, position and movement of the arms, distance between the feet, both in forward direction (stride) and in lateral direction (width), regularity of movements, ability to walk in a straight line, ease of turning, and ease of stopping. Along with

these observations, the examiner should note any changes in the six major determinants of gait.

Following are descriptions of several neurologic gait patterns.

Hemiplegic gait. In hemiplegic gait the leg is usually stiff, with loss of flexion at the hip and knee joints. The patient leans to the affected side and throws the whole leg outward from the body before bringing it back toward the trunk, producing a circumduction movement. The shoe is dragged against the floor, and there is usually an accompanying affected arm that does not swing but is held in fixed position against the abdomen with the elbow flexed.

High steppage gait. High steppage gait can be divided into two characteristic patterns. In the first pattern the toe touches the floor first, a foot drop due to paralysis of pretibial or peroneal muscles. The leg is raised high by abnormal knee and hip flexion. The toe touches the ground first, followed by a slapping noise as the foot strikes the floor.

In the second pattern the heel touches the floor first, owing to loss of sense of position. The high steppage gait is bilateral, with ataxia and side-to-side reeling. The heel touches the floor first and a stomp of the foot is heard. Romberg's sign is present, caused by a dysfunction of the afferent portion of peripheral nerves or posterior roots.

Carcinoma, diabetic neuropathy, tabes dorsalis, Friedreich's ataxia, subacute combined degeneration of the cord, compression lesions of the posterior columns, and multiple sclerosis that affects the posterior columns may all produce a high steppage gait.

Shuffling gait. Shuffling gait can be described as small, flat-footed shuffling steps; the foot does not clear the ground. In parkinsonism, rigidity, tremor, paucity of movement, shuffling with haste, and difficulty in starting, stopping, or turning are noted. The patient is in flexion, with lack of extension movements at the hips, knees, and elbows. The thorax and pelvis rotate in the same direction in swing phase. The amplitude of vertical excursions of the head is lessened in forward motion. The first noticeable motor signs in parkinsonism may be a nonrhythmic pattern with random or poorly timed activity of the arms in gait.

The shuffling gait seen in arteriosclerosis is due to loss of confidence and equilibrium. The patient stands erect, takes small shuffling steps with a wide base, and seems to stare at a distant point. Turning is achieved through a series of small steps made by one foot, the other foot acting as a pivot.

Ataxic gait. Ataxic gait is a reeling, unsteady gait with a wide base and a tendency to fall toward the side of lesion. Vertigo may accompany ataxia. It may be found in cerebellar disease, multiple sclerosis, and sometimes myxedema. Ataxic gait must be differentiated from drunken and staggering gait, in which the subject reels, totters, tips forward and backward, and may lose balance and fall. This gait is seen in alcohol or barbiturate poisoning, drug reaction, polyneuritis, or general paresis.

Scissors gait. In scissors gait the legs are adducted, crossing alternately in front of one another. Both lower limbs are spastic, and there is spasm of the adductor muscles at the hip joints, often accompanied by pronounced compensatory motions of the trunk and upper extremities. Bilateral upper motor neuron lesions, advanced cervical spondylosis, or multiple sclerosis may produce this gait pattern.

Waddling gait. Waddling gait can be described as rolling from side to side. The pelvic rotation

and tilt on the swing side are increased (penguin walk). Muscular dystrophy with weakness of hips, exaggerated lordosis, and pot-bellied posture can produce this gait.

Hysterical gait. Hysterical gait may simulate any paralysis or may be bizarre. There may be inability to walk, but in bed the subject may lose the characteristic spasticity.

When outlining therapy for the neurologic patient, the clinician must discuss all problems with him. Many of these patients hope that osteopathic manipulation will cure their problems, and they must be advised of the limitations of the expected results. Some have, as a secondary complaint, severe pain and dysfunction of the low back area. These symptoms can be relieved greatly. Some have asymptomatic somatic dysfunctions of the upper cervical vertebrae, which should be treated.

Musculoskeletal Gait Patterns
Several musculoskeletal gait patterns are described below.

Antalgic gait. Antalgic gait is characterized by a short stance phase and a rapidly executed swing phase: the patient tries to avoid standing on a painful extremity. Most musculoskeletal dysfunctions of gait are antalgic. The physician must evaluate where the pain is located. A simple question such as, When you put your weight on that foot, where does it hurt?, may assist in accurate diagnosis.

Gluteus medius gait. A gluteus medius gait is characterized by a shift of the body toward the deficient side, indicating a weakness of that gluteus medius muscle. It can be evaluated by finding a Trendelenburg sign in the upright position.

Gluteus maximus gait. In gluteus maximus deficiency, the trunk and pelvis are hyperextended backward over both hips to maintain the center of gravity behind the involved hip joint.

Short lower extremity. In short lower extremity, the pelvis and trunk depress in stance phase.

Elevated pelvis gait. In elevated pelvis gait, there is a hiking or elevation of the pelvis on the swing side if that hip or knee joint has motion limitation from any cause.

Congenital hip dislocation. Congenital dislocation of the hip creates a waddling gait.

Osteoarthrosis gait. Severe osteoarthrosis of the hip or knee joints will produce the scissors gait.

Foot problems. Any dysfunction of the foot may alter normal mechanics. These could include Morton's foot (neuroma), corns, calluses, bunions, hallux rigidus, plantar warts, or poorly fitting shoes. If plantar flexion is absent, there is no push-off and the heel and forefoot come off the floor together.

Pediatric Gait Patterns

Pediatric musculoskeletal problems should be evaluated and treatment instituted before the onset of weight-bearing. Equinus, calcaneus valgus, pronation, flatfoot, tibial torsion, metatarsal varus, clubfoot, and congenital dislocation of the hips should all be diagnosed and treated properly before the child begins to walk.

In one study, 64% of limping children with no history of gait dysfunction or trauma had primary involvement of the hip joint. Most cases were due to transient synovitis and resolved with rest. Many children with hip-related gait dysfunction have had a recent upper respiratory tract infection. Other causes include osteitis, rheumatic fever, rheumatoid arthritis, and Perthes' disease.

Gait Patterns in Low Back Dysfunction

An initial diagnosis of somatic dysfunction may often be made by evaluating the patient's gait. The most obvious problems are those relating to low back dysfunction.

A psoas dysfunction secondary to lumbar vertebral osteopathic somatic dysfunctions will produce the typical psoatic limp. The patient bends forward and toward the side of the dysfunction, and that hip will be in abduction. The somatic dysfunction is usually found in the upper lumbar area. Neglecting this site and treating the lower back or sacroiliac articulation is usually a futile effort.

Unilateral erector spinae contraction will cause lateral flexion to the side of contraction, scoliosis with convexity to the opposite side, and extension of the spine. The patient walks with a stiff back, with no lumbar rotation or flexion. The spinal areas involved are usually at the fourth or fifth lumbar and first sacral segments. An acute ante-rior sacrum dysfunction on the same side may also be present. If findings include a raised iliac crest height, lumbar scoliotic convexity, and sciatic pain distribution, all on the same side, the prognosis for a speedy recovery is often good. If the pain is on the other side, the cause may be a prolapsed disk or some other serious pathologic condition, and both physician and patient may be in for a difficult time.

Gait Patterns in Lower Extremity Dysfunction

Sciatica is associated with an antalgic, erector spinae gait pattern as the patient tries to avoid weight-bearing on the affected side. A common somatic dysfunction pattern in these patients comprises unilateral sacral flexion and flexion of the fifth lumbar vertebra, with rotation and side bending to the painful side, accompanied by trigger points at the piriformis, gluteus maximus, and gluteus medius muscles.

Observation of an asymmetric pelvic swing or tilt noted should be followed by a hip drop test. The findings on this test often concur with the gait observations, pointing toward lumbar lateral flexion restriction.

Somatic dysfunctions involving the lower extremity usually manifest with an antalgic gait. The clinician can use observation to determine the area involved, but then must depend on palpation and motion testing to establish the diagnosis.

The skill of observation can be improved if the physician is aware of the alterations of motion commonly produced by localized somatic dysfunction. At the hip joint, look for limitation in internal and external rotation in the swinging lower extremity. In the knee joint, there will be a restriction of femoral medial rotation on the tibia when attempting a close-packed position in extension of the stance lower extremity. At the ankle, the subtalar joint will be limited in eversion-inversion as the leg rotates internally-externally in stance phase. Lateral weight-bearing of the foot will shift toward the medial arch, with cuboid dysfunction during stance phase.

POSTURAL IMBALANCE AND LIFT THERAPY
Eileen L. DiGiovanna
Joseph A. DiGiovanna

Human bipedal posture has made balance extremely important to musculoskeletal function. In the erect human, gravity pulls on all parts of the body. While a column of vertebrae stacked evenly on top of each other would have been well balanced given little motion, anteroposterior curves developed in the spine to promote flexibility and increase strength. The transitions between spinal curves are well suited to meet the force of gravity. Correct posture is essential to keep the force of gravity centered on those vertebrae designed for this function.

Few persons are totally symmetric, and therefore postural imbalance is a significant source of musculoskeletal problems.

The body has certain automatic compensatory mechanisms that tend to right the body and maintain it in a state of equilibrium. For example, if, while standing, the left leg is lifted off the ground, the body's center of gravity will automatically move to the right, and the spine will shift and curve in the frontal plane to maintain the body in balance. Similarly, if the arms are held in front of the body, the spine will shift and curve in the sagittal plane, increasing lumbar lordosis to maintain balance. If a weight is held in the outstretched arms, the lordosis will exaggerate further to maintain body equilibrium. Thus, the body will make any adjustments necessary in order to maintain its balance and upright posture.

Numerous conditions can produce asymmetry in body mechanics and lead to functional postural imbalance. They include:

1. Trauma
2. Degenerative processes
3. Habit or occupation
4. Genetic tendencies
5. Mental attitude
6. Pregnancy
7. Obesity
8. Loss of muscle tone
9. Disease processes such as osteoporosis and polio
10. Congenital anomalies

Short Leg Syndrome

A source of postural imbalance in a large percentage of the "normal" population is the short leg syndrome. In 1977, Myron Beal reported the results of some studies on the short leg syndrome; included in his review were two earlier studies performed by Pearson et al on rural schoolchildren in 1947 and 1949. In the 1947 study, of 736 children, 410 had a difference of 0.5 mm in the lengths of the two legs, 152 had a difference of 5 to 10 mm, and 32 had a difference of 10 to 15 mm. The 1949 study, done on 710 students, found that 385 had a leg length difference of 0.5 mm, 194 a difference of 5 to 10 mm, and 17 a difference of 10 to 15 mm. Beal also reported on a study by Denslow that was done on asymptomatic young male students: 146 had a leg length difference of 5 to 10 mm, 28 a difference of 10 to 15 mm, one a difference of 15 to 20 mm, and two a difference of 20 mm.

The frequency of short leg syndrome is higher in persons with low back pain than in persons without low back pain, and the patients tend to be older.

DIAGNOSIS

I. History

The patient commonly reports bending over and feeling pain in the back, or feeling as though the back had locked. The patient may notice that he wears out one shoe faster than the other, or that one pant leg or shirt sleeve seems longer than the other.

Screening for scoliosis is often required by the school system and may allow early recognition of a postural problem.

Physical Examination

Scoliosis is often discovered during a routine physical examination. It must be determined if the scoliosis is due to a short leg (nonstructural or functional) or is developmental or congenital in origin (structural). A structural examination for asymmetry may yield important clues to solving the problem. A difference in leg length is assessed by measuring with a tape measure from the anterior superior iliac spines to the medial malleolus of each leg.

Radiologic Assessment

Once the diagnosis of short leg is suspected, the patient may be further evaluated with standing postural radiographs of the low back and femoral heads. These films are made with the patient standing erect, toes pointing forward and the feet approximately six inches apart. Equilibrium must be maintained as much as possible.

The iliac crests, sacral base, and femoral heads are measured bilaterally. This may be done with use of a specially gridded film or by use of a T-square to draw horizontal lines. The most important measurement is the sacral base (Fig. 15-2).

The scoliotic curve of the lumbar spine should also be evaluated. Normally the lumbar spine is convex on the side of the short leg as the spine side bends back toward the midline. Occasionally a compensatory curve will develop in the thoracic spine in the opposite direction from that in the lumbar spine. Sacral base leveling with straightening of the scoliotic curve is the goal of therapy.

Various types of unleveling of the femoral heads and sacral base may be found, as follows:

1. Parallel unleveling: sacral base unleveling equal and on the same side as the low femoral head.
2. Femoral head unleveling greater than sacral base unleveling: both low on same side.
3. Sacral base unleveling greater than femoral head unleveling: both low on same side.
4. Femoral head unleveling without sacral tilt.
5. Sacral base tilt without a short leg.
6. Sacral base low on one side with short leg on the opposite side.
7. Sacral base low on one side, lumbar spine convex on the side of the long leg.

PHYSICAL MANIFESTATIONS

A short leg has numerous effects on the body. The sacral base tilts toward the side of the short leg. The iliac crest is generally low on the short leg side. The lumbar spine develops a convexity toward the side of the short leg, and once the problem has existed for sufficient time, a compensatory curve will develop in the thoracic spine. The shoulder will be low on one side, depending on whether or not a secondary thoracic

Figure 15-2. Postural radiograph showing short right leg with marked sacral base unleveling. Note spinal convexity on the side of the short leg.

curve is present; the scapula will be low on the same side as the shoulder. The cervical angle will be more acute as the head is tilted toward the midline.

Asymmetric tensions are palpable in the paravertebral muscles. The muscles on the side of the convexity are stretched and those on the side of the concavity are shortened. There is usually a gapping of the medial knee compartment on the side of the short leg and an approximation of the medial knee compartment on the side of the longer leg. Stress is also created in the hip and ankle joints of the long leg.

TREATMENT

1. **Osteopathic manipulative treatment:**
   a. Relaxes and stretches contracted muscles
   b. Corrects somatic dysfunctions

   c. Increases mobility
   d. Normalizes tissues
2. **Exercises:** Exercises should be designed to stretch and tone the asymmetric muscles.
3. **Lift therapy:** A lift placed in the heel of the shoe on the side of the short leg, lifts the short leg and corrects the postural imbalance. The lift should be made of a firm, comfortable substance such as leather, cork, or hard rubber. Foam rubber is not satisfactory because it flattens, and height cannot be correctly measured.

When a heel lift is prescribed, the patient must be informed of the need to wear the lift at all times when walking. Once he is out of bed in the morning, he must wear shoes or slippers with the lift. The strain on the back is too great if the lift is worn only occasionally. The only exception is when walking on sand, where the surface is soft, giving, and already uneven.

When considering whether or not to prescribe a heel lift, several factors must be considered:

1. **Sacral base unleveling:** determined by radiographic assessment. Sacral base unleveling rather than femoral head heights has been deemed most significant. Most osteopathic physicians are of the opinion that anything over a quarter inch should be lifted. In certain cases, even an eighth inch should be treated.
2. **Length of time present:** period may be short, as in the case of a fractured lower extremity, or longer, as in the case of a developmental shortening.
3. **Amount of compensation:** includes such factors as the degree of side bending and rotation of the spine, wedging of vertebrae, and alteration of facets. Generally, the longer the condition has been present, the more compensation will have occurred.

David Heilig has developed a formula useful for determining the amount of lift to be used:

$$\text{Lift required} = \frac{\text{Sacral base unleveling}}{\text{Duration} + \text{Compensation}}$$

$$L = \frac{SBU}{D + C}$$

Duration is graded on a scale of 1 to 3:

    $1 =$ 1–10 years
    $2 =$ 10–30 years
    $3 =$ over 30 years
    $0 =$ side bending without rotation

Compensation is graded on a scale of 0 to 2:

    $1 =$ rotation toward the convexity
    $2 =$ wedging, altered facets

Except in the very young or in cases of acute shortening, it is best to begin by adding half the total difference. In older persons or in cases of greater compensation, it is best to start with no more than one-eighth inch. The lift is slowly increased over time, with manipulative treatment used to aid in adaptation to the lift. After the lift has been worn for a period of time and the patient is comfortable with it, the postural study should be repeated with the lift in place to determine if the correction is adequate.

If the lift is more than one-quarter-inch thick, it will have to be added to the outside of the heel. Lifts may also be added to orthotic devices. If the total lift required is greater than one-half inch, half the amount of heel lift will have to be added to the sole of the shoe as well. For example, if one-half inch is added to the heel, one-quarter inch should be added to the sole.

Before adding a lift it is important to ascertain that short leg is not due to a pronated foot on one side. In this case, an orthotic device to correct the pronation will probably correct the leg shortening.

Correcting a shortened extremity will correct many other postural defects, as it is the key to many musculoskeletal abnormalities. Besides correction of the postural deficits mentioned in the structural evaluation, a whole shift of body weight will occur. The pelvis will shift back to the midline, realigning the center of gravity and the weight-bearing portions of the body. The new position will affect the biomechanics of the entire musculoskeletal system.

References

Adams RD, Victor M. 1985. Principles of Neurology. New York: McGraw-Hill Book Co.

Basmajian JV. 1987. Muscles Alive, 4th ed. Baltimore: Williams & Wilkins Co.

Beal M. 1977. The short leg problem. J Am Osteopath Assoc 76(10):745–751.

Bickerstaff RE. 1968. Gait. In: Neurological Examination in Clinical Practice, 2nd ed. Oxford: Blackwell Scientific Publications.

Cailliet R. 1968. Foot and Ankle Pain. Philadelphia: F.A. Davis Co.

———. 1981. Low Back Pain Syndrome, 3rd ed. Philadelphia: F.A. Davis Co.

Forssberg H, Grillner S, Rossignol S. 1977. Phasic gain control of reflexes from the dorsum of the paw during spinal locomotion. Brain Res 132:121–139.

Heilig D. 1978. Principles of lift therapy. J Am Osteopath Assoc 77(6):466–472.

Henszinger RN. 1977. Limp. Pediatr Clin North Am 24:723–730.

Hoppenfeld S. 1976. Physical Examination of the Spine and Extremities. New York: Appleton-Century-Crofts.

Illingworth CM. 1978. 128 limping children with no fracture, sprain, or obvious cause. Clin Pediatr 17:139–142.

Kappler RE. 1973. Role of psoas mechanism in low-back complaints. J Am Osteopath Assoc 72(8):794–801.

———. 1982. Postural balance and motion patterns. J Am Osteopath Assoc 81(9):598–606.

Mann RA, Hagy JL, White V, et al. 1979. The initiation of gait. J Bone Joint Surg [Am] 61:232–239.

Merrifield HH. 1971. Female gait patterns in shoes with different heel heights. Ergonomics 14:411–417.

Michelle AA. 1962. Iliopsoas. St. Louis: Charles C Thomas, Publisher.

Mitchell FL. 1965. Structural pelvic function. In: Academy of Applied Osteopathy, 1965 Year Book. Vol II.

Morris JM. 1977. Biomechanics of the foot and ankle. pp. 178–199. Carmel, California: The Academy of Applied Osteopathy. Clin Orthop Rel Res 122:10–17.

Murray MP, Sepoc SB, Gardner GM, et al. 1978. Walking patterns of men with parkinsonism. Am J Phys Med 57:278–294.

Rasch PJ, Burke RK. 1978. Kinesiology and Applied Anatomy, 6th ed. Philadelphia: Lea & Febiger.

Roaf R. 1977. Posture. Orlando, Fla: Academic Press.

Saunders JB, Inman VT, Eberhart HD. 1953. The major determinants in normal and pathological gait. J Bone Joint Surg [Am] 35:543–558.

Schwartz RP, Heath AL, Misiek W, et al. 1933. Kinetics of Human Gait. Rochester, NY: University of Rochester Medical Society.

Simon RB. 1979. A neurologic screening exam in six minutes. Diagnosis 1(1):44–58.

Smidt GL. 1974. Methods of studying gait. Phys Ther 54:13–17.

Soderberg GL, Dostal WF. 1978. Electromyographic study of three parts of the gluteus medius muscle during functional activities. Phys Ther 58:691–696.

Strachan WF. 1941. Lateral imbalance and the use of lifts. J Am Osteopath Assoc 41:190–192.

Wells KF, Luttgens K. 1976. Kinesiology, 6th ed. Philadelphia: W.B. Saunders Co.

Winter DA, Robertson DGE. 1978. Joint torque and energy patterns in normal gait. Biol Cybernet 29:137–142.

Zarrugh MY, Radcliff CW. 1979. Computer generation of human gait kinematics. J Biomech 12:99–111.

Zohn DA, Mennell JMcM. 1987. Musculoskeletal Pain: Diagnosis and Physical Treatment. Boston: Little, Brown & Co.

16   Evaluation of the Thorax

APPLIED ANATOMY AND BIOMECHANICS

Dennis J. Dowling

Anatomic Relationships

LANDMARKS

On palpation, several landmarks may be noted and their relations to specific ribs established. The first rib is attached to the manubrium of the sternum just inferior to the clavicle anteriorly; posteriorly, it is cephalad to the superior border of the scapula. The second rib articulates with both the manubrium and the body of the sternum at the sternal angle anteriorly. Posteriorly, the third rib is located at approximately the median aspect of the spine of the scapula. The costal cartilage of the seventh rib attaches to the sternal body and xiphoid process ventrally while the angle of the rib rests near the tip of the scapula's inferior angle. The cartilage of the tenth rib is palpated at the lowest aspect of the thoracic cage in the midclavicular line. The 12th rib is almost horizontal and is found by palpating in the soft tissues posteriorly above the iliac crests.

STRUCTURE

The ribs are often classified as true or false. The cartilage of the true ribs, the first through seventh ribs, attaches to the sternum. The false ribs, ribs 8 through 12, are further divided into vertebrochondral ribs (eighth through tenth ribs) and floating ribs. The cartilage of the vertebrochondral ribs unites with the cartilage of the seventh ribs. The floating ribs lack cartilage and float freely.

Typical Ribs

The third through ninth ribs are typical ribs. The round, knoblike rib head is followed by the neck and tubercle, a body that arcs at the region of the rib angle, and a distal concavity where the cartilage attaches. The body of a typical rib is thin and flat, with interior and exterior surfaces and a costal groove on the inferior edge.

Each rib head has two facets for articulation with the body of the next superior vertebra and the same-numbered vertebral body. These articulations jointly constitute the costovertebral articulation. The tubercle articulates with the transverse process of the same vertebra via a facet and is known as the costotransverse articulation.

Atypical Ribs

The first, second, tenth, 11th, and 12th ribs are considered atypical ribs. The first rib is flat, has the greatest curvature and the shortest length of all the ribs, and has no angle or costal groove. Its superior surface has grooves for passage of the subclavian vessels and elevations for the attach-

239

ment of the anterior and middle scalene muscles. The single facet of the head articulates with the body of the T1 vertebra.

The second rib is similar to the first but longer and not as flat. The two demifacets on the rib head articulate with the T1 and T2 vertebrae.

The tenth rib is typical in every respect expect its costovertebral articulation. The single articular facet on the head forms a joint with the facet on the body of the T10 vertebra.

The 11th and 12th ribs have neither neck nor tubercles. As in the tenth rib, the heads have single facets corresponding to facets on the same-numbered vertebral bodies. The ventral ends float freely. The 12th rib does not possess a costal groove.

Supporting Structures
The clavicle is located at the anterosuperior aspect of the thoracic cage. Its medial end articulates with the manubrium and the cartilage of the first rib.

The sternum is composed of three parts: the xiphoid, body, and manubrium. The lateral edges of the sternum are scalloped for the attachment of costal cartilage.

The posterior portion of the thoracic cage and much of its motion are defined by the shape of the thoracic vertebrae. The bodies of the thoracic vertebrae have costal facets for articulation with the heads of the ribs. The long, thick, transverse processes have facets on their bulbous tips for articulation with the rib tubercles.

ARTICULATIONS
The **sternoclavicular joint,** one of the true joints of the shoulder girdle, may affect rib cage motion either primarily, via the manubrium and ligamentous attachments to the costal cartilage, or secondarily, owing to the position of the upper extremity.

The **costovertebral joint** is the articulation of the rib head with the bodies of one or two vertebrae. For a typical rib, the costovertebral joint includes the bodies of the vertebra at the same level and the vertebra immediately above, the annulus fibrosus of the intervening disk, and the costal facets. It is a synovial joint with a single capsule. The facets of the costovertebral joint are slightly convex and form an angle that fits into the depression formed by the vertebral facets and the disk.

Several ligaments are associated with the costovertebral joint, including the interosseous ligament and the superior, intermediate, and inferior bands of the radiate ligament.

The **costotransverse articulation** is likewise a simple synovial joint surrounded by a capsule. Three ligaments—the superior, posterior, and interosseous costotransverse ligaments—connect the transverse process to the neck of tubercle. The superior costotransverse ligament also connects the transverse process to the neck of the next lower rib.

Together, the costotransverse and costovertebral joints form a complex coupled joint. An imaginary line drawn between the two articulations is the axis that defines the direction of rib motion (Fig. 16-1).

The **costochondral region** of a rib consists of a concave pit on the end of the bony portion, to which is attached the cone-shaped cartilage.

The **sternochondral articulation** is formed by the costal cartilage and the triangular notches of the sternum. Small synovial joints are present. The apex of each notch faces medially, with an anteroposterior axis that allows freedom of motion along the coronal plane. The joints are supported by radiate ligaments.

MUSCLES
The major muscle of inspiration is the diaphragm, which is responsible for at least 60% of the generated thoracic cage pressure change. The muscular portion inserts onto the xiphoid process, the lower six ribs, and the upper lumbar vertebrae. All of these muscular portions converge on the aponeurotic central tendon (Fig. 16-2).

The diaphragm is a dome-shaped muscle with two lateral hemidiaphragms whose shape is influenced by the viscera. In addition to inspiration and expiration, the diaphragm is important in micturition, defecation, parturition, circulation of blood, lymphatic pumping, and speech.

Other inspiratory muscles include the external intercostals, levator costarum, and the accessory muscles. The accessory muscles are called into action for forced inspiration, such as is needed during exercise, or in pathologic states, including attacks of asthma. These auxillary inspiratory muscles include the sternocleidomastoid, scalenes, serratus posterior superior, pectoralis, inferior fibers of the serratus anterior, the latissimus

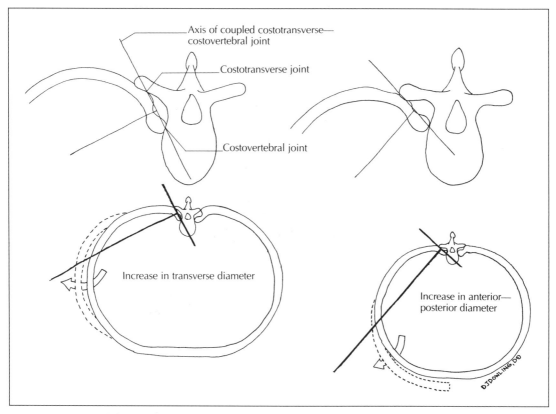

Figure 16-1. Axes of the costotransverse-costovertebral joints.

dorsi, and the superior fibers of iliocostalis muscles.

Expiration is primarily produced by recoil of the diaphragm and the energy stored in the costal cartilage. The sternocostalis and internal intercostalis muscles are also involved. The accessory expiratory muscles include the rectus abdominis, external oblique, internal oblique, transversus abdominis, serratus posterior inferior, transversus thoracic, pyramidalis, subcostalis, quadratus lumborum, iliocostalis, longissimus, and latissimus dorsi muscles (the latissimus may play a role in either expiration or inspiration, depending on the fixed position of the arm).

INNERVATION

The vertebral region is supplied primarily by dorsal rami while the ventral rami form the 11 pairs of intercostals and the pair of subcostals. They begin in the intercostal space, then enter the costal groove of the first through 11th ribs at the level of the angle. The intercostals connect to the sympathetic chain via the rami communicantes. The sympathetic trunks are located anterior to the heads of the ribs.

The diaphragm is innervated by the phrenic nerve, which consists of the ventral rami of the third, fourth, and fifth cervical nerves. Sensory input is also conducted through the phrenic nerve, with contributions from the intercostals.

Biomechanics

MUSCULAR ACTION

During inspiration, the diaphragm descends as it contracts. Movement is checked by the stretching of the mediastinal contents and by resistance of the abdominal organs. Simultaneous descent and contraction of the diaphragm decreases intrathoracic pressure and thereby increases the volume of the thoracic cavity. As the central tendon be-

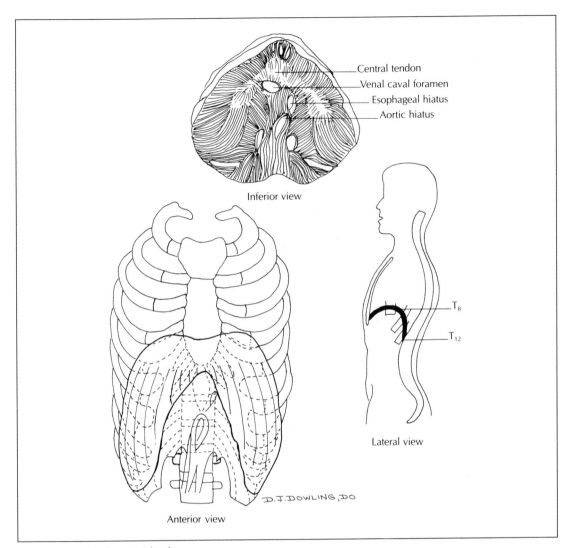

Central tendon
Venal caval foramen
Esophageal hiatus
Aortic hiatus

Inferior view

T_8

T_{12}

Lateral view

D.J.DOWLING,DO

Anterior view

Figure 16-2. The thoracic diaphragm.

comes fixed, continued contraction of the muscular fibers causes elevation of the lower ribs. Elevation of the upper ribs is assisted by the sternum.

Diaphragmatic movement increases the thoracic volume in three dimensions. Depression of the central tendon alters the vertical dimension, elevation of the ribs increases the transverse dimension, and elevation of the sternum and upper ribs changes the anteroposterior dimension (Fig. 16-3). Both the external intercostals and the levator costarum assist in inspiration by elevating the ribs.

The sternocostalis and internal costalis muscles depress the ribs during expiration. The accessory expiratory muscles can be divided into abdominal muscles, thoracic cage muscles, and thoracolumbar muscles. The abdominal muscles strongly depress the thoracic floor and increase intraabdominal pressure. Thoracic cage muscles such as the serratus posterior inferior act directly on rib attachments to draw the ribs downward. The thoracolumbar muscles also depress the ribs and possibly the scapula.

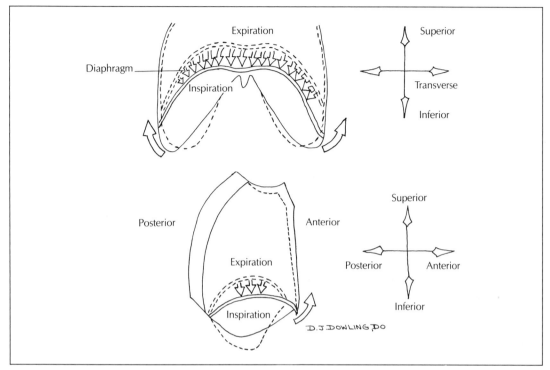

Figure 16-3. Diameter changes that occur during diaphragmatic motion.

RIB MOTION

The axis formed by the coupled costovertebral and costotransverse joints determines the primary direction of rib movement. This is influenced by the angle between the vertebral body and the transverse process and by the distance between the costal articulations with the vertebra. The axes of the ribs permit three basic types of motion: pump handle, bucket handle, and caliper motion (Fig. 16-4).

Pump handle motion. The term *pump handle motion* is derived from the similarity between the rib motion and that of an old-fashioned water pump. One end is fixed, the free end describes an arc. The costovertebral-costotransverse axis of the upper ribs lies close to the coronal plane. As the ribs move about this axis, they increase the anteroposterior diameter of that portion of the rib cage.

Bucket handle motion. The handle on a bucket is fixed at both ends. The axis is closer to a sagittal plane in the lower ribs. With one end of the bucket handle fixed at the vertebral end, the ma-

jority of the rib elevation occurs through upward excursion of the lateral portion. This motion increases the transverse diameter of the rib cage.

Mixed pump and bucket handle motion. The costovertebral-costotransverse axis for the middle ribs lies at a roughly 45-degree angle to the sagittal and coronal planes. The motion of these ribs is of a mixed pump and bucket handle type with an increase in both the transverse and anteroposterior dimensions.

Caliper motion. The 11th and 12th ribs have only costovertebral articulations. Since there are no transverse process limitations, the motion of these ribs is caliper-like along a horizontal plane. This motion produces slight changes in both the anteroposterior and the transverse dimensions.

ANTEROPOSTERIOR SHAPE CHANGES

During inhalation, the first through tenth ribs elevate. The sternum moves upward and forward. The small amount of motion possible at the sternal angle—since it is usually a symphysis—al-

Figure 16-4. Rib motions: (**A**) bucket handle motion, (**B**) pump handle motion, (**C**) caliper motion.

lows the angle to flatten. The upper ribs move farther forward than the lower ribs because of the greater pump handle motion that occurs in this region.

COSTAL CARTILAGE ELASTICITY

The costal cartilage is hyaline. It is basically unossified embryonic cartilaginous rib and contributes significantly to thoracic cage mobility. During inspiration, the sternum has a greater superior excursion than the ribs. The ribs initially move inferiorly relative to the sternum. Since the cartilage is basically fixed at the sternal end, it twists along the long axis and behaves as a torsion rod and stores potential energy. As the diaphragm relaxes and ascends, this energy is released as the cartilage recoils (Fig. 16-5).

Osteopathic Diagnosis

Palpation and visual observation are used during osteopathic examination. Knowledge of the structure and biomechanics of the area under evaluation is integral to this process. Somatic dysfunctions restrict motion of the thoracic cage and its components. The bucket handle and pump handle movements may be limited when examined at the greatest extent of inspiration and expiration. Asymmetric excursion and difficulty in movement imply restriction of the region examined.

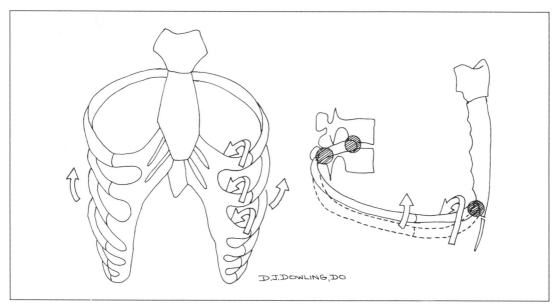

Figure 16-5. Elasticity of the costal cartilage.

LYMPH: THE FLUID OF LIFE
Paula D. Scariati

Natural defenses are often suboptimal and variable because they have been hindered by inheritance and/or abnormal structure-function relationships. These natural defenses are found predominantly within the fluids of the body, especially the blood and the lymphatics, so the "first and wisest step" for the physician to take is to act to improve circulation and drainage, allowing the body's defenses to combat disease and carry away its debris.

Tenets of Osteopathic Philosophy
Student Doctor, December 1986

Anatomy

The lymph vascular system has both deep and superficial vessels. The **deep vessels** generally follow the deepest veins, which often travel with companion arteries and nerves. The **superficial vessels** travel through the superficial fascia, and their related lymph nodes are usually found where large superficial veins flow into the deeper veins. Certain areas are devoid of lymphatic vessels and nodes; these areas include the brain, spinal cord, bone marrow, and structures that receive their nutrition by diffusion (i.e., cartilage, epidermis).

The **superficial lymph system** drains the skin. This drainage goes to three main groups of lymph nodes: the axillary nodes, cervical nodes, and inguinal nodes. In addition to receiving lymph from the total body skin, these nodes also receive lymph from the deeper tissues of the upper extremities, the lower extremities, and the head and neck. Drainage of the skin is rather symmetric (Fig. 16-6). Eventually, lymph collected in the superficial system is drained off into the deeper lymphatic system.

The **deep lymph system** drains the deeper structures of the thorax, abdomen, pelvis, and perineum directly, without passing through the superficial system. Deep in the body, lymph channels lie around all the major organs. In general, these lymph channels with their associated nodes drain along the major arteries and veins toward one central trunk, either the right lymphatic duct or the thoracic duct (Fig. 16-7). Lymph from either of these two lymphatic vessels enters the venous

Figure 16-6. Symmetric drainage of the skin by the superficial lymph system.

superior surface of the spleen, the diaphragmatic surface, sits against the diaphragm. The normal-sized spleen does not extend below the left costal margin and thus is not normally palpable.

The functions of the spleen include the following:

1. Clearance of microorganisms and particulate antigens.
2. Synthesis of immunoglobulins, opsons, etc.
3. Destruction of red blood cells.
4. Removal of poorly opsonized bacteria (the liver clears well-opsonized bacteria).

Physiology

Embryologically, the lymphatics begin as closed endothelial tubes that are permeable to fluid and high molecular weight compounds. Once fully developed, the function of the lymphatic system is to remove from the interstitium the fluid, albumin, and macromolecules that have escaped from the microcirculation.

Four major forces act at the capillary membrane to promote the movement of fluid into and out of the capillary:

1. The capillary pressure (Pc), which tends to move fluid out through the capillary membranes.
2. The interstitial fluid pressure (Pif), which tends to move fluid in through the capillary membrane when the Pif is positive but outward when the Pif is negative.
3. The plasma colloid osmotic pressure (π p), which tends to cause osmosis of fluid inward through the membrane.
4. The interstitial fluid colloid osmotic pressure (πif) which tends to cause osmosis of fluid outward through the membrane.

The major function of the lymphatic pump is to remove extracellular proteins and thereby regulate the osmotic pressure of the extracellular space.

Once in the interstitium, the lymph is drawn into the lymphatic capillaries. It may be difficult to understand how fluid can flow out of the interstitial spaces into the lymphatic capillaries in the face of negative pressure in the interstitial spaces, which average about 5 mm in size. Whenever a tissue is compressed, interstitial fluid pressure in

system at the point where the jugular vein and the subclavian vein meet to become the brachiocephalic vein. The thoracic duct only enters the left venous circulation; thus, most of the body lymph empties on the left side. Some conception of the two main interconnecting components of the lymphatic circulation and of the motion of lymph with and against gravity will help the clinician understand what occurs when the lymphatic system fails or is overloaded.

The spleen is the largest single mass of lymphoid tissue in the body. (The lymph nodes are smaller aggregates of lymphoid tissue.) The spleen is located deep to ribs 9 to 11 on the left side. The

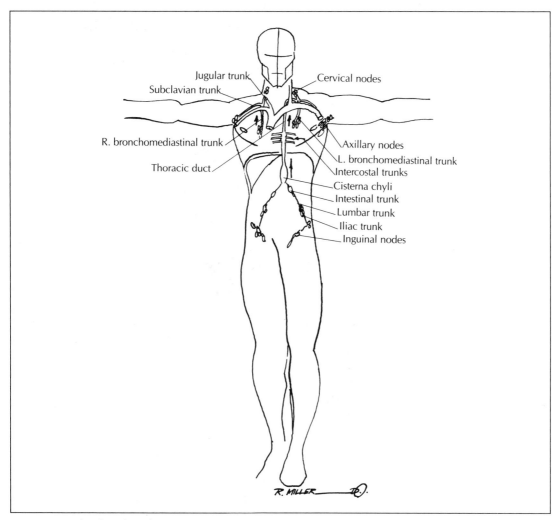

Figure 16-7. The deep lymph system.

the local area of compression rises temporarily to a positive value. This pressure differential causes minute amounts of fluid to move into the lymphatics and subsequently to be pumped away from the tissue. Recoiling of the space after the fluid is pumped away reestablishes the initial negative pressure.

Lymph is mobilized by the contraction of large lymphatics and contiguous skeletal muscle. The lymphatics have an extensive system of one-way valves to maintain the flow of lymph toward the heart. Normal lymph flow is 2 litres per day for the entire body. This volume contains approximately 200 grams of protein lost from the microcirculation. Most lymph comes from the gastrointestinal tract and the liver. The lymphatic system is the *only* mechanism for returning interstitial proteins to the circulatory system.

The faster lymph moves, the faster excess extracellular proteins, debris, and bacteria can be cleared from the body and vital proteins returned to the circulatory system. Four major factors determine the rate of lymph flow, as follows:

1. **Interstitial fluid pressure:** Elevation of interstitial free fluid pressure above the normal 5.3 mm Hg increases the flow of fluid into the lymphatic capillaries and increases the rate of lymph flow. Factors that help elevate the interstitial free fluid pressure include

a. Increased capillary pressure

b. Decreased plasma colloid osmotic pressure

c. Increased interstitial fluid protein

d. Increased capillary permeability

2. **The lymphatic pump:** Valves in the lymph channel prevent the backflow of lymph.

3. **Intrinsic pumping by the lymph vessels:** When a lymph vessel becomes stretched with fluid, the smooth muscle in the wall of the vessel contracts. Furthermore, each segment of the lymph vessel between successive valves functions as a separate, automatic pump. To reiterate, filling of a segment of a lymphatic vessel causes it to contract, and the fluid is pumped through a downstream valve into the next lymphatic segment. This new segment of lymph vessel now stretches and contracts in response to the lymph accumulation. This process continues until the lymph is emptied back into the venous system.

Many physiologists also believe that the lymphatic capillary (the smallest lymphatic vessel that adheres to the surrounding tissue) is also capable of pump action. This prevents the fluid that escapes from the capillary vessels from back-diffusing and causing edema. In this case, it is the endothelial cells of the circulatory system's capillaries that overlap and act like valves. Thus the lymph must move forward.

4. **Pumping caused by external compression of the lymphatics:** Extrinsic or external factors that compress the lymph vessels can also cause pumping. In order of importance, these factors include:

a. Contraction of muscle

b. Movement of the parts of the body

c. Arterial pulsations

d. Compression of the tissue by objects outside the body

THE THORAX AS A FLUID PUMP

Muscular contraction and movement of body parts are forceful external stimuli that act on the lymphatic pump. In particular, respiration is a major stimulator of the lymphatic pump.

Respiration has two components, inspiration and expiration. During inspiration the diaphragm contracts and descends, creating a more negative intrathoracic pressure that draws air into the lungs. The increased pressure on the lymphatic walls results in compression of the lymphatic plexuses so that lymph is propelled. Again, inspiration is intimately associated with the propulsion of lymph. During inspiration, the descending diaphragm compresses the hepatic system and prevents hepatic drainage.

During expiration, opposite movements occur. The diaphragm relaxes and moves back up. The lymphatic plexuses expand and the lymph pools. The hepatic system drains during this phase of respiration.

Two final points must be made about respiration and its effect on lymphatic flow. First, deep, long breaths maximize lymphatic motion. Second, structure governs function. If respiratory/thoracic motion is restricted, the ability to move lymph will be impaired.

EDEMA

Edema represents fluid overload on the lymphatic pump system. Once tissues become edematous, the lymphatic capillaries dilate tremendously. The flaps between the endothelial cells of the capillaries become separated from one other, so that they are no longer reliable, and the lymphatic pump begins to fail. Edema does not occur until the lymphatic pump has reached its maximum capabilities and is overwhelmed.

EVALUATION OF THE THORAX

Eileen L. DiGiovanna

There are several reasons for evaluating the thorax during a structural examination. The status of the rib cage is an important clue to the status of the respiratory mechanism. Free motion of

the ribs is necessary for full expansion of the lungs. Conversely, pulmonary diseases cause secondary changes in rib motion.

The ribs may also be a source of chest wall or

upper back pain. Rib dysfunction may result in shoulder, arm, or neck pain. Finally, rib dysfunctions may be primary or secondary to thoracic spine dysfunction.

Observation of the chest wall will reveal any asymmetry, the typical barrel chest of chronic pulmonary diseases, increased or decreased rate of respiration, or the degree to which the patient uses abdominal versus thoracic breathing.

The thorax is palpated to detect static asymmetries as well as asymmetries or restrictions of rib motion. Static asymmetries represent anterior or posterior ribs. Palpation for static asymmetries is particularly helpful when localized pain is due to rib dysfunction. Ribs may be palpated along the posterior thorax at the angle of the ribs with the patient prone. A posterior rib on palpation appears to lie more posteriorly than the rib above or below it. Posterior ribs are frequently due to posterior rotation of the transverse process with which the rib articulates. As with any somatic dysfunction, there will be associated tissue changes in the area of the rib head.

Palpation along the sternal border anteriorly will reveal ribs that have moved anteriorly, a common cause of anterior chest wall pain. Rib dysfunction on the left side may be mistaken by the patient for cardiac pain. Tenderness and tissue changes may be palpated along the sternal border at the costochondral junction.

Palpation of the anterior chest wall may disclose elevated or depressed ribs. In the case of a depressed rib, the space between it and the rib below will be narrowed, while the space between it and the rib above will be widened. These differences are reversed for an elevated rib: the space between it and the rib above will be narrowed, while the space between it and the rib below is widened. A single rib or a group of ribs may be elevated or depressed. Motion testing is necessary for diagnosis, as the findings on static palpation may be misleading.

Diagnostic Terminology

Various authors use different terms to describe rib dysfunctions. Some common terms are:

1. Anterior or posterior ribs
2. Elevated or depressed ribs
3. Ribs in a position of inspiration or expiration (inhalation or exhalation dysfunctions)

4. Ribs restricted in inspiration or expiration (inhalation or exhalation restrictions)

When reading literature, note whether the author states that a rib is in a *position of inspiration* (elevated) or *restricted* in inspiration (depressed). An inspiration restriction denotes a rib that does not move into a position of inspiration but is held in a depressed or expiratory position. Inspiratory and expiratory restrictions are restrictions of motion of the rib on its respiratory axis; that is, during inspiration the anterior portion of the rib is elevated and during expiration the rib is depressed.

Evaluation of the First Rib

The first rib is unlike the other ribs because of its attachments to the scalene muscles and its functional relationship to the clavicle. It is customarily palpated at three sites:

1. The posterior superior surface, through the trapezius
2. The anterior superior surface in a depression behind the clavicle
3. The anterior articulation just below the clavicle at the sternal border.

The technique for motion testing of the first rib is described below.

1. Patient position: supine.
2. Physician position: seated at the head of the table.
3. **Technique:**
   a. The physician places her thumbs or finger pads on the anterior surface in the supraclavicular depression and evaluates the static position of the first ribs. Is one rib higher than the other?
   b. Tissue texture and muscle tone over the rib are examined for abnormalities.
   c. The physician places her thumbs on the posterior surface just anterior to trapezius and springs the ribs lightly, evaluating the resistance of the ribs (Fig. 16-8). If resistance is felt when the rib is sprung, that rib is dysfunctional.
   d. The physician evaluates rib motion by placing her thumbs or finger pads on the

Figure 16-8. Position for evaluating the first rib.

Figure 16-9. Pump handle motion testing of the upper ribs.

anterosuperior surface of the first ribs and asking the patient to make a full inspiratory and expiratory effort.

e. **Significance:**
   i. If one rib stops moving before the other rib during inspiration, that rib has an *inspiratory restriction.*
   ii. If one rib stops moving before the other rib during exhalation, that rib has an *expiratory restriction.*

Gross Motion Testing of the Ribs

This section describes a general screening test for evaluating motion of groups of ribs.

Figure 16-10. Bucket handle motion testing of the upper ribs.

1. Patient position: supine.
2. Physician position: standing at the side of the table, facing the patient's head.
3. **Technique:**
   a. **Upper ribs (1–3)**
      i. Pump handle motion
         a. The physician places her fingers flat along the sternal border bilaterally, with the fingertips touching the inferior surface of the clavicle (Fig. 16-9).
         b. Motion is evaluated as the patient inhales and exhales deeply.
      ii. Bucket handle motion
         a. The physician places her fingers flat on the upper chest wall and at a 45-degree angle to the sternal border,

with the index finger lying just below clavicle (Fig. 16-10).
         b. Motion is evaluated in full inhalation and exhalation.
   b. **Middle ribs (4–7)**
      i. The physician places her thumbs along the sternal border with the tips toward the patient's head.
      ii. The fingers are placed laterally along the middle ribs, each finger covering one rib (Fig. 16-11).

Figure 16-11. Gross motion testing of the middle ribs.

Figure 16-12. Gross motion testing of the lower ribs.

Figure 16-13. Gross motion testing of ribs 11 and 12.

iii. As patient inhales and exhales fully,
   a. Evaluate pump handle motion with the thumbs.
   b. Evaluate bucket handle motion with the fingers.
iv. In a female patient it may be preferable to evaluate pump handle and bucket handle motions individually by placing the fingers along the sternal border first and then along the ribs at the midaxillary area.

c. **Lower ribs (8–10)**
   i. The physician places her thumbs along the costochondral border and spreads the fingers along the ribs laterally (Fig. 16-12).
   ii. The evaluation of the lower ribs follows that for the middle ribs.

d. **Ribs 11 and 12**
   These ribs are evaluated with the patient prone. Their caliper-type motion is evaluated.
   i. The physician forms a C with her thumb and second and third fingers. The thumb is placed at the area of the rib heads and the fingers along the ribs (Fig. 16-13).
   ii. Rib motion is evaluated in full inhalation and exhalation.
   iii. **Significance:**
      a. If a group of ribs stops moving on one side before the other during inhalation, one or more ribs in that group have an inhalation restriction. The restriction may be of pump handle motion, bucket handle motion, or both.
   b. If a group of ribs stops moving on one side before the other during exhalation, one or more ribs in that group have an exhalation restriction. The restriction may be of pump handle motion or bucket handle motion.
   c. Occasionally bilateral restrictions may be present. Their identification requires knowledge of normal rib excursions, which comes with experience and concentration on full ranges of motion.

Individual Rib Motion Testing

The individual ribs are tested in the manner just described for each level of ribs, but only one rib on each side is tested and compared. Individual ribs may be tested if one rib is painful or if restriction of motion is found on gross motion testing. If a group inhalation restriction has been found, usually the top rib in the group is responsible for the restriction. If a group exhalation restriction has been found, usually the lowest rib in the group is responsible.

Evaluation of the Sternum

Because of the close association of the sternum with the ribs, the sternum must be evaluated when respiratory excursion appears limited. The sternum is evaluated by placing the thumb of one hand on the manubrium and the other thumb on the body of the sternum (Fig. 16-14). By applying pressure with each thumb alternately, the physician can determine if sternal motion is free at the angle of Louis.

Figure 16-14. Evaluation of the sternum.

Evaluation of the Clavicle

Evaluation of the clavicle is discussed in Chapter 19 (Diagnosis and Treatment of the Upper Extremity—Shoulder). Because of the close relationship between the clavicle and the first rib, when first or second rib restriction is found, the clavicle must be evaluated.

THE DIAPHRAGM
Paula D. Scariati

The major muscles of respiration are the diaphragm, the internal and external intercostal muscles, the parasternal muscles, and the scalenes. Abdominal muscles that participate in respiration include the external and internal oblique muscles and the transverse and rectus abdominis muscles. The diaphragm generates two thirds of the inspiratory effort. Nevertheless, a person with a paralyzed diaphragm may still have good respiratory function.

The diaphragm is composed of muscular portions and an aponeurotic portion, the *central tendon*. The muscular portion is divided into three parts, based on origin:

1. Sternal part
   Origin: Posterior aspect of the xiphoid process of the sternum
   Insertion: Central tendon
2. Costal part (forms the right and left hemidiaphragms)
   Origin: Internal surface of the inferior six ribs at their costal margins
   Insertion: Central tendon
3. Lumbar part
   Origin: Arises from the lumbar vertebrae via two crura and arcuate ligaments
   a. Left crus: attaches to L1–L2 and the associated intervertebral disk on the left side of the aorta.
   b. Right crus: attaches to L1–L3 and the associated intervertebral disks on the right side of the aorta.
   c. Median arcuate ligament: unites the medial side of the two crura. It passes over the anterior surface of the aorta and gives origin to some of the fibers of the right crus.
   d. Medial arcuate ligament: a thickening of the anterior layer of thoracolumbar fascia over the superior part of the psoas major muscle. It forms a fibrous arch from the crus of the diaphragm to the transverse process of L1.
   e. Lateral arcuate ligament: a thickening of the anterior layer of thoracolumbar fascia over the superior part of the quadratus lumborum muscle. It forms a fibrous arch that runs from the transverse process of L1 to the 12th rib.

Embryology

The splanchnic mesenchyme surrounding the laryngotracheal tube forms the connective tissue, cartilage, muscle, and the blood and lymphatic vessels of the lung. The diaphragm, the dome-shaped, musculotendinous partition between the thoracic and abdominal cavities, originates in four different structures: (1) the *septum transversum*, which develops into the central tendon of the diaphragm in the adult, (2) the *pleuroperitoneal membranes*, which form a part of the musculature of the main part of the diaphragm, (3) the *dorsal mesentery of the esophagus*, which contributes to the formation of the crura of the diaphragm, and (4) the *body wall*, which contributes to the peripheral portions of the diaphragm and forms the costodiaphragmatic recesses, giving the diaphragm its dome shape.

Structure, Function, and Innervation of the Diaphragm and Associated Muscles

The central tendon is a strong, C-shaped aponeurosis that is the insertion site for all the muscular fibers of the diaphragm. The middle portion of the central tendon lies just inferior to the heart and fuses with the fibrous pericardium here.

The motor innervation of the diaphragm is provided by the phrenic nerve, which originates in nerve roots C3–C5. During embryogenesis, the diaphragm migrates caudad relative to the vertebral column. The sensory innervation of the diaphragm is mainly provided by the phrenic nerve, with intercostal nerves providing sensory innervation to the fringes of the diaphragm that develop from the lateral body wall.

The function of the diaphragm is to contract during inspiration. This causes the dome of the diaphragm to move inferiorly and compress the abdominal viscera (through increased intraabdominal pressure). Intrathoracic pressure decreases as a consequence of the increased volume of the thoracic cavity. Air is drawn into the lungs; venous and lymphatic motion are facilitated.

All of the structures that pierce the diaphragm are affected by the integrity of the muscle. The three main apertures in the diaphragm allow passage of the venae cavae, esophagus, and aorta. The right phrenic nerve passes via the vena caval foramen. The superior epigastric vessels pass through the sternocostal hiatus. The musculo-phrenic vessels pass near the ninth costal cartilage. The subcostal nerves and vessels pass posterior to the lateral arcuate ligament. The sympathetic trunk passes posterior to the medial arcuate ligament. Splanchnic nerves pierce the crura. The hemiazygous vein passes through the left crus.

Owing to its varied origins and insertions, the diaphragm acts in a number of ways during inspiration. The **crural diaphragm** contracts and moves the central tendon caudad, increasing intraabdominal pressure and pushing the abdominal wall outward. Simultaneously, it contributes to decreasing the intrapleural pressure and inflating the lungs. The **costal diaphragm** has a similar action, but as it exerts a caudal force on the central tendon, it concomitantly exerts a cephalic force on the costal margin. Thus, it both expands the rib cage and assists in lung inflation with abdominal motion.

Increased intraabdominal pressure secondary to diaphragmatic contraction also acts to expand the rib cage. This is achieved by the transmission of abdominal pressure through an area of apposition of the costal diaphragm to the inner surface of the lower rib cage.

The different actions of the crural and costal portions of the diaphragm on respiratory effort indicate that the tension developed by one portion of the muscle is not transmitted to the other portion. Thus, these muscles are linked mechanically in parallel at the start. However, as lung volumes increase, the costal and crural parts become linked in series. Thus, with progressive hyperinflation, the diaphragm becomes a less effective force generator because its costal and crural parts develop the same tensions; they then have the same action.

RIB CAGE MUSCLES DURING RESPIRATION

In addition to the diaphragm, the rib cage muscles contribute to respiration. The parasternal muscles act to decrease the angle between the upper border of the ribs and the sternum. Because the ribs are fixed in their anteroposterior positions by bony attachments, these muscles facilitate the bucket handle motion of the rib cage. The primary action of the scalene muscles is to elevate the first and second ribs by decreasing the angle between the upper border of the rib and the vertebral column, thus facilitating the pump handle motion of the ribs.

Normally, the parasternals and scalenes contract with the diaphragm. If the diaphragm were to contract alone, it would displace the abdomen more than the rib cage. Working together, these forces counterbalance each other and vary according to position (e.g., erect versus supine) and postural compliance (e.g., kyphosis with decreased rib compliance).

INTERACTING SYSTEMS OF CONTROL

The anatomical and mechanical events described are often regulated by and interact with other systems of control, including neural control, humoral influences, and mechanical factors such as the mucous coat of the respiratory passageways, cilial clearance, and the muscle and cartilage incorporated into the various parts of the respiratory passageways.

Physiology

Inhaled air passes through the nose and pharynx and is distributed to the lungs by way of the trachea, bronchi, and bronchioles. The trachea is the first-generation respiratory passageway; the right and left main-stem bronchi are second-generation passageways. Each division thereafter constitutes another generation. After passing through 20 to 25 generations of airways, inhaled air reaches the alveoli, where exchange of oxygen and carbon dioxide takes place.

The process of respiration can be divided into four events:

1. **Pulmonary ventilation,** defined as the inflow and outflow of air between the atmosphere and the alveoli.
2. **Diffusion** of oxygen and carbon dioxide between the lungs and the alveoli.
3. **Transport** of oxygen and carbon dioxide in the blood and body fluids to and from the cells.
4. **Regulation** of ventilation.

In pulmonary ventilation, the lungs move in two planes: (1) up and down, facilitated by diaphragmatic contraction, and (2) anteriorly-posteriorly, facilitated by rib motion. Normal, quiet breathing entails mostly motion in the vertical plane. Maximal respiratory efforts recruit anteroposterior lung motion, which increases lung volume by 20%.

During inspiration, intraalveolar pressure becomes negative with respect to the atmospheric pressure. This effect is secondary to diaphragmatic contraction, and air is drawn into the lungs. Expiration is passive. Intraalveolar pressures increase and air flows out.

In normal, quiet respiration, the chest wall always tends to expand, whereas the lungs tend to collapse. This recoil tendency of the lungs is due to two factors:

1. Elastic fibers in the lung which are stretched and in response tend to shorten (the stretch reflex).
2. Surface tensions caused by intermolecular attractions between the surface molecules of alveolar fluid. This tension is countered to a great extent by lung surfactant.

Under resting conditions, a negative pressure of about 4 mm Hg is required to keep the lung expanded. This is known as the pleural pressure or the lung recoil pressure.

Compliance is defined as the expansibility of the lungs and the thorax. The muscles of respiration use energy to expand the lungs and the thoracic cage around the lungs during respiration.

The interactions of respiration are far greater than the musculo-osseous-thoracic interactions described here. The ability to manipulate the muscle, fascia, bone, and the cranial rhythmic impulse allows the osteopathic physician to address respiratory dysfunctions at a variety of levels.

References

Cathie AG. 1965. Physiologic motions of the spine as related to respiratory activity. In: Academy of Applied Osteopathy—1965 Yearbook. Carmel, California: Academy of Applied Osteopathy.

Guyton AC. 1986. Textbook of Medical Physiology, 7th ed. Philadelphia: W.B. Saunders Co.

Kapandji IA. 1974. The Physiology of the Joints. Vol III. Edinburgh: Churchill Livingstone.

Langley L, Telford IR, Christensen JB. 1980. Dynamic Anatomy and Physiology, 5th ed. New York: McGraw-Hill.

Moore KL. 1985. Clinically Oriented Anatomy, 2nd ed. Baltimore: Williams & Wilkins Co.

———. 1988. The Developing Human: Clinically Oriented Embryology, 4th ed. Philadelphia: W.B. Saunders Co.

Pansky B. 1984. Review of Gross Anatomy, 5th ed. New York: Macmillan Publishing Co.

Robbins SL, ed. 1984. Pathologic Basis of Disease, 3rd ed. Philadelphia: W.B. Saunders Co.

Sabiston DC. 1986. Textbook of Surgery: The Biological Basis of Modern Surgical Practice. Philadelphia: W.B. Saunders Co.

Schiowitz S, DiGiovanna E, Ausman P. 1983. An Osteopathic Approach to Diagnosis and Treatment. Old Westbury, NY: New York College of Osteopathic Medicine.

17

Treatment of the Thoracic Cage

MUSCLE ENERGY TECHNIQUES FOR THE RIBS
Eileen L. DiGiovanna

Muscle energy treatment of the ribs is used to correct inspiratory and expiratory restrictions. Each treatment entails the following general principles:

1. Patient contracting a muscle to move a rib.
2. Patient providing respiratory assistance.
3. Force applied by physician to assist motion.

Techniques are described separately for the first rib, the second through tenth ribs, and the 11th and 12th ribs.

Inspiratory Restrictions
FIRST RIB: PUMP HANDLE MOTION
1. Patient position: supine.
2. Physician position: standing at the side of the table, facing the patient's head.
3. **Technique:**
   a. The patient places his hand, palm up, on his forehead.
   b. The physician reaches under the patient with her near hand and grasps the posterosuperior surface of the first rib with her fingers.
   c. The physician places her other hand, palm down, on top of the patient's hand.
   d. The patient is asked to raise his head off the table and simultaneously take a deep breath.
   e. As the patient lifts his head, the physician resists motion by pressing down on patient's hand and simultaneously pulling caudad on the back of the rib (Fig. 17-1).
   f. Repeat the above steps three times.
4. Three mechanisms have aided in moving the rib in an elevated, or inspiratory, pump handle motion:
   a. Patient's contraction of the anterior scalene elevated the rib, since the head is fixed.
   b. The deep inspiration assisted the rib into a position of inspiration.
   c. The physician's pull on the posterior part of the rib flipped the anterior part upward.

FIRST RIB: BUCKET HANDLE MOTION
1. Patient position: supine, with his head turned 40 degrees from the midline, toward the rib being treated.
2. Physician position: standing at the side of the table, facing the patient's head.
3. **Technique:**
   a. The technique is as for treating pump handle motion of the first rib, except that the middle scalene muscle instead of the anterior scalene muscle is used (Fig. 17-2).

Figure 17-1. Muscle energy technique for treatment of inspiratory restriction of the first rib (pump handle motion).

Figure 17-2. Muscle energy technique for treatment of inspiratory restriction of the first rib (bucket handle motion.)

RIBS 2–10: PUMP HANDLE MOTION
1. Patient position: supine.
2. Physician position: standing at the side of the table, facing the patient's head.
3. **Technique:**
   a. The patient places his hand, palm up, on his forehead.
   b. The physician reaches behind the patient with her near hand and grasps the superoposterior part of the rib being treated.
   c. The physician places her hand on top of the patient's hand.
   d. The patient is instructed to lift his hand toward the ceiling. The physician provides resistance (Fig. 17-3).
   e. At the same time, the physician pulls down on the posterior rib and the patient inhales deeply.
4. In this technique, the patient uses the serratus anterior muscle to elevate the anterior part of the rib as the physician pulls down on the posterior rib to aid elevation at the anterior part.

RIBS 2–10: BUCKET HANDLE MOTION
1. Patient position: supine.
2. Physician position: standing at the side of the table, facing the patient's head.
3. **Technique:**
   a. The technique is the same as for treating

Figure 17-3. Muscle energy technique for treatment of inspiratory restriction of the second through tenth ribs (pump handle motion).

pump handle motion of these ribs, except that the patient is instructed to move his arm up and out at a 45-degree angle. The lateral part of the serratus will then elevate the lateral part of the ribs to improve bucket handle motion.

RIBS 11 AND 12
1. Patient position: prone.
2. Physician position: standing at the side of the table, opposite the rib being treated.
3. **Technique:**
   a. The patient's legs are pulled toward the physician.
   b. The patient's arm on the involved side is placed above his head.

c. The physician grasps the anterior inferior iliac spines and rotates the pelvis.

d. The palm of the physician's opposite hand is placed over the involved rib(s).

e. The patient is asked to inhale deeply.

f. As the patient inhales, the physician pushes laterally on the rib, separating it from its articulation to allow the breath to carry it into inhalation (Fig. 17-6).

Expiratory Restrictions

RIB 1: PUMP HANDLE MOTION

1. Patient position: supine.

2. Physician position: standing or seated at the head of the table.

3. **Technique:**

   a. The patient's neck is bent forward.

   b. The physician places her thumb on the rib between the two heads of the sternocleidomastoid muscle.

   c. The patient inhales, then exhales completely.

   d. The physician presses down on the rib, following it into exhalation.

   e. The physician holds the rib down as the patient takes a shallow breath and exhales again.

RIB 1: BUCKET HANDLE MOTION

1. Patient position: supine, with the head side bent slightly toward the affected rib.

2. Physician position: standing or seated at the head of the table.

3. **Technique:** The technique is the same as for treating expiratory restriction of the pump handle motion of the first rib, except that the physician's thumb is placed lateral to the sternocleidomastoid muscle.

RIBS 2–5: PUMP HANDLE MOTION

1. Patient position: supine.

2. Physician position: standing or seated at the head of the table.

3. **Technique:**

   a. The physician places her fingers on the superior surface of the costal cartilage of the rib being treated and the one below it.

   b. The patient's neck is bent forward fully.

   c. The patient exhales fully as the physician encourages the rib to move into a position of expiration.

Figure 17-4. Muscle energy technique for treatment of expiratory restriction of the second through fifth ribs (pump handle motion).

d. The physician holds down the rib as the patient inhales, then moves it farther into expiration as the patient exhales forcefully (Fig. 17-4).

   Note: The intercostal muscles are thus used to pull down on the ribs as the physician forces them down with her finger.

RIBS 2–5: BUCKET HANDLE MOTION

1. Patient position: supine, with the shoulders and neck side bent toward the affected side.

2. Physician position: standing or seated at the head of the table.

3. **Technique:** The technique is the same as for treating pump handle motion expiratory restriction of ribs 2–5, except that the physician's fingers are placed in the midaxillary line above and below the rib being treated.

RIBS 6–10: PUMP HANDLE MOTION

1. Patient position: supine, with the shoulders lifted up by the physician's hand placed between the scapulae or with the upper back resting on the physician's thigh. The upper trunk is thus bent forward.

2. Physician position: standing at the head of the table, supporting the patient.

Figure 17-5. Muscle energy technique for treatment of expiratory restriction of the sixth through tenth ribs (bucket handle motion).

Figure 17-6. Muscle energy technique for treatment of expiratory restriction of the 11th and 12th ribs (arm at side for treating expiratory restrictions and above head for inspiratory restrictions).

3. **Technique:**
   a. The rib is forced into expiration as the patient exhales forcefully.
   b. The rib is held down during inhalation.
   c. The maneuver is repeated twice more.

RIBS 6–10: BUCKET HANDLE MOTION
1. Patient position: same as for treating pump handle motion, except that the upper trunk is side bent toward the affected rib as well as forward bent (Fig. 17-5).
2. Physician position: standing at the head of the table, supporting the patient.
3. **Technique:** same as for treating pump handle motion.

RIBS 10–12
1. Patient position: prone.
2. Physician position: at the side of the table, opposite the involved rib.
3. **Technique:**
   a. The patient's legs are pulled toward the physician.
   b. The patient's arm remains at his side (the only position difference from the treatment of inspiratory restrictions).
   c. The physician grasps the anterior inferior iliac spine and pulls it posteriorly.
   d. With the thenar eminence on the involved rib, the physician pushes it away from its articulation as the patient exhales forcefully (Fig. 17-6).

COUNTERSTRAIN TECHNIQUES FOR THE RIBS

Eileen L. DiGiovanna

This section describes counterstrain techniques for somatic dysfunctions of the anterior and posterior ribs. In most of these techniques the patient's head or thorax is bent to the side, with additional rotation into or away from the tender point.

Anterior Tender Points

RIBS 1 AND 2 (DEPRESSED)
The locations of the tender points of the anterior rib cage are shown in Figure 17-7. The tender point for the first rib is lateral to the sternum, at the level of the angle of Louis, just below the ster-

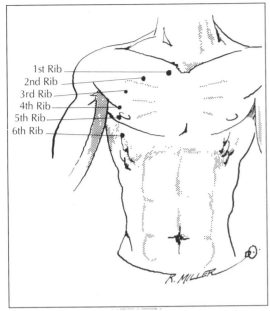

Figure 17-7. Tender point locations, anterior rib cage.

noclavicular joint. The tender point for the second rib is in the midclavicular line at the level of the second rib interspace.

1. Patient position: supine.
2. Physician position: standing at the patient's side near the head of the table.
3. **Technique:**
   a. The tender point is monitored with the physician's finger.

Figure 17-8. Counterstrain technique for a depressed first rib.

Figure 17-9. Counterstrain technique for somatic dysfunction of ribs 3–6 (depression).

   b. The patient's head is slightly flexed, rotated, and side bent toward the tender point (Fig. 17-8).
   c. Slightly more flexion is required for the second rib than for the first.
   d. When the point is no longer tender, the position is held for 120 seconds. The patient is slowly returned to neutral.

RIBS 3–6 (DEPRESSED)
The anterior tender points for the third through sixth ribs lie along the anterior axillary line on the ribs, or more medially along the sternal border at the rib interspaces.

1. Patient position: seated on the table.
2. Physician position: standing behind the patient.
3. **Technique:**
   a. The physician places her foot on the table opposite the side of the tender point and drapes the patient's arm over her thigh.
   b. The physician moves her thigh laterally so that the patient, who is leaning on the thigh, side bends to the side of the tender point.
   c. The patient is asked to curl his legs onto the table toward the side of the tender point (Fig. 17-9).
   d. When the point is no longer tender, the position is held for 120 seconds. The patient is then slowly returned to a neutral position.

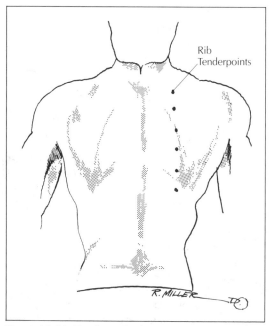

Figure 17-10. Tender point locations, posterior rib cage.

Posterior Tender Points

The posterior tender points lie along the angles of the ribs. Their locations are shown in Figure 17-10.

RIB 1 (ELEVATED)
1. Patient position: seated.

2. Physician position: standing behind the patient.
3. **Technique:**
   a. The physician places her foot on the table on the side of the tender point and drapes the patient's arm over her thigh.
   b. The patient leans on the physician's thigh, which is moved laterally, causing elevation of the first rib.
   c. The head is side bent toward the tender point. It is then bent forward or backward, whichever gives maximal softening of the tissues (Fig. 17-11).

RIBS 2–8 (ELEVATED)
1. Patient position: seated.
2. Physician position: standing.
3. **Technique:**
   a. The physician places her foot on the table on the side of the tender point and drapes the patient's arm over her thigh.
   b. The thigh is moved laterally with the patient leaning on it, further elevating the ribs on that side.
   c. For upper ribs the head is side bent and rotated away from the tender point.
   d. For lower ribs the patient is asked to curl his legs onto the table on the side opposite the tender point (Figs. 17-12, 17-13).
   e. When the point is no longer tender, the position is held for 120 seconds. The patient is then returned to a neutral position.

Figure 17-11. Counterstrain technique for an elevated first rib.

Figure 17-12. Counterstrain technique for elevation of the second through eighth ribs.

Figure 17-13. Lateral view of counterstrain technique for elevated ribs.

HIGH VELOCITY, LOW AMPLITUDE THRUSTING TECHNIQUES FOR THE RIBS
Barry Erner

Posterior Rib Head Somatic Dysfunction

1. Patient position: supine.
2. Physician position: standing at the side of the table opposite the side of the dysfunction.
3. **Technique:**
   a. The patient crosses the arm closest to the physician over his chest and grasps his opposite shoulder. With his far arm, the patient reaches across and grasps the opposite iliac crest (Fig. 17-14).
   b. The physician places the thenar eminence of his localizing hand under the posterior rib head being treated.
   c. The physician rests his other hand over the anterior chest wall, stabilizing the rib cage.
   d. After the patient has exhaled completely, the physician exerts a rapid thrust through the patient's crossed arms toward his thenar eminence, which is resting on the posterior rib head dysfunction (Fig. 17-15).

   Note: As with high velocity, low amplitude thrusting techniques of the thoracic spine, flexion of the spine down to the segment of dysfunction may be necessary for rib dysfunctions lower in the thorax. Flexion is achieved by the physician grasping the patient behind the shoulders with his nonlocalizing hand, then hugging the patient to create localized flexion down to the necessary point.

Figure 17-14. Patient position for high velocity, low amplitude thrusting technique for a posterior rib head somatic dysfunction.

Figure 17-15. High velocity, low amplitude thrusting technique for a posterior rib head somatic dysfunction.

Upper Rib Somatic Dysfunction (Ribs 1–4)

This technique is used for restricted motion at the costovertebral junction.

1. Patient position: prone.
2. Physician position: standing at the side of the table, opposite the dysfunction.
3. **Technique:**
   a. The patient cups his chin with the palm of his hand on the same side as the rib dysfunction.
   b. The patient's head is rotated into the motion barrier.
   c. The physician crosses his hands, placing one hand over the rib head dysfunction and the other on the side of the patient's occiput on the same side as the somatic dysfunction.

Figure 17-16. High velocity, low amplitude thrusting technique for upper rib somatic dysfunction, patient prone.

Figure 17-17. Alternative technique 1 for treatment of upper rib somatic dysfunction, patient prone.

Figure 17-18. Alternative technique 2 for treatment of upper rib somatic dysfunction, patient in lateral recumbent position.

d. The physician exerts rotational and lateral flexion forces on the patient's head, creating a locking at the cervicothoracic spinal junction.

e. Additional rotation and lateral flexion are induced by the physician until spring is noted under the hand placed over the rib head somatic dysfunction.

f. The physician exerts a rapid thrust on the dysfunctional rib. The force vector exaggerates the lateral cephalic springing motion noted in e (Fig. 17-16).

Alternative 1

1. Patient position: prone.
2. Physician position: standing at the head of the table, facing the patient.
3. **Technique:**
   a. The patient cups his chin with the palm of his hand on the same side as the rib dysfunction.
   b. The physician's hand placement is the same as previously described, except that the hands are not crossed.
   c. The localization and thrust are medial-caudal (Fig. 17-17).

Alternative 2 (Ribs 1–3)

1. Patient position: lateral recumbent position with the side of the rib dysfunction up.
2. Physician position: standing at the side of the table, facing the patient.
3. **Technique:**
   a. The physician cups the patient's head with one hand.
   b. The pads of the index and middle fingers of the physician's other hand are placed over the heads of the dysfunctional ribs.
   c. The physician uses his axilla and palpating hand to apply a caudal traction to the patient's arm and shoulder.
   d. The physician flexes the patient's head laterally toward the dysfunctional side until motion is felt in the palpating finger pads.
   e. The physician simultaneously exerts a rapid lateral flexion force on the patient's cervical spine and a caudal traction through the patient's upper shoulder and arm (Fig. 17-18).

First Rib Somatic Dysfunction (Expiratory Restriction)

1. Patient position: sitting on a stool or the treatment table, feet flat on floor.
2. Physician position: standing behind the patient with his knee and hip flexed and placed on the stool opposite the side of the rib dysfunction.
3. **Technique:**
   a. The patient drapes his arm on the side opposite the dysfunction over the physician's flexed knee.
   b. The patient leans on the physician's knee, allowing his torso to become limp.
   c. The patient places his arm on the same side as the rib dysfunction between his legs.
   d. The physician flexes the cervical spine laterally toward the dysfunction until all the slack is removed from the cervicothoracic junction.
   e. The physician places his thrusting hand with the metacarpophalangeal border (between the thumb and index finger) in the crease created by the patient's neck and the trapezius muscle.

Figure 17-19. High velocity, low energy thrusting technique for a first rib somatic dysfunction.

   f. The physician simultaneously applies a downward and medial thrust while rapidly exaggerating full cervical spine lateral flexion (Fig. 17-19).

RIB-RAISING TECHNIQUES
Eileen L. DiGiovanna

In certain pulmonary diseases it is helpful to loosen tenacious mucus and to articulate the ribs to improve their motion. Rib raising techniques achieve both these goals as the physician purposefully elevates groups of ribs. This section describes a few of these techniques.

The Bed-ridden Patient

This technique is especially useful for the patient who is unable to sit-up, for a weakened, sick patient, or for a comatose patient.

1. Patient position: supine.
2. Physician position: standing or seated at the side of the table or bed.
3. **Technique:**
   a. The physician places her hands, palm up, on the bed, with her fingers under the patient's rib cage.
   b. With the wrist as a fulcrum, the physician uses her fingers to raise and lower the ribs (Fig. 17-20).
   c. This process is repeated up and down the thorax.

Rib Raising and Thoracic Pump in the Bed-Ridden Patient

1. Patient position: supine.
2. Physician position: standing at the head of the table or bed.
3. **Technique:**
   a. The patient raises her arms above her head and clasps her hand behind the physician's thighs.

Figure 17-20. Rib raising in the bed-ridden patient.

b. As the physician rocks back and forth, doing the thoracic pump, the patient's chest is elevated through the pull on her arms.

The Seated Patient

This technique is applicable to patients who are able to sit upright, and especially to patients who have difficulty breathing and prefer to be upright.

1. Patient position: seated on the edge of the bed or on a chair.
2. Physician position: standing in front of the patient.
3. **Technique:**
   a. The patient crosses his arms in front of him with the elbows resting on the physician's upper arms.

b. The physician reaches behind the patient's back, with the fingers of each hand grasping a group of ribs (Fig. 17-21).
c. The physician rocks back while pressing down on the posterior ribs. At the same time the patient falls forward onto his arms, which elevates the anterior rib cage.
d. The physician repeats this maneuver rhythmically, moving her hands up and down the thoracic spine.
e. The patient may assist in the treatment by inhaling deeply as the physician rocks back and exhaling fully as the physician moves forward.

Alternative Technique

1. Patient position: seated straddling the table.
2. Physician position: standing behind the patient.
3. **Technique:**
   a. The physician places the thumbs of each hand pointing toward the spine and spreads her fingers over the ribs bilaterally.
   b. The patient places his hands on the table in front of him.
   c. The physician pushes forward on the rib cage as the patient inhales and leans forward between his arms (Fig. 17–22).
   d. This maneuver is repeated rhythmically as the physician moves her hands up and down the thorax.
   e. The patient's inhalation elevates the ribs anteriorly as the physician depresses them posteriorly.

Figure 17-21. Rib raising for the seated patient.

Figure 17-22. Alternate approach to rib raising in the seated patient.

LYMPHATIC PUMP
Eileen L. DiGiovanna

Movement of the lymph depends on muscular movement. A bed-ridden patient loses considerable muscular motion. Since the movement of lymph is necessary to carry immune cells and phagocytes to their sites of action, aid should be given to patients who have decreased active motion. One of the best ways the osteopathic physician can help such a patient is with some form of lymphatic pump.

Thoracic Pump
PATIENT PASSIVE

This technique may be used in comatose patients or patients who are too weak to aid in treatment.

1. Patient position: supine.
2. Physician position: standing at the head of the table or bed.
3. **Technique:**
   a. Physician places her hands on either side of the patient's anterior chest wall with her fingers pointing toward the patient's feet. The heel of the physician's hand just touches the inferior border of the clavicle (Fig. 17-23).
   b. For a female patient, the physician's hands may point toward the midline and slightly overlap on top of the sternum.

c. The physician maintains her elbows in a locked position.
d. The physician leans her body weight forward, gently compressing the patient's chest. Care should be taken that the pressure is not too great.
e. The physician initiates a rhythmic motion by rocking back and forth, compressing and releasing. The motion should cause the patient's feet to move.
f. The rhythmic movement is continued for two or three minutes.

PATIENT RESPIRATORY ASSIST

This technique uses the patient's respiration to assist, through sudden intrathoracic pressure changes, the movement of lymph through the thoracic duct and cysterna chyli.

1. Patient position: supine.
2. Physician position: standing at the head of the table or bed.
3. **Technique:**
   a. The physician's hands are placed on the patient's chest in the same manner as in the previous technique.
   b. The patient is instructed to inhale deeply, then exhale slowly. At the end of exhalation, the patient is told to inhale deeply.

Figure 17-23. Thoracic pump for lymphatic drainage.

Figure 17-24. Pedal pump for lymphatic drainage.

   c. As the patient inhales and exhales, the physician's hands follow the respiratory motion.

   d. At the end of exhalation, the physician gently compresses the chest and provides a resistance to the patient's next inhalation.

   e. When the physician feels the patient is using force to inhale, she quickly releases the resistance. The patient will gasp with a sudden intake of air.

Pedal Pump

In some patients it is difficult to use the thoracic pump. Some difficulties that might preclude its use include the following:

1. The physician cannot get to the head of the bed.
2. The patient may be on a respirator or may have tubes or wires in the thorax.
3. The patient may be too osteoporotic for pressure to be applied to the chest.
4. The patient may have had chest trauma or surgery.

In these instances, a pedal pump rather than a thoracic pump may be used to mobilize lymph.

The technique described below should not be used in patients suspected of having phlebothrombosis or who are at high risk of clot formation.

1. Patient position: supine.
2. Physician position: standing at the foot of the table or bed.
3. **Technique:**
   a. The physician grasps the patient's feet by placing her hands or the dorsum or on soles of the feet.
   b. The patient's feet are pumped up and down so that the leg muscles are used to move the lymph (Fig. 17-24).
   c. This technique should produce a gentle rocking of the body.

References

Jones, Lawrence. 1981. Strain and Counterstrain. Colorado Springs, Colo.: American Academy of Osteopathy.

Mitchell F Jr., Moran P, Pruzzo N. 1979. An Evaluation and Treatment Manual of Osteopathic Muscle Energy Procedures. Valley Park, Mo: Mitchell, Moran, and Pruzzo Associates.

18

The Upper Extremity

THE SHOULDER
Eileen L. DiGiovanna

Functional Anatomy

The shoulder is the articulation between the head of the humerus and the glenoid fossa of the scapula. It is the most mobile joint in the body as well as the most unstable. The glenohumeral articulation functions within the setting of the shoulder girdle. The shoulder girdle consists of three bones (the clavicle, humerus, and scapula), three true, synovial joints (glenohumeral, sternoclavicular, and acrominoclavicular), two functional joints, two accessory joints, and the muscles that move the three bones.

SYNOVIAL JOINTS

The sternoclavicular joint has sellar articular surfaces, frequently with an interposed meniscus. This joint affords movement of the clavicle in a frontal and horizontal plane as well as rotation on its long axis.

The acromioclavicular joint is a plane joint. Occasionally there is an intraarticular plate between the surfaces. The acromioclavicular joint permits motion of the clavicle in an anteroposterior or cephalic-caudal direction, as well as rotation. More motion is possible at the lateral end of the clavicle, owing to the crank shape of the bone.

The glenohumeral joint allows greater freedom of motion than any other joint in the body. The humeral head is convex and has a larger surface area than the concave glenoid fossa on which it moves. The humeral head slides along the surface of the fossa and rolls in various angular motions.

The capsule of the glenohumeral joint is loose and pleated. The ligaments, which are merely thickenings in the capsule, provide little support. Most of the support of the joint is provided by the rotator cuff muscles, which snug the head into the fossa. These muscles include the supraspinatus, infraspinatus, teres minor, and subscapular muscles.

FUNCTIONAL JOINTS (PSEUDOJOINTS)

The two functional joints in the shoulder girdle are the suprahumeral joint and the scapulothoracic joint. Both figure prominently in shoulder biomechanics and pathology. The suprahumeral joint is formed by the articulation of the head of the humerus with the coracoacromial arch, composed of the acromium, the coracoid process, and the ligament between them. Articulation occurs during abduction. At rest, there is a space in the joint through which pass the tendon of the long head of the biceps, the supraspinatus muscle and supraspinatus tendon, the subacromial bursa, and the capsule—all important and sensitive structures.

Figure 18-1. Impingement on the coracoacromial ligament.

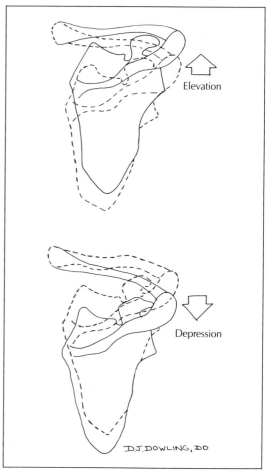

Figure 18-2. Elevation and depression of the scapula.

These soft tissues are compressed during abduction around 90 degrees (Fig. 18-1). Internal rotation of the humerus causes impingement to occur at about 60 degrees. During external rotation, the head of the humerus glides posteriorly and impingement does not occur until 120 degrees of abduction. For this reason, persons with habitually slouched shoulders and internally rotated arms are more prone to degenerative processes such as tendinitis and bursitis.

The second functional joint is the scapulothoracic joint. Because muscle and fascia lie between the articulating surfaces, it is not a true joint.

ACCESSORY JOINTS

The accessory joints are the costosternal joints anteriorly, especially those of the first and second ribs, and the costovertebral joints posteriorly. The accessory joints are not anatomically involved in the shoulder joint or shoulder girdle, but dysfunction of these joints can interfere with free shoulder motion.

Motion of the Shoulder Bones

HUMERUS

The humerus moves in the following ways:

1. **Flexion** to 180 degrees.
2. **Extension** to 45 degrees.
3. **Abduction** to 180 degrees, placing the arm in the same position as flexion to 180 degrees.
4. **Adduction,** achieved with slight flexion or extension to clear the trunk.
5. **Horizontal flexion and extension,** after the arm has been abducted to 90 degrees.
6. **Internal and external rotation** around the long axis of the humerus, for a total of 180 degrees.
7. **Circumduction,** a combination of movements causing the arm to describe an irregular cone.

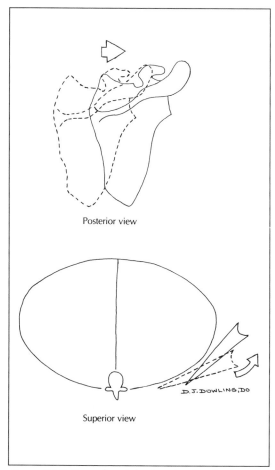

Figure 18-3. Scapular abduction (protraction).

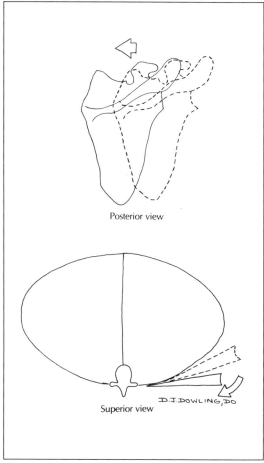

Figure 18-4. Scapular adduction (retraction).

SCAPULA

The motions of the scapula are the following:

1. **Elevation,** upward and parallel to the spine, and **depression,** a return from elevation (Fig. 18-2).
2. **Abduction** or **protraction** away from the spine, which is combined with a lateral tilt around the thorax (Fig. 18-3).
3. **Adduction** or **retraction,** moving closer to the spine (Fig. 18-4).
4. **Upward or forward tilt,** turning on a horizontal axis so that the posterior surface faces upward and the inferior angle protrudes. This motion is accompanied by a longitudinal axis rotation of the clavicle (Fig. 18-5).
5. **Upward and downward rotation** in relation to the glenoid fossa's elevation or depression; a frontal plane rotation (Fig. 18-6).

The glenoid fossa rotates upward during abduction and this accomplishes several important functions:

1. The humerus impinges on the acromion at 90 degrees. To prevent impingement and permit abduction to 180 degrees, the scapula must rotate.
2. The fossa moves under the head of the humerus and increases the stability of the joint when the arm is elevated, preventing a downward dislocation.

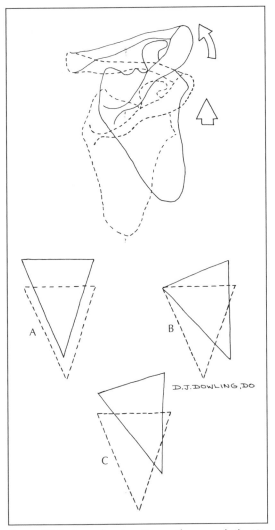

Figure 18-5. Scapular elevation with upward tilt: (**A**) pure elevation, (**B**) pure tilt, (**C**) coupled motions.

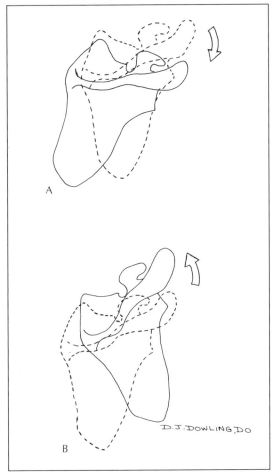

Figure 18-6. Rotation of the scapula: (**A**) downward, (**B**) upward.

3. The fibers of the deltoid, attached from the scapula to the humerus, contract to abduct the arm to 90 degrees, at which point they are maximally contracted. As the fossa rotates upward, it maintains the deltoid in position for maximal contraction.

JOINT RHYTHMS AND MECHANISMS

The scapulohumeral rhythm is free-flowing and synchronous movement of the scapula and humerus. During abduction, the scapula rotates as the humerus elevates. For every 15 degrees of abduction, humeral elevation accounts for 10 degrees and scapular rotation for 5 degrees. Dysfunction of humeral elevation or of scapular rotation can disturb this rhythm and interfere with shoulder function. Dysfunction of clavicular motion can also interfere with this rhythm.

Glenohumeral movement requires a synchronous posterior downward glide of the humeral head during abduction to prevent impingement on the coracoacromial arch. This necessitates an external rotation of the humerus to turn the greater tuberosity away from the arch.

Another mechanism indirectly involved in shoulder function is the bicipital mechanism. The tendon of the long head of the biceps passes through a groove between the greater and lesser tuberosities of the humerus and attaches to the rim of the glenoid. The tendon glides through the groove whenever the humerus is moved. Contraction of the muscle does not move the tendon. Biceps tendinitis, capsulitis, or adhesions may prevent free gliding of the tendon and interfere with normal motions.

The clavicle moves during most shoulder activity. Dysfunctions in clavicular motion can interfere with normal shoulder movement.

Evaluation of the Shoulder

Observation is the first step in evaluating the shoulder. The physician should look for a smooth contour and symmetry between the two shoulders. Blemishes or signs of trauma should be noted.

The shoulder should then be palpated. This is best done by the physician standing behind the patient. Symmetry, smoothness of contour, swelling, and tenderness should be noted.

The range of motion should be tested passively and actively, with any restrictions noted. A general motion screening is done by asking the patient to raise both arms slowly and touch the backs of his hands over the head. The physician observes scapular motion and symmetry of shoulders, elbows, and wrist angles.

The Apley scratch test is a good method to test active range of motion. The patient is instructed to reach across his chest, over the shoulder, and touch the opposite scapula. Then he reaches behind his back and touches his opposite scapula. Finally, he reaches behind his head and touches the opposite scapula. These maneuvers test all the ranges of motion in the shoulder joint.

Muscle strength and sensation should be tested. There are no specific reflexes at the shoulder. These are found at the elbow.

TESTS FOR SHOULDER DYSFUNCTION

Several specific tests may be used to detect shoulder dysfunction; these are described below.

Arm drop test. The patient's arm is elevated to 90 degrees of abduction and released. If there is a tear in the rotator cuff muscles, the arm will drop.

If the tear is partial, by tapping on the arm the physician will cause it to drop.

Apprehension test. This test is for a chronically dislocating shoulder. The arm is abducted, extended, and externally rotated. At the point where the shoulder is about to dislocate, the patient will appear apprehensive.

Yergason test. The Yergason test is performed to assess the stability of the biceps tendon in the bicipital groove. The physician applies traction to the elbow and externally rotates the arm. The patient attempts to internally rotate the arm against resistance. If the tendon is unstable in the groove, it will pop out with a snap, and the patient will experience pain (Fig. 18-7).

All patients with chronic shoulder problems must be evaluated for dysfunctions of the cervical spine, upper thoracic spine, and upper ribs.

Shoulder Pathology

TENDINITIS

The two tendons of the shoulder most commonly involved by an inflammatory process are those of the long head of the biceps and the supraspinatus tendon. Both pass through the suprahumeral space and are compressed during abduction of the shoulder.

The tendons lack adequate circulation at the area where a gap occurs between vessels entering the tendon from the muscle and vessels entering from the bone. This area is known as the *critical zone.* The critical zone is also the most likely site of deposition of calcium in calcific tendinitis. About 90% of nontraumatic shoulder pain is due to tendinitis.

BURSITIS

Although bursitis is a common diagnosis in shoulder pain, only a small percentage of shoulder pain is actually due to bursitis. The most commonly affected bursa is the subacromial bursa, owing to its location in the suprahumeral space. Occasionally, a calcium deposit in a tendon will rupture through into the bursa, leading to calcific bursitis.

FROZEN SHOULDER

Also known as adhesive capsulitis, frozen shoulder results from prolonged immobilization of the shoulder. Frozen shoulder may result from appli-

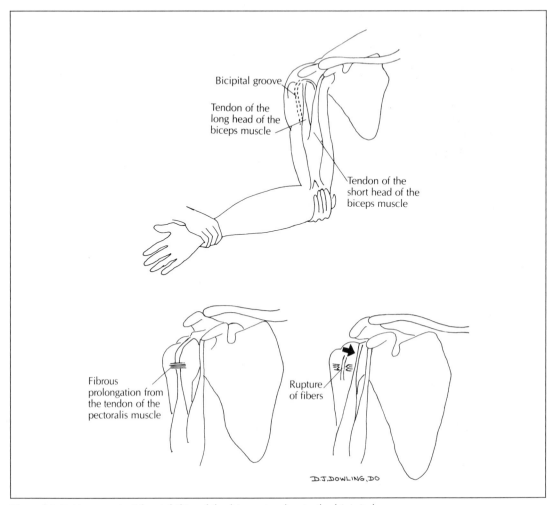

Bicipital groove

Tendon of the
long head of the
biceps muscle

Tendon of the
short head of the
biceps muscle

Fibrous
prolongation from
the tendon of the
pectoralis muscle

Rupture
of fibers

D.J.DOWLING,DO

Figure 18-7. Yergason test for stability of the biceps tendon in the bicipital groove.

cation of a splint or sling, or from failure to move the shoulder because of pain from trauma or an inflammatory process in the shoulder. Inflammatory and fibrous changes occur in all the periarticular soft tissues. The range of motion of the shoulder can be markedly restricted, with abduction and internal rotation usually the most affected. Patients should be instructed to exercise the shoulder. Complete immobilization should not be continued for more than 48 hours. Prevention is the best treatment.

ARTHRITIS

Any type of arthritis may involve any of the shoulder girdle joints. The sternoclavicular joint is most commonly affected.

TRAUMA

The shoulder sustains trauma from direct blows, from falls on an outstretched arm, or from twisting injuries. Fractures commonly involve the clavicle. The neck of the humerus is another common site of fracture.

The humeral head may dislocate from the fossa since support of this joint is so poor. Anterior dislocations, under the clavicle or under the coracoid, are the most common. Posterior dislocations are less common but are more difficult to evaluate without radiography. In both fractures and dislocations, the physician must be alert to nerve compression or vascular compromise, since many important nerves and muscles lie in this area.

Occasionally the biceps tendon is unstable in

its groove, usually when the transverse ligament has been damaged by trauma or worn by repeated microtrauma. The tendon then will snap out of the groove on certain motions, such as the Yergason test.

ACROMIOCLAVICULAR SEPARATION

Following a blow to the acromion, the scapula may torque around the corocoid and tear ligaments at the acromioclavicular joint, producing acromioclavicular separation. The injury may be graded as first degree, second degree, or third degree, depending on the amount of ligamentous injury. Acromioclavicular separation is best diagnosed with radiographs of the patient holding a weight in his hand to pull the acromion away from the end of the clavicle.

SOMATIC DYSFUNCTION

Most articular somatic dysfunctions of the shoulder occur at the sternoclavicular or acromioclavicular joints. These dysfunctions are characterized by pain at the involved joint and restricted motion in one or more of the planes of joint motion.

THE ELBOW
Eileen L. DiGiovanna

Functional Anatomy

The elbow links the forearm with the upper arm and, in concert with the shoulder, allows motion of the hand through space. The elbow functions as a ginglymus or hinge joint. It is formed by the articulation of the proximal ends of the radius and ulna with the distal end of the humerus.

The motions observed in the elbow joint are flexion, extension, and rotation (supination and pronation). Flexion and extension are the only motions that involve the true elbow joint. Flexion may be active or passive. Active flexion ends at about 145 degrees and is primarily limited by opposition of the contracting muscles of the arm and forearm. The range of passive flexion is slightly larger as the muscles relax and are flattened. Bony opposition and tension in the triceps and posterior capsular ligaments also limit flexion. The primary flexor muscle is the biceps brachii, which is assisted by the brachialis and the brachioradialis.

Extension of the elbow from the anatomic position is limited (5 to 10 degrees) by contact of the olecranon process with the fossa, tension in the anterior ligament, and resistance of anterior muscles. The triceps brachii is the only elbow muscle that functions in extension. Since most elbow extension is accomplished by gravity, the triceps functions primarily against resistance.

Besides flexion and extension, the forearm can rotate around its longitudinal axis. Rotation involves the superior radioulnar joint of the elbow and the inferior radioulnar joint, which lies above the wrist. These motions are observed with the forearm flexed to 90 degrees.

Supination is the rotary motion that turns the palm of hand toward the ceiling; pronation is the rotary motion that turns the palm toward the floor. In neutral rotation the palm faces medially with the thumb up. The total range of rotation is about 180 degrees.

During supination, the interosseous membrane between the radius and ulna becomes taut. Supination involves the supinator and biceps muscles; pronation involves the pronator quadratus and pronator teres. The pronators are less powerful than the supinators.

When the arm is in the anatomic position, the upper arm and the forearm form an angle at the elbow, with the forearm directed away from the body in a valgus position. This is known as the *carrying angle* and is normally greater in women than in men (10 to 15 degrees in women, 5 degrees in men). If the carrying angle exceeds 15 degrees, it is called *cubitus valgus*. A decrease is known as *cubitus varus* or "gunstock" deformity.

Evaluation

The elbow should be examined first by observation. The carrying angle should be noted, as should any swelling, which may be diffuse or localized to the olecranon bursa posteriorly. Signs of old or new trauma should be noted, such as scars, abrasions, bruises, and the like.

The soft tissues and bony structures are then palpated to evaluate the integrity of the bones and the presence of any swelling, tenderness, masses, asymmetries, or crepitus. The ulnar nerve may be palpated in the groove between the medial epicondyle and the olecranon. The physician checks for scar tissue around the nerve that might compromise it. The Tinel test (tapping the nerve gently) may disclose a neuroma. The olecranon bursa should not be palpable unless it is filled with fluid or thickened.

Range of motion should be checked actively and passively. Both muscle strength and sensation should be tested.

There are three reflexes of the upper extremity, all deep tendon reflexes:

1. **Biceps reflex:** elicited by tapping the biceps tendon in the antecubital fossa; tests primarily C5.
2. **Brachioradialis reflex:** elicited by tapping the tendon on the lateral aspect of the lower forearm above the wrist; tests C6.
3. **Triceps reflex:** elicited by tapping the triceps tendon on the posterior arm just above the olecranon; tests C7.

Although these are upper extremity reflexes, they are tests for cervical nerve root dysfunction.

It may be necessary to test the elbow for ligamentous stability. This is done by placing first a valgus stress and then a varus stress on the elbow, using one hand as a fulcrum and the other as an opposing force.

Elbow Pathologies

EPICONDYLITIS

Epicondylitis is a common elbow problem, generally called tennis elbow if the lateral epicondyle is involved and golfer's elbow if the medial epicondyle is involved. This is an overuse syndrome that is associated with any activity that requires repetitive pronation and supination, such as gripping a tennis racquet, golf club, screwdriver, or doorknob. The wrist extensor muscles are involved in lateral epicondylitis. Tennis elbow is tested by having the patient make a fist and hold it in extension while the physician tries to force it into flexion. A positive test will reproduce the patient's pain over the lateral epicondyl.

Whenever the elbow is evaluated the shoulder and wrist should be examined as well, since symptoms may be referred.

SOMATIC DYSFUNCTION

The most common articular somatic dysfunction at the elbow involves the head of the radius. Restriction in anterior or posterior motion is tested by moving the radial head in an anteroposterior direction. This condition often mimics the pain of tennis elbow. The anterior slide of the radial head is coupled with supination/flexion, and the posterior slide with pronation/extension.

THE WRIST AND HAND
Eileen L. DiGiovanna

Functional Anatomy

THE WRIST

The wrist or carpus is the distal articulation of the radius and the articular disk with the proximal row of carpal bones. The disk joins the ulna and radius and lies between the ulna and the proximal row of carpal bones. Laterally to medially, these bones are the scaphoid (navicular), lunate, and the triquetrum. A small bone, the pisiform, lies slightly anterior to the triquetrum.

A midcarpal joint lies between the proximal and distal rows of carpal bones. The distal row is made up of the trapezium, the trapezoid, the capitate, and the hamate. The third functional joint at the wrist is the distal radioulnar joint.

The wrist moves in two planes. In the *sagittal*

plane it flexes to approximately 85 degrees and extends to approximately 45 degrees. Flexion and extension appear to occur around more than one axis. In the *coronal plane* the wrist moves into abduction (radial deviation) and adduction (ulnar deviation). Abduction is about 15 degrees and adduction 45 degrees.

Pronation and supination occur at the radioulnar joint and, combined with flexion, extension, abduction, and adduction, permit circumduction so that the hand can lie in any plane.

The wrist is moved by four groups of muscles:

1. **Flexor carpi ulnaris:** flexes the wrist and adducts the hand.
2. **Extensor carpi ulnaris:** extends the wrist and adducts the hand.
3. **Flexor carpi radialis and palmaris longus:** flex the wrist and abduct the hand.
4. **Extensor carpi radialis longus and brevis:** extend the wrist and abduct the hand.

The bodies of these muscles lie close to the elbow and the corresponding tendons are long, passing down the forearm to attach to the wrist.

The carpal bones form an arch spanned by the flexor retinaculum. The concavity of the arch lies on the palmar surface between the bones and the transverse ligament (the flexor retinaculum) and is called the *carpal tunnel*. Through this tunnel pass the tendons of the wrist and finger flexors and the median nerve. It is the site of origin of the thenar and hypothenar muscles.

Another tunnel, the tunnel of Guyon, is formed by the ligament attaching the hook of the hamate and the pisiform. Through this tunnel pass the ulnar nerve and artery.

On the lateral aspect of the wrist is a small depression known as the anatomic snuffbox. The floor of the snuffbox is the scaphoid or navicular bone. It lies distal to the radial styloid and becomes prominent when the thumb is forcefully extended. It is bounded by the abductor pollicis longus, extensor pollicis brevis, and the extensor pollicis longus tendons.

THE HAND

The human hand is prehensile to a degree not attained in other species. Only in man can the thumb be brought into opposition with each of the other fingers. This is a remarkable organ of sense, capable of measuring thickness and distance as well as perceiving light touch and temperature. The delicate movements of the hand allow grasping and fine movements.

The hand consists of five metacarpal bones that articulate proximally with four carpal bones in the distal row. The second and third metacarpals remain relatively fixed while the first, fourth, and fifth move around this fixed segment. The five metacarpals articulate distally with the proximal phalanges of the fingers. These are usually considered hinge joints. They permit flexion/extension, abduction, adduction, and circumduction.

An extensor tendon lies along the dorsal aspect of each joint, and there are fibrocartilaginous plates over the palmar surface, known as palmar or volar plates. These plates lie between the joint and the flexor tendons.

Each finger, except the thumb, has a proximal and a distal interphalangeal joint. Since there are only two bones in the thumb, there is only one joint. The interphalangeal joints are hinge joints, allowing flexion and extension and some axial rotation.

The skin over the palm of the hand is thicker than over the dorsum and is firmly attached to the fascia at the palmar creases. This permits the hand to grasp objects securely. Also important to grasp is the ability of the hand to change shape to conform to the object being grasped. It can flatten and spread out to conform to a flat surface or it can form a hollow cuplike depression.

The muscles of the fingers lie in the forearm. The tendons cross the wrist with the wrist muscle tendons. The flexor muscles cross the palm through numerous fibroosseous tunnels. The extensor tendons pass along the dorsum of the hand through fewer tunnels. The flexor and extensor muscles are all extrinsic muscles.

Intrinsic muscles include the interosseous and lumbrical muscles. In addition to assisting with flexion and extension, they abduct and adduct the fingers.

At the base of the thumb on the palmar surface is the thenar eminence, which is made up of the intrinsic muscles of the thumb: the adductor pollicis, opponens pollicis, abductor policis brevis, and flexor pollicis brevis. These muscles are innervated by the median nerve. The thenar eminence atrophies when the median nerve is trapped, as in carpal tunnel syndrome.

On the medial aspect of the palm, at the base of the fifth digit, is the hypothenar eminence, which contains three muscles: the flexor digiti minimi, abductor digiti minimi, and opponens digiti minimi.

PREHENSILE MOTIONS OF THE HAND

According to Kapandji, there are six ways in which the hand can grasp objects; the thumb is involved in four kinds of prehensile motions.

1. **Prehension by terminal opposition** is the finest and most precise form of grasp. The tip of the finger pad or fingernail makes contact when the thumb and index finger grasp a thin object.
2. **Prehension by subterminal opposition** is the most common form of grasp. The object is held between the pads of the thumb and index fingers.
3. In **prehension by subterminolateral opposition,** the pad of the thumb holds an object, such as a coin, pressed against the radial surface of the first phalanx of the index finger.
4. **Palmar prehension** is used to grasp heavy, relatively large objects. The entire hand is wrapped around the object. The thumb opposes the force of the other four fingers.
5. **Prehension by digitopalmar opposition** entails grasp of a small-diameter object by the fingers pressing against the palm. The thumb is not involved.
6. **Prehension between lateral aspects of the fingers** is exemplified by holding a cigarette. This grip is weak, and the object must be small. The thumb is not involved.

Evaluation

OBSERVATION

The hand should be observed while in use, such as unbuttoning a shirt, and at rest. At rest the hand should lie in slight flexion. The fingers should be counted.

Any joint or soft tissue swelling should be noted. Infection may spread rapidly through the soft tissues of the hand. Fusiform swelling of the proximal interphalangeal joints is indicative of rheumatoid arthritis. Discrete bony nodules on the distal interphalangeal joints are called Heberden's nodes and are indicative of osteoarthritis.

The arthritides may cause painful swelling of the hand and wrist joints and may result in specific deformities. A "swan's neck" deformity occurs when the proximal interphalangeal joint is hyperextended and the distal interphalangeal joint is flexed. Various joints may sublux, and ulnar deviation may develop.

If the tendon of the extensor digitorum communis avulses from the base of the middle phalanx, the proximal interphalangeal joint will hyperflex and the distal interphalangeal joint will extend, producing the "boutonniere" deformity. A mallet finger is one in which the distal interphalangeal joint is flexed and will not extend, owing to avulsion of the distal insertion of the extensor digitorum communis.

The nails should be inspected for clubbing, color (abnormal pallor or cyanosis), or infection around the edges (paronychia). Any atrophy of the thenar or hypothenar areas should be noted.

PALPATION

The wrist and hand joints should be palpated for swelling, asymmetries, temperature changes, and tenderness. The skin of the wrist and hand should be evaluated for temperature and moisture changes. Calluses should be noted. The anatomic snuffbox may be palpated. In case of trauma, any tenderness in this area should be noted, as the navicular is the most commonly fractured of the carpal bones.

The tunnels across the dorsum of the wrist should be palpated for swelling or tenderness. The volar tunnels should be similarly evaluated. Ganglia may occur in the tendon sheaths.

RANGE OF MOTION

All joints should be put through their passive range of motion and the patient asked to demonstrate active range of motion. The digits are evaluated together and individually. The fingers and thumb should be flexed and extended, and finger abduction and adduction should be tested. When the patient touches the thumb to the tip of each of the other fingers, the wrist should flex, extend, abduct, and adduct.

MUSCLE STRENGTH TESTING

A general screening of hand strength is to ask the patient to squeeze two or three of the examiner's fingers. If a weakness is found, each finger flexor is tested individually. The extensors are checked by trying to force the fingers into flexion.

To test the intrinsic muscles, the patient spreads his fingers while the examiner tries to close them. Then the patient tries to close his fingers against the examiner's resistance.

The pinch mechanism is tested by having the

Figure 18-8. Phalen's test.

Figure 18-9. Tinel sign of the wrist and elbow.

patient form an O with his thumb and index finger as the examiner hooks his fingers into the O and tries to pull it apart.

Wrist flexion and extension strength should be tested with the hand made into a fist.

SENSATION TESTING
The peripheral nerves may be tested by sensation testing the following sites:

1. **Radial nerve:** dorsum of web space between thumb and index finger.
2. **Median nerve:** tip of index finger.
3. **Ulnar nerve:** tip of fifth finger.

The dermatome levels are the following:

1. C6: thumb and index finger and lateral palm.
2. C7: middle finger.
3. C8: fourth and fifth fingers and medial palm.

SPECIAL TESTS
Bunnel-Littler test. This test evaluates the tightness of the intrinsic muscles of the hand. The metacarpophalangeal joint is held in extension and the patient tries to move the proximal interphalangeal joint into flexion. If the proximal interphalangeal joint does not flex, then the intrinsic muscles are tight or the joint capsule is contracted. The metacarpophalangeal joint is

rested briefly, then retested. If the proximal interphalangeal joint still cannot flex, the problem is in the joint capsule.

Allen test. This test evaluates functioning of the medial and ulnar arteries. Occlude the two arteries and have the patient open and close his fist. The palm should be pale. Release one artery and the hand should flush. Repeat with the other artery.

Phalen's test. This test is for carpal tunnel syndrome. The patient flexes the wrists and presses the backs of his hands together. He holds this position for a minute. In carpal tunnel syndrome this will produce pain or paresthesias in the affected hand (Fig. 18-8).

Tinel sign. By tapping over the volar carpal ligament, pain or paresthesias may be produced over the distribution of the median nerve in a case of carpal tunnel syndrome (Fig. 18-9).

Finkelstein test. This test is used to rule out de Quervain's disease. The patient closes his fingers around his thumb and then ulnar deviates his wrist. Pain along the lateral wrist is a positive test.

Pathology of the Wrist and Hand
CARPAL TUNNEL SYNDROME
In carpal tunnel syndrome the median nerve is compressed in the tunnel by fibrous bands, scar tissue from chronic inflammation or micro-trauma, arthritis, or myxedema due to hypothyroidism. The syndrome is characterized by pain or paresthesias such as tingling in the hand, particularly along the distribution of the median nerve. Numbness may be the presenting symptom. Weakness of the hand frequently occurs. On examination the thenar eminence may be atrophied. The flexor tendons might be slightly swollen. The Tinel sign and a positive Phalen test are valuable diagnostic clues.

Osteopathic treatment should be aimed at loosening tense fascia, freeing the area of edema fluid, and stretching fibrous bands. Any joint restrictions should be corrected.

DE QUERVAIN'S DISEASE
This condition is a stenosing tenosynovitis of the thumb. It is more common in women than in men and is related to repetitive movements of the thumb that cause inflammation within the tendon sheath. The main symptoms are pain and difficulty moving the thumb. Swelling around the anatomic snuffbox may be noted. There is pain on circumduction of the thumb. The specific test for this condition is the Finkelstein test. Injection with steroids may be necessary.

Osteopathic treatment is aimed at relieving edema and freeing motion of the joints and fascia. Counterstrain treatment of tender points may be helpful.

DUPUYTREN'S CONTRACTURE
This condition is characterized by contracture of the palmar fascia and nodule formation. There appears to be a genetic predisposition to the disease. It is frequently found in alcoholics. It can be triggered or aggravated by trauma. The nodules are tender. The palmar fascia contracts, flexing the fingers, particularly on the ulnar side. Finger and hand function can be severely limited.

Osteopathic treatment is aimed toward keeping the palmar fascia as free as possible; the metacarpophalangeal and proximal interphalangeal joints should be mobilized to prevent secondary joint immobilization and tethering of the flexor tendons. Surgical intervention may be required.

ARTHRITIS
Rheumatoid arthritis and osteoarthritis may involve the joints of the wrist and hand. Psoriatic arthritis and gouty arthritis may also affect this area. Many of the findings and specific deformities were mentioned earlier. In the arthritides, the small accessory motions of the joint are lost first. The osteopathic physician must articulate all joints once the acute inflammation has subsided. The patient should be encouraged to exercise the joints greatly to maintain mobility.

References

Arminio JA. 1982. DeQuervain's disease: The forgotten syndrome. Resident Staff Physician 28(6):84–88.

Bateman JE. 1978. The Shoulder and Neck. Philadelphia: W.B. Saunders Co.

Cailliet R. 1966. Shoulder Pain. Philadelphia: F.A. Davis Co.

———. 1976. Hand Pain and Impairment, 2nd ed. Philadelphia: F.A. Davis Co.

DiGiovanna E. 1981. Shoulder kinetics. Osteopath Ann 9(3):75–79.

Hoppenfeld S. 1976. Physical Examination of the Spine and Extremities. Norwalk, Conn: Appleton-Century-Crofts.

Janecki CJ, Field JH. 1984. Washerwoman's sprain, working woman's pain. Aches Pains 14:20.

Kapandji IA. 1972. The Physiology of the Joints. Vol 1. Upper Limb. Edinburgh: Churchill Livingstone.

Leddy JP, Hamilton JJ. 1984. Tennis elbow: Not just a case for the courts. Aches Pains 14:21.

Lipscomb PR. 1984. Carpal tunnel syndrome: Guide to office diagnosis. J Musculoskel Med 35:41.

Moseley HF. 1972. Shoulder Lesions. Edinburgh: Churchill Livingstone.

Nirschl RP. 1984. The prevention and management of tennis elbow. Pain Analg 6:10.

Paletta, FX. 1981. Dupuytren's contracture. AFP 23: 85–90.

Polley HF, Hunder GA. 1987. Physical Examination of the Joints. Philadelphia: W.B. Saunders Co.

Quiring DP. 1960. The Extremities. Philadelphia: Lea & Febiger.

Rasch PJ, Burke RK. 1978. Kinesiology and Applied Anatomy. Baltimore: Lea & Febiger.

Roland AC, Cawley PW. 1984. Common elbow injuries. Family Practice Recertifications, MRA Publications, Inc., September 1984.

Weiss TE. 1984. Painful hands: Differential diagnosis by physical examination only. Consultant 24(12): 51–65.

19

Diagnosis and Treatment of the Upper Extremity

THE SHOULDER GIRDLE
Eileen L. DiGiovanna

The two major goals of osteopathic manipulation of the shoulder girdle are to restore function and to prevent motion loss. This section describes several active, passive, and isometric techniques.

Spencer Techniques
The Spencer techniques are seven gentle stretching maneuvers used to treat shoulder restriction caused by hypertonic muscles, early adhesive capsulitis, healed fractures and dislocations, and any other traumatic or degenerative condition in which improved motion is needed. Motion testing is done passively or by using the Apley scratch test, described in Chapter 18. The general guidelines for performing all seven techniques are as follows:

1. Patient position: lateral recumbent position with the affected shoulder up. The patient's knees and hips are flexed, his back is straight and perpendicular to table, his lower arm is down and comfortable, and his head is supported by a pillow.
2. Physician position: standing at the side of the table, facing the patient.
3. **Technique:** The physician grasps the patient's forearm with one hand, flexing the patient's el-

bow. The physician's other hand is placed on top of patient's shoulder to lock the shoulder girdle, limiting scapular movement.

Each technique is repeated six to eight times, stopping when it becomes painful to patient or motion is restricted. With each movement, the physician tries to exceed the point reached in the previous excursion.

1. **To increase extension:** The physician moves the patient's arm in a horizontal plane, extending the shoulder and returning it to neutral position, gently increasing the excursion. The patient's elbow is kept in flexion (Fig. 19-1).
2. **To increase flexion:** The physician flexes the patient's shoulder, straightening the elbow, until the arm is over the patient's ear (Fig. 19-2). This maneuver is gently repeated in rhythmic motion, with the shoulder returned to neutral position each time. The physician may have to change the position of the hand locking the scapula in order to be comfortable during this maneuver.
3. **To increase circumduction:** The patient's elbow is flexed sharply and the shoulder is abducted to a 90-degree angle. The physician locks the patient's shoulder in this position

Figure 19-1. Spencer technique to increase shoulder extension.

Figure 19-2. Spencer technique to increase shoulder flexion.

Figure 19-3. Spencer technique to increase shoulder circumduction.

and, using the patient's elbow as a pivot, gently rotates the shoulder in gradually increasing circles, clockwise and then counterclockwise (Fig. 19-3).

4. **Circumduction with traction:** The physician extends the patient's elbow and abducts the arm to 90 degrees. The physician then locks the patient's scapula in this position and, using the patient's forearm as a pivot, gently rotates the humerus in gradually increasing circles, clockwise and then counterclockwise, maintaining a traction force at the patient's wrist (Fig. 19-4).

5. **To increase abduction:** The physician places her upper hand on the patient's shoulder. The patient's elbow is flexed and his hand rests on the physician's forearm below the elbow joint. The physician's lower arm gently exerts an upward pressure on the patient's flexed elbow, bringing the shoulder into abduction (Fig. 19-5).

6. **To increase internal rotation:** The patient's hand, with the elbow flexed, is placed behind his lower ribs. The physician's upper hand locks the scapula; her lower hand gently draws the patient's elbow forward and down (Fig. 19-6). The patient's elbow is released and the maneuver is repeated. An external rotation force may also be used in this position.

7. **Traction stretch:** The patient's hand is placed on the physician's shoulder with his elbow straight. The physician clasps her hands around the patient's shoulder over the humerus. The physician may then provide a gentle pull on the patient's shoulder. By leaning back, the physician uses her body weight rather than muscular force (Fig. 19-7).

ISOMETRIC VARIATIONS
OF SHOULDER THERAPY

The positions used in the Spencer techniques may also be used to treat the shoulder with isometric therapy. The physician moves the arm to a barrier. The patient actively moves his arm against resistance in extension, flexion, abduction, adduction, and internal or external rotation.

For example, in the case of restricted motion in extension, the patient first assumes a position of maximum comfortable extension. The patient then tries to move his arm into flexion while the physician applies a mild isometric resistive force. This position is held for 4 seconds, then the patient relaxes. The physician increases the patient's arm extension and the maneuver is repeated.

Figure 19-4. Spencer technique to improve circumduction, with traction.

Figure 19-5. Spencer technique to increase shoulder abduction.

Figure 19-6. Spencer technique to increase internal rotation of the shoulder.

Figure 19-7. Spencer technique for traction stretch.

Figure 19-8. Test for abduction of the clavicle.

Figure 19-9. Test for flexion of the clavicle.

Muscle Energy Treatment of the Clavicle

TEST FOR CLAVICULAR MOTION

In **abduction,** the distal end of the clavicle moves superiorly and the proximal end moves inferiorly. The physician tests motion in abduction by placing her index finger on the clavicular head next to the sternum while the patient is supine and asking the patient to shrug (Fig. 19-8).

In **flexion,** the distal end of the clavicle moves anteriorly and the proximal end moves posteriorly on the sternum. The physician tests motion in flexion by placing her index finger on the clavicular head next to the sternum and asking the patient to flex his shoulder to 90 degrees and to reach up to the ceiling forcefully (Fig. 19-9).

Figure 19-10. Muscle energy treatment for restricted abduction of the sternoclavicular joint.

Figure 19-11. Muscle energy treatment for restricted flexion of the sternoclavicular joint.

RESTRICTED ABDUCTION
OF THE STERNOCLAVICULAR JOINT

1. Patient position: supine.
2. Physician position: standing at the side of the table, next to the affected shoulder.
3. **Technique:** The physician places one hand on the proximal clavicular head. With her other hand she grasps the patient's wrist and holds the arm extended and internally rotated (Fig. 19-10). The patient is instructed to raise his arm against the physician's hand, hold it in position, then relax. The technique is repeated twice more.

RESTRICTED FLEXION OF THE
STERNOCLAVICULAR JOINT

1. Patient position: supine.
2. Physician position: standing at the side of the table, next to the affected shoulder.
3. **Technique:** The physician places one hand on the restricted clavicle and with the other reaches behind the axilla to cover the scapula. The patient holds the physician's shoulder with the hand of the affected side (Fig. 19-11). The physician flexes the clavicle toward the manubrium until movement is palpated in the sternoclavicular joint. This is done by straightening the body and pulling the scapula anteriorly. The patient is instructed to pull his shoulder down, hold this position for 2 to 3 seconds, then relax. The maneuver is repeated twice more.

High Velocity, Low Amplitude Thrusting Techniques for the Shoulder Girdle

GLENOHUMERAL SOMATIC DYSFUNCTION

1. Patient position: prone.
2. Physician position: standing at the side of the table, on the side of the dysfunction.
3. **Technique:**
   a. The physician grasps the patient's glenohumeral joint by encircling the joint with both hands.
   b. The physician's thumbs rest in a crossed pattern on the posterior aspect of the patient's glenohumoral joint.
   c. The physician exerts a rapid downward and slightly lateral force through the patient's glenohumeral joint (Fig. 19-12).

SUPERIOR CLAVICULAR SOMATIC DYSFUNCTION

1. Patient position: supine.
2. Physician position: standing at the side of the table, on the same side as the dysfunction.
3. **Technique:**
   a. The physician grasps the superior surface of the restricted clavicle with the fingers of his monitoring hand.
   b. With his other hand, the physician flexes the patient's arm to 90 degrees (ipsilateral to the dysfunction).
   c. The physician exerts a simultaneous

Figure 19-12. High velocity, low amplitude thrusting technique for somatic dysfunction of the glenohumeral joint.

Figure 19-13. High velocity, low amplitude thrusting technique for somatic dysfunction of the superior clavicle.

downward thrust on the clavicle and lateral traction on the patient's arm to produce the corrective force (Fig. 19-13).

STERNOCLAVICULAR SOMATIC DYSFUNCTION

1. Patient position: supine.
2. Physician position: standing at the head of the table.
3. **Technique:**
   a. The physician rests the thenar eminence of his monitoring hand over the sternoclavicular joint which is restricted.
   b. The physician grasps the patient's arm on the side of the dysfunction and exerts a cephalad traction force on the arm.
   c. The physician achieves correction by exerting a downward thrust through the sternoclavicular joint while simultaneously inducing a rapid traction force through the patient's arm (Fig. 19-14).

ARTICULATORY TECHNIQUES FOR CLAVICULAR RESTRICTIONS

The clavicle may be elevated or depressed at the sternal end. The techniques described are for an elevated clavicle.

Technique 1
1. Patient position: supine.
2. Physician position: seated at the head of the table.
3. **Technique:** The patient's neck, fully flexed,

rests against the physician's chest. This position locks out spinal motion. The physician places her thumb over the sternal end and exerts a downward and caudal pressure on the clavicle (Fig. 19-15). The patient is instructed to inhale and exhale fully. During exhalation the physician springs the clavicle to release the restriction.

Technique 2
1. Patient position: seated.
2. Physician position: standing close behind the patient.
3. **Technique:** The physician reaches under affected arm and grasps the abducted humerus. With her other hand she reaches over the patient's shoulder and places the thumb or hypothenar eminence on the sternal end of the clavicle. The hand holding the humerus applies a lateral traction. The other hand provides a downward force on the clavicle (Fig. 19-16). This may be an articulatory or a high velocity, low amplitude force.

Counterstrain Techniques for the Shoulder

TENDER POINT LOCATIONS

The anterior tender points for the shoulder (Fig. 19-17) are the following:

1. Anterior acromioclavicular: anterior surface of distal clavicle.

Figure 19-14. High velocity, low amplitude thrusting technique for somatic dysfunction of the sternoclavicular joint.

Figure 19-15. Articulatory technique for an elevated clavicle, patient supine.

Figure 19-16. Articulatory technique for an elevated clavicle, patient seated.

2. Long head of biceps: over the tendon.
3. Short head of biceps: inferolateral to the coracoid process.

The posterior tender points (Fig. 19-18) are the following:

1. Posterior acromioclavicular: behind the lateral end of the clavicle.
2. Supraspinatus: in the supraspinatus fossa.

In the axilla lie:

1. Subscapularis tender point: on the anterior surface of the scapula.
2. Latissimus dorsi tender point: deep in the axilla on the medial surface of the humerus.

TREATMENT

Anterior Acromioclavicular Tender Point
1. Patient position: supine.
2. Physician position: at the side of the table opposite the tender point.
3. **Technique:** The tender point is monitored as the arm is adducted across the chest. The physician applies traction by pulling on the arm at the wrist (Fig. 19-19).

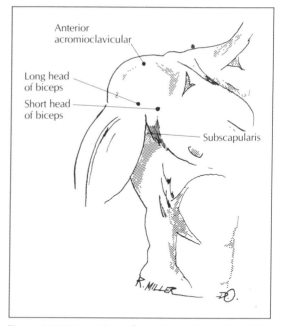

Figure 19-17. Location of anterior tender points of the shoulder girdle.

Long Head of Biceps Tender Point
1. Patient position: supine.
2. Physician position: at the side of the table, next to the tender point and facing the head of the table.

Figure 19-18. Location of posterior tender points of the shoulder girdle.

Figure 19-19. Counterstrain treatment for an anterior acromioclavicular tender point.

Figure 19-20. Counterstrain treatment for a tender point of the long head of the biceps.

3. **Technique:** The patient's arm is flexed to 90 degrees at the elbow and shoulder. The physician applies downward pressure at the elbow along the humerus to the monitoring finger (Fig. 19-20).

Short Head of Biceps Tender Point
1. The short head of biceps tender point is treated in same manner as the long head, except that some fine tuning into adduction is needed.

Posterior Acromioclavicular Tender Point
1. Patient position: prone.
2. Physician position: at the side of the table opposite the tender point.
3. **Technique:** The patient's arm is adducted across his back. The physician applies traction by pulling at the wrist (Fig. 19-21).

Figure 19-21. Counterstrain treatment for a posterior acromioclavicular tender point.

Supraspinatus Tender Point
1. Patient position: supine.
2. Physician position: at the side of the table next to the tender point.
3. **Technique:** The patient's arm is flexed and abducted to 120 degrees. The humerus is markedly externally rotated. The muscle should become very soft in this position (Fig. 19-22).

Subscapularis Tender Point
1. Patient position: supine.
2. Physician position: at the side of the table next to the tender point.
3. **Technique:** The patient's arm is held posteriorly over the side of the table and toward his feet. His arm is internally rotated. No traction is applied.

Latissimus Dorsi Tender Point
1. The latissimus dorsi tender point is treated in the same manner as the subscapularis tender point except that traction is applied along the length of the arm.

Figure 19-22. Counterstrain treatment for a supraspinatus tender point.

THE ELBOW
Eileen L. DiGiovanna

Adduction/Abduction

Adduction and abduction are accessory rocking motions of the upper part of the ulna on the trochlea of the humerus. Abduction is an accessory motion of pronation. Adduction is an accessory motion of supination.

MOTION TESTING
The patient's elbow is semiflexed about 45 degrees. The physician palpates the articulation by placing a finger on the dorsal aspect of the radial and ulnar sides of the olecranon, then tries to palpate into the trochlea. With his other hand the physician grasps the patient's forearm and, starting from a neutral position, fully supinates the forearm, inducing a rocking, adduction motion of the ulna. Reversing the forearm motion into full pronation induces a rocking abduction motion. The elbow is tested for restriction of either motion.

MUSCLE ENERGY TREATMENT
Adduction (Supination) Restriction
1. Patient position: supine.
2. Physician position: standing at the side of the table.
3. **Technique:**
   a. The physician places the patient's elbow into full supination.
   b. The patient gently tries to pronate his forearm against the physician's equal, restraining, isometric force.
   c. This position is held for 4 seconds, then the patient relaxes.
   d. The technique is repeated.

Abduction (Pronation) Restriction
1. To treat an abduction restriction, the position of the arm is reversed.

Figure 19-23. High velocity, low amplitude thrusting technique for adduction restriction of the elbow.

Figure 19-24. High velocity, low amplitude thrusting technique for anterior radial head.

HIGH VELOCITY, LOW AMPLITUDE THRUSTING TECHNIQUE FOR ABDUCTION/ADDUCTION RESTRICTION

1. Patient position: seated.
2. Physician position: standing facing the patient.
3. **Technique:**
   a. The physician grasps the patient's elbow. The fingers of his monitoring hand are on either side of the olecranon. The other hand is used to hold and stabilize the patient's forearm, in supination/extension.
   b. The physician tests the motion of the radioulnar joint in adduction and abduction.
   c. If restriction of motion is noted in abduction, the physician places the patient's elbow into abduction and exerts a hyperabduction corrective thrust. This is done with the elbow locked in extension.
   d. If restriction of motion is noted in adduction, the physician places the patient's elbow into adduction and exerts a hyperadduction corrective thrust. This is done with the elbow locked in extension (Fig. 19-23).

Radial Head Dysfunctions

MOTION TESTING
1. Patient position: seated or supine.
2. Physician position: standing facing patient. The radial head is palpated by flexing and extending the elbow.

3. **Technique:**
   a. The physician grasps the radial head between his thumb and index finger.
   b. The radial head is moved in a ventral and dorsal direction; any restriction of motion noted.

   Note: The most common dysfunction of the radial head is a posterior radial head. This is diagnosed from ability to move the radial head dorsally with restriction of motion ventrally. An anterior radial head is restricted in motion dorsally and has free motion ventrally. Posterior glide of the radius is coupled with pronation/extension, and anterior glide is coupled with supination/flexion.

HIGH VELOCITY, LOW AMPLITUDE THRUSTING TECHNIQUE FOR ANTERIOR RADIAL HEAD

1. Patient position: seated.
2. Physician position: standing facing patient.
3. **Technique:**
   a. The physician grasps the patient's dysfunctioned arm, flexing it at the elbow and pronating it at the wrist.
   b. The physician places the second and third digits of his other hand into the crease of the patient's elbow, directly over the radial head.
   c. The physician exerts a rapid hyperflexion force on the elbow while simultaneously thrusting the radial head dorsally with the fingers of the other hand (Fig. 19-24).

Figure 19-25. High velocity, low amplitude thrusting technique for posterior radial head.

POSTERIOR RADIAL HEAD SOMATIC DYSFUNCTION

1. Patient position: seated.
2. Physician position: standing facing the patient.
3. **Technique:**
   a. The physician encircles the patient's dysfunctioned elbow with both hands and extends it.
   b. The physician places his thumbs over the head of the radius anteriorly and the phalanx of his index finger over the radial head posteriorly.
   c. The physician exerts a rapid hyperextension force on the patient's elbow while simultaneously inducing a ventral counterforce through the radial head (Fig. 19-25).

Counterstrain Treatment of the Elbow

The tender points associated with the elbow are shown in Figure 19-26. Radial head or lateral epicondyle tender points may be treated in the same manner.

1. **Radial head/lateral epicondyle tender points**
   a. The elbow is held in full extension. This may be over a fulcrum of the table edge or the physician's knee.
   b. The arm is then supinated and abducted with varying amounts of force.

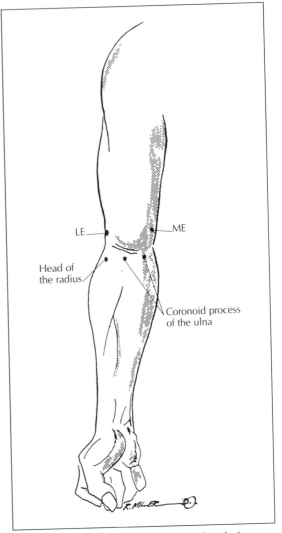

Figure 19-26. Tender points associated with the elbow. *LE*, lateral epicondyle; *ME*, medial epicondyle.

c. The position is maintained for 90 seconds, then the arm is returned slowly to a neutral position (Fig. 19-27).

2. **Coronoid tender points**
   a. The elbow is fully flexed.
   b. The forearm is pronated and abducted gently.
   c. The position is held for 90 seconds, then the arm is slowly returned to a neutral position.

Figure 19-27. Counterstrain treatment of lateral epicondyle tender point.

THE WRIST AND HAND
Eileen L. DiGiovanna

The Wrist

TESTS FOR SOMATIC DYSFUNCTION
Somatic dysfunction of the wrist permits motion toward the dysfunction; motion away from the dysfunction will be restricted. The technique described below may be used to test motion of the radionavicular joint and each of the intercarpal joints. It may also be used to test the carpometacarpal and metacarpophalangeal joints.

1. Physician position: seated facing the patient.
2. **Technique:**
   a. The physician grasps the bones adjacent to the joint to be tested between his thumb and forefinger.
   b. The bones are moved through their range of motion and any restriction is noted.
   c. The motions tested are gliding in all directions and long-axis traction.

Gross motion is tested in flexion, extension, and radial and ulnar deviation. Both passive and active techniques may be used.

MUSCLE ENERGY (ISOMETRIC) TECHNIQUES
As in muscle energy techniques for treating dysfunction of any other joint, the wrist is moved to its barrier to motion and the patient is asked to push isometrically back toward the freedom of motion. The technique described below is used for wrist restriction in ulnar deviation.

1. **Technique:**
   a. The joint is moved into ulnar deviation to the barrier to motion.
   b. The patient is asked to push toward the radial aspect as the physician provides resistance.
   c. This position is held for 4 seconds, then released.
   d. The joint is moved to its new barrier.
   e. The maneuver is repeated three or four times.

HIGH VELOCITY, LOW AMPLITUDE THRUSTING TECHNIQUE FOR CARPAL SOMATIC DYSFUNCTION
1. Patient position: seated on the table.
2. Physician position: standing facing the patient.
3. **Technique:**
   a. The physician grasps the patient's hand on the side of the dysfunction and localizes the dorsal radiocarpal joint with his thumbs.
   b. The physician exerts a whiplike thrust on the hand, moving it into rapid hyperflexion

Figure 19-28. High velocity, low amplitude thrusting technique for carpal dysfunction.

while simultaneously exerting a downward counterforce through the carpal somatic dysfunction (Fig. 19-28).

COUNTERSTRAIN TREATMENT

The locations of the tender points associated with the wrist are shown in Figures 19-29 and 19-30. All of these tender points respond to flexing or extending the wrist over the tender points (Figs. 19-31, 19-32).

The Hand

TESTS FOR SOMATIC DYSFUNCTION

1. Physician position: seated facing the patient.
2. **Technique:**
   a. The physician grasps the bones adjacent to the joint being tested between his thumb and index finger.
   b. The bones are moved through their range of motion as gentle traction is applied.

ARTICULATION TREATMENT

Intersegmental Articulations

1. Physician position: seated or standing, facing the patient.
2. **Technique:**
   a. The physician locks one metacarpal between the thumb and index finger of one hand.
   b. With the thumb and index finger of his other hand, the physician maneuvers the neighboring metacarpal into anterior or posterior glide or rotation, as desired.

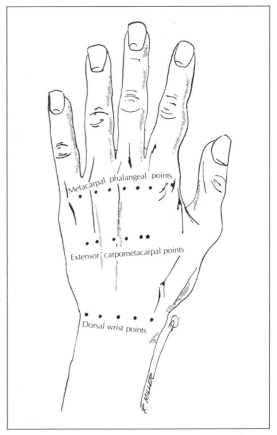

Figure 19-29. Dorsal tender points of the wrist and hand.

Fingers

1. Physician position: seated or standing, facing the patient.
2. **Technique:**
   a. The physician locks the metacarpal, in this instance the second, between the thumb and index finger of one hand.
   b. The physician places the thumb of his other hand on the dorsum of the first phalanx and the index finger on the volar surface of the first phalanx.
   c. The physician applies long-axis extension (straight-line traction) or rotation or anterioposterior glide.

Figure 19-30. Ventral tender points of the wrist and hand.

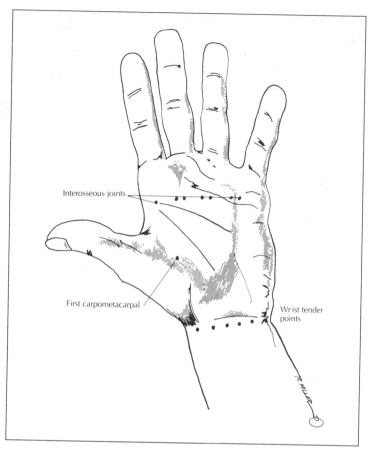

Interosseous joints

First carpometacarpal

Wrist tender points

Figure 19-31. Counterstrain treatment of ventral tender point of the wrist by flexion of the wrist.

Figure 19-32. Counterstrain treatment of dorsal wrist tender points by extension of the wrist.

HIGH VELOCITY, LOW AMPLITUDE THRUSTING TECHNIQUE FOR PHALANGEAL DYSFUNCTION

1. Patient position: seated on the table.
2. Physician position: standing facing the patient.
3. **Technique:**
   a. With one hand, the physician holds and stabilizes the patient's wrist.
   b. The physician localizes the dysfunctioned joint and exerts a simultaneous traction and hyperflexion thrust through the somatic dysfunction (Fig. 19-33).
   c. To treat the second or third phalanges, the physician holds the phalanx above the articulation being treated and maneuvers the distal phalanx through the desired motion.

Figure 19-33. High velocity, low amplitude thrusting technique for phalangeal dysfunction.

COUNTERSTRAIN TREATMENT

The locations of the tender points associated with the hand are shown in Figures 19-29 and 19-30. A tender point of the first carpometacarpal joint that is associated with pain and weakness of the thumb is treated by markedly rotating the thumb toward the palm, with a slight amount of flexion. The interossei tender points are treated by flexing the joint and applying some traction. An extension carpometacarpal tender point is treated by extending the joint and applying traction.

EXERCISE THERAPY FOR THE UPPER EXTREMITY

Stanley Schiowitz
Albert R. DeRubertis

The Shoulder Girdle

The function and biomechanics of the shoulder girdle were reviewed in Chapter 18. The physician prescribing exercise therapy must take into account the three true articulations, the two pseudoarticulations, and the origins and insertions of all the muscles used in joint function.

GLENOHUMERAL JOINT

A. Pendulum exercise, acute phase—passive (Fig. 19-34)

1. Patient position: bent forward, body supported by the good arm holding onto support, the back comfortable.
2. **Instructions:**
   a. Allow your painful arm to hang down, away from your body.
   b. Move your body forward and backward, then side to side. This creates shoulder joint motion without active participation of the shoulder muscles.

Figure 19-34. Pendulum exercise, acute phase—passive motion.

Figure 19-35. Pendulum exercise with active use of the shoulder.

c. Gradually increase body motion. Do not create pain. Start with 5 to 10 seconds of exercise.
d. Slowly bring your body back to an upright position. Passively move the painful arm back to your side, using your good arm to move it if necessary.
e. Relax, rest, and repeat.

B. Pendulum exercise, after acute phase—active (Fig. 19-35)
1. Patient position: bent forward, body supported by the good arm holding onto support, the back comfortable.
2. **Instructions:**
   a. Allow your painful arm to hang down, away from your body.
   b. Swing your arm forward and backward, side to side, and in circles.
   c. Gradually increase the excursion of the arm motion. A weight may be held in your hand to increase the force used.
   d. Continue for 5 to 15 seconds, then slowly bring your body into the upright position.
   e. Relax, rest, and repeat.
   Note: Do not increase or create pain when performing this exercise.

C. Flexion stretch (Fig. 19-36)
1. Patient position: Standing facing a wall, an arm's length away.

2. **Instructions:**
   a. Place the hand of the arm to be exercised against the wall with the elbow fully extended.
   b. Walk your fingers up the wall slowly, increasing flexion at the shoulder.
   c. After reaching the limit of painless flexion, hold your arm in this position for 10 to 15 seconds. Then slowly walk your fingers higher on the wall, one inch at a time, to increase flexion. Hold your arm for 10 to 15 seconds at each new plateau of flexion, then walk the fingers higher.
   d. At the end of two or three minutes, or if fatigued, slowly walk the arm down the wall.
   e. Relax, rest, and repeat.

D. Abduction stretch (Fig. 19-37)
1. Patient position: standing with the side of the painful arm toward the wall.
2. **Instructions:** Repeat the technique described for flexion stretch, walking the arm up into abduction.
   Note to physician: If the cause of the dysfunction is supraspinatus impingement, do not prescribe this exercise.

E. Abduction–external rotation stretch (Fig. 19-38)

Figure 19-36. Flexion stretch.

Figure 19-37. Abduction stretch.

Figure 19-38. Abduction—external rotation stretch.

1. Patient position: standing or sitting with both hands clasped behind the head and the elbows brought together in front of the body.
2. **Instructions:**
   a. Slowly separate your elbows as far back as they can be painlessly stretched.
   b. Hold this position for 5 to 15 seconds.
   c. Return to the starting position.
   d. Relax, rest, and repeat.
F. Adduction—internal rotation stretch (passive) (Fig. 19-39)
   1. Patient position: standing with the arms at the sides.
   2. **Instructions:**
      a. Turn the hand of the arm to be treated inward (internal rotation).
      b. Grasp that wrist with your other hand and pull it slowly across your chest to shoulder height.
      c. Gradually increase your pull to maximum painless stretch. Hold for 5 to 15 seconds.
      d. Return arm to the starting position.
      e. Relax, rest, and repeat.
G. Adduction—internal rotation stretch (active) (Fig. 19-40)
   1. Patient position: standing with both arms at the sides.

Figure 19-39. Adduction—internal rotation stretch (passive).

2. **Instructions:**
   a. Bring the arm that is to be treated across your body and up over the opposite shoulder. Keep your palm pointing down.
   b. Reach back over your shoulder and touch your scapula.
   c. Walk your fingers down the scapula to achieve maximum painless stretch. Hold for 5 to 15 seconds.
   d. Return your arm to the starting position.
   e. Relax, rest, and repeat.

Figure 19-40. Adduction—internal rotation stretch (active).

Figure 19-41. Forced flexion stretch.

Figure 19-42. Forced rotation stretch.

FROZEN SHOULDER FORCED STRETCH EXERCISES

These exercises are not performed during the acute phase of injury. Moderate wet heat should be applied as an aid to muscle relaxation before the patient begins exercising. If analgesics or non-steroidal anti-inflammatory drugs are prescribed, they should be taken 20 minutes before exercise. At the conclusion of these exercises, an ice pack should be applied for 20 minutes.

A. Forced flexion stretch (Fig. 19-41)
  1. Patient position: seated facing a table, with the elbow on the side of the shoulder to be treated on the table.
  2. **Instructions:**
     a. Place the back of the elbow joint on the table, making a 90-degree angle between the forearm and the elbow.
     b. Drop your body forward and downward, increasing shoulder flexion. Remain in this position for 15 seconds.
     c. Allow your entire weight to rest on your elbow joint. With the increased flexion (stretch), you may feel mild pain.
     d. Hold this position for 15 seconds. Raise your body up.
     e. Relax, rest, and repeat.
     f. Attempt to increase flexion motion with each repetition.

B. Forced rotation stretch (Fig. 19-42)
  1. Patient position: seated facing a table, with the elbow on the side of the shoulder to be treated on the table. Hold a three- to five-pound weight in your hand.
  2. **Instructions:**
     a. Allow your arm to pivot on the elbow inward, toward the table. The weight you are holding should slowly create forced internal rotation.
     b. Remain in this position for 10 seconds, then pivot the arm outward, creating external rotation.
     c. Return your arm to midline.
     d. Relax, rest, and repeat.
     e. Increase the weight held in your hand gradually, in order to force the rotation.

Figure 19-43. Forced extension stretch.

Figure 19-44. External rotator strengthening.

C. Forced extension stretch (Fig. 19-43)
  1. Patient position: stand with your back to a table. Bring your shoulder back with the elbow bent, until your fist rests upon the table.
  2. **Instructions:**
     a. Gently do a deep knee bend, resting your weight on your fist. This maneuver increases shoulder extension.
     b. Gradually increase the deep knee bend, resting all your weight on your fist.
     c. Hold this position of forced extension for 15 seconds.
     d. Return to the upright position.
     e. Relax, rest, and repeat.

STRENGTHENING EXERCISES WITH MECHANICAL AIDS
A. External rotators (Fig. 19-44)
  1. Patient position: standing, both arms at the sides, elbows bent to 90 degrees, holding a length of rubber tubing in both hands.
  2. **Instructions:**
     a. Pull the tubing horizontally between your hands as far as possible. Keep your elbows and arms against your body.
     b. Hold this position for 5 to 15 seconds.
     c. Return to the starting position.
     d. Relax, rest, and repeat.
B. Extensors (Fig. 19-45)
  1. Patient position: standing, both arms at the

sides, holding a length of rubber tubing in both hands.
  2. **Instructions:**
     a. Pull the rubber tubing horizontally as far as possible, while simultaneously raising both arms to shoulder height. Try to stretch out the arms fully.
     b. Hold this outstretched position for 5 to 15 seconds.
     c. Return to starting position.
     d. Relax, rest, and repeat.
C. Flexors (Fig. 19-46)
  1. Patient position: standing, one hand holding a length of rubber tubing firmly below the waist at the midbody line.

Figure 19-45. Extensor strengthening.

Figure 19-46. Flexor strengthening.

Figure 19-47. Abductor strengthening.

Figure 19-48. Internal rotator strengthening.

2. **Instructions:**
   a. Grasp the other end of the rubber tubing with the arm to be treated.
   b. Pull on the tubing in a forward direction until your elbow is fully extended.
   c. Swing your fully extended arm over your head into full flexion.
   d. Hold this position for 15 seconds.
   e. Slowly return to the starting position.
   f. Relax, rest, and repeat.
D. Abductors (Fig. 19-47)
   1. Patient position: standing, one hand holding a length of rubber tubing firmly below the waist at the midbody line.
   2. **Instructions:**
      a. Grasp the other end of the rubber tubing with the arm to be treated.
      b. Pull sideways, stretching the tubing, until your elbow is fully extended.
      c. Swing your fully extended arm over your head into full abduction.
      d. Hold this position for 15 seconds.
      e. Slowly return to the starting position.
      f. Relax, rest, and repeat.
E. Internal rotators (Fig. 19-48)
   1. Patient position: seated next to a table with the side to be treated beside a leg of the table.
   2. **Instructions:**
      a. Place a length of rubber tubing around

the table leg and grasp it with the hand next to the table leg.
   b. Keep that elbow flexed to 90 degrees and held firmly against your body.
   c. Pull and stretch the tubing by rotating your hand toward the midbody line. This creates internal rotation.
   d. Hold this position for 15 seconds.
   e. Slowly return to the starting position.
   f. Relax, rest, and repeat.

Elbow Joint

The exercises described in this section stretch the agonist muscles while strengthening the antagonist muscles. Each motion is performed slowly. The difficulty of the exercise is enhanced as the patient increases the weight used. To ensure maximum stretch, the patient uses his other arm to increase passively the motion after the extreme of voluntary stretch has been reached.

A. Flexion-extension pronation stretch (Fig. 19-49)
   1. Patient position: seated, with the side to be exercised next to a table. The elbow is placed near the edge of the table, with a towel or small pillow between it and the table.
   2. **Instructions:**
      a. Hold three- to five-pound weight in your

Figure 19-49. Flexion-extension pronation stretch.

Figure 19-50. Flexion-extension supination stretch.

hand. Turn your hand so that the palm faces down (*pronation*).

b. Allow the elbow to extend down to the table with the weight creating extension off the table. The elbow acts as a fulcrum. Use your other hand to gently push the elbow into forced extension. Hold this position for 5 seconds.

c. Bring your arm up off the table into full elbow flexion. With your other hand, gently push the elbow into forced flexion. Hold for 5 seconds.

d. Repeat the entire motion. Remember to keep your palm down in full wrist pronation at all times.

B. Flexion-extension supination stretch (Fig. 19-50)

1. Patient position: seated, with the side to be exercised beside a table. The elbow is placed near the edge of the table, with a folded towel or small pillow between it and the table.

2. **Instructions:**

a. Hold a three- to five-pound weight in your hand. Turn your hand so that the palm faces up (*supination*).

b. Allow the elbow to extend down to the table with the weight creating extension off the table. The elbow acts as a fulcrum. With your other hand, gently push the elbow into forced extension. Hold this position for 5 seconds.

c. Bring your arm up off the table into full elbow flexion. With your other hand, gently push the elbow into forced flexion. Hold for 5 seconds.

d. Repeat the entire motion. Remember to keep your palm up in full wrist supination at all times.

Wrist
WRIST STRETCH

A. Extension–dorsiflexion stretch (Fig. 19-51)

1. Patient position: standing, with the side to be treated next to a wall but far enough away to allow full elbow extension.

2. **Instructions:**

a. Place your palm, fingers pointing up, flat on the wall so that the elbow is fully extended.

b. Lean onto the wall, causing extension stretch of the wrist. Hold for 5 seconds.

c. Relax, rest, and repeat.

B. Extension–palmar flexion stretch (Fig. 19-52)

1. Patient position: standing, with the side to be treated next to a wall but far enough away to allow full elbow extension.

2. **Instructions:**

a. Place your palm, fingers pointing down, flat on wall so that the elbow is fully extended.

b. Lean onto the wall, causing extension stretch of the wrist. Hold for 5 seconds.

c. Relax, rest, and repeat.

C. Flexion–palmar flexion stretch (Fig. 19-53)

1. Patient position: standing, with the side to be treated next to a wall but tar enough away to allow full elbow extension.

2. **Instructions:**

a. Place the back of your hand, fingers pointing up, flat on the wall so that the elbow is fully extended.

Figure 19-51. Wrist extension—
dorsiflexion stretch.

Figure 19-52. Wrist extension—
palmar flexion stretch.

Figure 19-53. Wrist flexion—
palmar flexion stretch.

Figure 19-54. Wrist flexion—
dorsiflexion stretch.

   b. Lean onto the wall, causing flexion
      stretch of the wrist.
   c. Hold for 5 seconds.
   d. Relax, rest, and repeat.
D. Flexion–dorsiflexion stretch (Fig. 19-54)
   1. Patient position: standing, with the side to
      be treated next to a wall but far enough
      away to allow full elbow extension.

2. **Instructions:**
   a. Place the back of your hand, fingers
      pointing down, flat on the wall so that
      the elbow is fully extended.
   b. Lean onto wall, causing flexion stretch of
      wrist.
   c. Hold for 5 seconds.
   d. Relax, rest, and repeat.

Figure 19-55. Wrist flexor strengthening.

Figure 19-56. Wrist extensor strengthening.

Figure 19-57. Wrist rotator strengthening.

WRIST STRENGTHENING

A. Wrist flexors (Fig. 19-55)
  1. Patient position: seated, with the side to be treated beside a table. The forearm rests on the table with elbow at about 90 degrees of flexion. The wrist is off the table.
  2. **Instructions:**
    a. Hold a three- to five-pound weight in your hand. The palm faces up, putting the wrist in *supination*.
    b. Move the hand holding the weight up toward the ceiling (flex the wrist). Your forearm remains flat on the table.
    c. Hold for 5 to 15 seconds.
    d. Slowly lower the weight off the table, extending the wrist fully.
    e. Relax, rest, and repeat.
B. Wrist extensors (Fig. 19-56)

  1. Patient position: seated, with the side to be treated beside a table. The forearm rests on the table with the elbow at about 90 degrees of flexion. The wrist is off the table.
  2. **Instructions:**
    a. Hold a three- to five-pound weight in your hand. The palm faces down, placing the wrist in *pronation*.
    b. Bring the hand holding the weight up toward the ceiling (extend the wrist). The forearm remains on the table.
    c. Hold this position for 5 to 15 seconds.
    d. Slowly lower the weight off the table, flexing the wrist fully.
    e. Relax, rest, and repeat.
C. Wrist rotators (Fig. 19-57)
  1. Patient position: seated, with the side to be treated beside a table. The forearm rests on the table with the elbow at about 90 degrees of flexion. The wrist is off the table.
  2. **Instructions:**
    a. Hold a three- to five-pound weight in your hand. The palm faces down.
    b. Slowly rotate your forearm, keeping the wrist stiff, until the palm faces up.
    c. Hold this position for 5 seconds.
    d. Slowly rotate your wrist back to the starting position.
    e. Hold this position for 5 seconds.
    f. Repeat the technique.
D. Ulnar-radial adduction
  1. Patient position: seated, with the side to be treated beside a table. The forearm rests on the table with the elbow at about 90 degrees of flexion. The wrist is off the table.

Figure 19-58. Finger stretch.

Figure 19-59. Finger coordination.

2. **Instructions:**
   a. Hold a three- to five-pound weight in your hand. The palm faces down. The wrist is held stiff.
   b. Bend your wrist to the side, trying to touch your thumb to your arm.
   c. Hold this position for 5 seconds.
   d. Bend your wrist to the side in the opposite direction, trying to touch your small finger to your arm.
   e. Hold this position for 5 seconds.
   f. Repeat the technique.

The Hand

A. Finger stretch (Fig. 19-58)
   1. Patient position: sitting or standing.
   2. **Instructions:**
      a. Make a tight fist and hold it for 5 seconds.
      b. Open your fist and stretch your fingers as far out as possible.
      c. Hold this position for 5 seconds.
      d. Repeat the procedure.
B. Finger coordination (Fig. 19-59)
   1. Patient position: sitting or standing.
   2. **Instructions:**
      a. Hold your hand with the palm down.
      b. Hold a card firmly between the thumb and fingertips. Let go suddenly, so that the card falls to the floor.
      c. Repeat, using the thumb and different fingers.
      d. Repeat the entire process.
C. Finger coordination (Fig. 19-60)
   1. Patient position: sitting or standing.

Figure 19-60. Finger coordination.

Figure 19-61. Finger–palm strengthening.

2. **Instructions:**
    a. Hold your hand with the palm down.
    b. Place a card between each of the fingers (four cards).
    c. Release one card at a time by separating the fingers.
    d. Repeat the technique, releasing the cards in different order.
D. Finger strengthening (Fig. 19-61)
    1. Patient position: sitting or standing.
    2. **Instructions:**
        a. Hold a rubber ball in the hand to be treated.
        b. Alternately squeeze the ball between your thumb and little finger, thumb and ring finger, thumb and middle finger, thumb and index finger.
        c. Squeeze the ball with all your fingers.
        d. Hold each squeeze for 3 to 5 seconds.
        e. Repeat the sequence.

References

Moran, PS, Pruzzo, NA, et al. 1973. An Evaluation and Treatment Manual of Osteopathic Manipulative Procedures, vol. I, Kansas City: Institute for Continuing Education in Osteopathic Principles.

Jones, Lawrence. 1981. Strain and Counterstrain. Colorado Springs: Amer. Academy of Osteopathy.

20

The Lower Extremity

THE HIP JOINT
Stanley Schiowitz

Functional Anatomy

The hip joint joins the pelvis to the lower extremity. It is a ball-and-socket articulation that allows motion in three planes and circumduction. Its bony components are the acetabulum, which is at the junction of the ilium, ischium, and pubic bones; and the head of the femur. The convex femoral head fits into the concave acetabulum. The articular surfaces are reciprocally curved but are not coextensive, nor are they fully congruent. The close-packed position of the hip joint is full extension, abduction, and medial rotation.

The hip joint is strongly maintained by its capsule and its ligaments—the iliofemoral ligament, the pubofemoral ligament, the ischiofemoral ligament, and the ligament of the head of the femur. The ligaments slacken or tauten with motion, thereby stabilizing and limiting hip movement. In an upright human the femoral head and neck face medially, anteriorly, and cephalad. Any change in direction will influence pelvic tilt and gait.

The shaft of the femur descends medially, creating a mechanical genu valgus. The femoral shaft also undergoes torsional osseous changes so that the femoral condyles can articulate with the tibial condyles in a frontal plane. The genu valgus is exaggerated with increased pelvic width and contributes to the unstable gait patterns in elderly women.

A major bony landmark is the greater trochanter, easily palpated on the lateral superior aspect of the shaft. The lesser trochanter is on the medial aspect of the inferior end of the femoral neck. This trochanter, though not palpable, is very important, as it is the site of attachment of the iliopsoas tendon. At its distal end, the femoral condyles and epicondyles are easily palpable at the knee joint.

Gross Motion

The gross motions of the hip joint are flexion/extension, abduction/adduction, internal and external rotation, and circumduction. All hip joint motions should be measured with one hand stabilizing the pelvis. Average normal measurements are as follows:

1. Abduction/adduction, hip and knee flexed: 70 to 75 degrees.
2. Abduction, hip and knee extended: 40 to 45 degrees.
3. Adduction, crossing the anterior aspect of the opposite extended leg: 20 to 30 degrees.
4. Rotation, hip and knee extended or flexed, should be similar: external rotation—about 45 degrees; internal rotation—about 35 degrees.
5. Flexion, knee flexed: 120 to 130 degrees.

305

6. Flexion, knee extended: usually less than 90 degrees, because it is limited by extensor muscle action.

7. Extension, subject prone: 20 to 30 degrees. If the opposite leg is placed in 90 degrees of flexion, hip extension is 90 to 120 degrees.

Major Muscles

1. **Iliopsoas.** The iliopsoas muscle is a major flexor of the hip upon the trunk. Its origins are very extensive, involving the vertebrae and their disks from the 12th thoracic vertebra to the sacrum, and the anterior ilium and sacrum. The iliopsoas muscle is affected by a wide variety of dysfunctions. Except in cases of nerve damage, it is always slightly hypertonic. The clinician should be aware of this when prescribing an exercise program and should avoid iliopsoas contracting and strengthening programs, especially for patients with low back pain. Athletes involved in major hip flexion sports, such as skating, soccer, and running, have overly developed iliopsoas muscles, creating an exaggerated lumbar-thoracic lordosis.

2. **Tensor fascia lata.** The tensor fascia lata originates in the anterior part of the external lip of the iliac crest and deep fascia lata and inserts onto the iliotibial tract of the fascia lata. This muscle flexes, medially rotates, and abducts the hip joint. Chronic dysfunction may manifest with a number of seemingly unrelated symptoms, including knee pain (especially at the fibular head) buttock pain, and a burning feeling in the lateral upper thigh.

3. **Gluteus medius.** The gluteus medius originates on the external surface of the ilium, below and between the iliac crest and the posterior gluteal line, and inserts onto the lateral surface of the greater trochanter. It is a major abductor of the hip joint and assists slightly in medial rotation and flexion. Hypotonic dysfunctions will affect stance and gait; hypertonic dysfunctions will usually be point sensitive and mimic sciatic nerve symptoms.

4. **Gluteus maximus.** The gluteus maximus originates at the posterior gluteal line of the ilium, the posterior lower sacrum and coccyx, the aponeurosis of the erector spinae, the sacrotuberous ligament, and the gluteal aponeurosis. The major actions of this muscle are to extend and laterally rotate the hip. Hypotonic dysfunctions will affect stance and gait. Hypertonic dysfunctions are usually greater in scope than those of the gluteus medius, involving sacral motion and ilial motion as well as hip joint motion.

The gluteus maximus follows the law of muscle detorsion. Therefore, to increase hip extension, as in ballet movement, the ilium must be rotated. Somatic dysfunction of the lumbar spine will limit lumbar regional motion, pelvic rotation, and hip extension.

5. **Hamstrings.** The hamstrings are three muscles, the semimembranosus, semitendinosus, and biceps femoris. All originate at the tuberosity of the ischium and insert onto various areas of the fibula and tibia. They are two-joint muscles that extend the hip and flex the knee. Both motions are interdependent and will affect each other's function. Dysfunctions are commonly found at the ischium, at the lateral aspect of the knee, and at the pes anserine bursa.

6. **Piriformis.** The piriformis muscle originates on the pelvic surface of the sacrum, at the margin of the greater sciatic foramen, and at the sacrotuberous ligament. It inserts onto the superior border of the greater trochanter. The piriformis muscle is a lateral hip rotator, and its proximity to the sciatic nerve makes it a common site for dysfunction. When hypertonic, it is readily palpable in the lateral rectal mucosa. The piriformis symptom complex follows a sciatic neuritic pain distribution. Specific point tenderness can usually be evoked at a point in the buttocks halfway between the posterosuperior iliac spine and the superolateral aspect of the greater trochanter.

Tests for Evaluating Hip Dysfunction

This section describes several tests for evaluating specific dysfunctions of the hip. Most of the tests are done with the active assistance of the patient.

Erichsen's test. Erichsen's test is a test for sacroiliac disease and early spondylitic arthritis. The clinician grasps the iliac bones and presses them together (Fig. 20-1). A positive test result is indicated by pain.

Ludloff's sign. Ludloff's sign indicates traumatic separation of the epiphysis of the lesser trochanter. Ecchymosis is found at the base of the

Figure 20-1. Erichsen's test for
sacroiliac dysfunction.
Compression in a frontal plane.

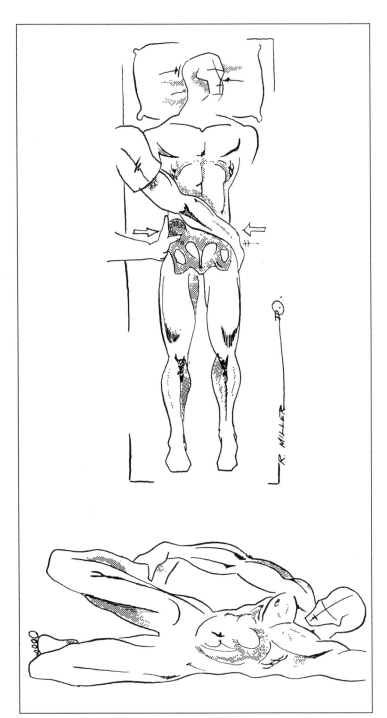

Figure 20-2. Ober's test for
contracture of the iliotibial fascia.

Figure 20-3. Patrick's (Fabere) test for hip joint motion restriction.

femoral triangle, and the subject cannot raise the thigh when seated.

Ober's test. Ober's test is a test for contracture of the iliotibial fascia. The patient lies on the good side with the knee and thigh flexed. The top leg is held by patient in hip abduction, hip extension, and knee flexion (Fig. 20-2). The patient then drops the leg to the table. If the leg remains abducted, the test is positive.

Patrick's (Fabere) test. This test evaluates hip motion restriction in flexion, abduction, external rotation, and extension. The supine patient flexes the hip and knee of one leg and places its lateral malleous on the other leg just above the patella. The clinician gently presses the knee toward the table (Fig. 20-3). Pain or limitation of motion on extension usually indicates hip joint dysfunction (arthritis, synovitis). The hip motions are compared on the two sides.

Trendelenburg test. The Trendelenburg test evaluates gluteus medius weakness or congenital hip joint dislocation. The subject stands on the leg to be tested and raises the other leg (flex hip and knee) (Fig. 20-4). The clinician observes the gluteal crease lines. The test is positive (stance leg) if the gluteal crease on the raised leg remains level or drops. Normally it should rise.

Thomas test. The Thomas test evaluates flexion contraction of the iliopsoas muscle. In a supine position, the patient flattens the lordotic curve by

Figure 20-4. Trendelenburg test for gluteus medius weakness or congenital hip joint dislocation.

Negative   Positive

Figure 20-5. Thomas test for hip flexion muscle contracture.

flexing both legs and knees to the abdomen, then releases one leg to the table without creating lordosis (Fig. 20-5). The clinician measures the extension of the leg. The maneuver is repeated with the other leg, and the two sides are compared. Inability to fully extend the leg may indicate iliopsoas contracture.

Common Musculoskeletal Hip Joint Disorders

CONGENITAL DISLOCATION OF THE HIPS (NEWBORN)

Cardinal Diagnostic Findings
1. Asymmetry of gluteal skin folds.
2. Leg seems shorter.
3. Limitation of abduction present.
4. Positive Ortolani's sign, hip "clicks" with reduction as it is flexed, abducted, and externally rotated.
5. X-ray evidence.

TRANSIENT SYNOVITIS

Cardinal Diagnostic Findings
1. Child 3 to 12 years old.
2. Males predominate in 4:1 ratio.
3. No history of trauma, but limp is present.
4. Hip held in flexion, abduction, and external rotation.
5. Low-grade temperature is present.
6. Hip is tender to touch.
7. X-ray evidence.

LEGG-CALVE-PERTHES' DISEASE (OSTEOCHONDRITIS DEFORMANS JUVENILIS; ASEPTIC NECROSIS OF OSSIFICATION CENTER OF FEMORAL HEAD)

Cardinal Diagnostic Findings
1. Males predominate, ages 4 to 12, usually unilateral.
2. Antalgic gait present.
3. Pain is in groin, thigh, and may radiate to knee.
4. Sedimentation rate may be elevated. All other tests are normal.
5. Thomas test is positive: contracture of psoas and adductor muscles.
6. Limitation of hip abduction, extension, and internal rotation.
7. Disuse atrophy may develop in upper part of thigh.
8. X-ray evidence.

SLIPPED CAPITAL FEMORAL EPIPHYSIS

Cardinal Diagnostic Findings
1. Most common in adolescents, aged 10 to 15 years.
2. Males more commonly affected, in 3:1 or 4:1 ratio.
3. In a female, will occur at an earlier age, owing to advanced skeletal maturity.
4. Bilateral involvement noted in 40% of patients.
5. Coxa vara will develop.
6. Antalgic gait present.
7. Limitation of hip motion.
8. Male may have female fat distribution with sexual underdevelopment.
9. X-ray evidence.

ISCHIOGLUTEAL BURSITIS

Common Diagnostic Findings
1. Adults with sedentary occupations.
2. Point tenderness over ischial tuberosity.
3. Pain relieved by local injection of anesthetic.
4. Pain relieved when patient takes weight off buttocks (stands up).
5. X-ray evidence usually not present.

TROCHANTERIC BURSITIS

Common Diagnostic Findings
1. Point tenderness on palpation of the greater trochanter.
2. Pain usually distributed down the lateral aspect of the leg; may mimic a neuritis.
3. Pain present with weight-bearing, walking.
4. X-ray evidence usually not present.

MERALGIA PARESTHETICA

Common Diagnostic Findings
1. Usually caused by pressure on nerve, usually about anterior superior iliac spine. Good history necessary.
2. Persistent paresthesia, anesthesia, or hypesthesia at lateral buttock, down lateral thigh to the knee, for no apparent reason.
3. No point tenderness or muscle dysfunction.
4. Gait, weight-bearing normal.
5. Tinel sign may be present.
6. No x-ray evidence.

PSOATIC DYSFUNCTION

Common Causes
1. Trauma to lumbar spine, lesser trochanter, or pubes.

2. Psoatic myositis due to local inflammation or infection.
3. Psoatic bursitis.
4. Visceral dysfunction causing psoasitis, such as
   a. Appendicitis
   b. Renal or urethral dysfunction
   c. Fallopian tube infection
   d. Retroperitoneal lymphadenopathy
   e. Iliac or femoral phlebitis

Common Diagnostic Findings
1. Psoatic gait present.
2. On standing, hip and knee are flexed on pathologic side.
3. On standing, downward pelvic tilt on pathologic side.
4. In supine position, exaggerated lordosis.
5. Thomas sign present.
6. Point tenderness in femoral triangle.
7. Pelvis shifts to opposite side.
8. Occasionally no x-ray evidence.

THE KNEE JOINT
Stanley Schiowitz

Functional Anatomy

The knee joint is the largest and most complicated articulation in the body. It is a compound joint comprised of medial and lateral femoral-tibial articulations and a patella-femoral articulation, all within one joint capsule. Positioned midway in each supporting limb of the body, the knee is subjected to severe stresses as it performs its functions of weight-bearing and locomotion. The anatomic description of this articulation is simplified by considering it as two separate joints. The larger one, the femorotibial joint, consists of two condylar joints between corresponding femoral and tibial condyles. The second one, the femoropatellar joint, is between the patella and the femur.

THE FEMOROTIBIAL JOINT

The femoral condyles are convex in both planes and, viewed laterally, are spiral shaped. The lateral condyle flattens more rapidly in the anteroposterior dimension than does the medial condyle, producing inequality in articular lengths. This is evident when the knee is placed in full extension. An automatic coupled rotation occurs to accommodate this inequality. Hoppenfeld describes a "screw home" motion in which the medial aspect of the tibia rotates laterally around the lateral femoral condyle, allowing the medial femoral condyle to complete its extension. This approximates a close-packed position, allowing prolonged periods of standing without relying on muscle function.

The tibial condyles are concave and end toward the midtibial line in intercondylar eminences. The condyles are separated by the intercondylar area.

The femorotibial joint is one of the few articulations with menisci. The medial meniscus is semicircular. Its anterior end is attached to the anterior intercondylar area in front of the anterior cruciate ligament. The lateral meniscus is almost a complete ring. Its anterior end is attached in front of the intercondylar eminence of the tibia, blending partially with the anterior cruciate ligament.

The femoral condyles roll and slide on the tibial condyles during flexion and extension, accompanied by similar motions of the menisci. During extension the menisci are pulled anteriorly; with flexion they are moved posteriorly.

The femorotibial joint is stabilized by the capsule and its related ligaments and muscular attachments. Laterally, these attachments comprise the fibular collateral ligament, biceps tendon, popliteus tendon, and the iliotibial tract; medially, they comprise the pes anserine, the medial head of the gastrocnemius, the tibial lateral ligament, and a portion of the quadriceps tendon. Posteriorly the joint is stabilized by both heads of the gastronemius, the semitendinous muscle, the biceps tendon, the oblique popliteal ligament, and the arcuate ligament. The anterior aspect is stabilized by the quadriceps muscles, the quadriceps tendon, the patella, the patellar tendon, and the medial and lateral retinacula.

The cruciate ligaments are intraarticular but extrasynovial. They stabilize the knee in the anteroposterior direction and allow the joint to function as a hinge while keeping the articular surfaces together. The *anterior cruciate ligament* arises from the tibia and runs backward, upward, and laterally to insert onto the lateral femoral condyle. During flexion, the anterior cruciate ligament slides the femoral condyle forward. The *posterior cruciate ligament* arises from the posterior aspect of the tibia and runs forward and upward obliquely to insert onto the lateral aspect of the medial femoral condyle. During extension the posterior cruciate ligament slides the femoral condyle posteriorly.

THE FEMOROPATELLAR JOINT

The femoropatellar joint is a sellar joint; the articulating surface of the patella is adapted to the patellar surface of the femur. This femoral articulation involves the anterior surface of both condyles. An oblique groove divides it into a large lateral and smaller medial area. The joint's stability is maintained by the quadriceps muscles, the quadriceps tendon, and the patellar tendon. Its major motions are vertical up-and-down movement on the femur, and movement in a sagittal plane with respect to the tibia. This allows a pulley function during flexion and extension of the knee.

Major Muscles

The quadriceps femoris is the extensor muscle of the knee. It consists of four muscles that have a common tendon of insertion onto the anterior tuberosity of the tibia. The rectus femoris arises from two tendinous heads, one from the anterior iliac spine and the second from a groove above the acetabulum and the hip joint capsule. It is directed downward along the anterior aspect of the thigh and ends in the common tendon. It functions as a two-joint muscle, producing both hip flexion and knee extension. The vastus lateralis is the largest part of the quadriceps. It arises from the upper intertrochanteric line and the anterior and inferior borders of the greater trochanter. The vastus medialis arises from the lower part of the intertrochanteric line, the spiral line, the medial lip of the linea aspera, the medial supracondylar line, and the tendons of the adductor longus and

magnus. The vastus intermedius arises from the front and lateral surface of the upper shaft of the femur.

The flexor muscles of the knee are located in the posterior compartment of the thigh. They are the hamstrings, the gracilis, the sartorius, the popliteus, and the gastrocnemius muscles. All of these muscles are biarticular with the exception of the popliteus and the short head of the biceps. Their action on knee flexion is related to the position of the hip. Rotation of the knee is also a function of these knee flexors.

Knee Movements

The active motions of the knee are classified as flexion/extension and medial/lateral rotation. Normally the knee flexes to 135 degrees; extension is a return from flexion to 0 degrees. Medial/lateral rotation, with the knee in flexion, is 10 degrees in each direction. With the foot on the ground, the last 30 degrees of extension is accompanied by a conjunct medial femoral rotation. With the foot off the ground, extension is accompanied by a conjunct lateral rotation of the tibia.

Accessary motions with the knee semiflexed are anteroposterior glide, abduction/adduction, and long-axis extension.

Special Tests

VARUS-VALGUS STRESS TEST

This test evaluates the medial and lateral collateral structures. With the patient supine, the ankle joint is held between the examiner's side and arm, thus freeing both hands. The knee is tested in full extension by applying a valgus and then a varus force to the proximal tibia (abduction/adduction motion of leg) (Fig. 20-6). The examiner notes any instability or increased motion on application of force in either direction. Then the test is repeated with the knee slightly flexed. If the cruciate ligaments are intact, motion can be stable with the knee in full extension, even with collateral ligament rupture.

ROTARY INSTABILITY TESTING

Anterior Draw Test

The anterior draw test evaluates anterior cruciate ligament dysfunction. The patient is supine, with his knee flexed 90 degrees and his foot on the ta-

Figure 20-6. Varus-valgus stress for collateral structure dysfunction.

Varus stress

Valgus stress

R. MILLER

Figure 20-7. Anterior draw test for anterior cruciate ligament dysfunction.

R MILLER

ble. The examiner sits on the patient's foot or otherwise holds it firmly to stabilize it. The examiner then grasps the back of the proximal tibia with one or both hands and pulls it forward (Fig. 20-7). The patient's leg and foot are internally rotated 30 degrees, then externally rotated 15 degrees, and in a neutral position. On internal rotation, anterior shift of the lateral tibial plateau in conjunction with medial rotation implies injury to the anterior cruciate and lateral ligament. On external rotation, anterior shift of the medial tibial plateau in conjunction with lateral rotation implies injury to the anterior cruciate and medial collateral ligaments. With the foot in neutral position (anterior drawer sign) an anterior tibial shift indicates anterior cruciate ligament dysfunction, probably accompanied by medial and lateral ligamentous injury.

Posterior Draw Test
The posterior draw test evaluates posterior cruciate ligament dysfunction. The patient's foot is placed in neutral position, as for the anterior draw test. The examiner applies force on the anterior tibia in a posterior direction (Fig. 20-8). The femoral condyles become prominent anteriorly as the tibia subluxates posteriorly, indicating posterior cruciate ligament dysfunction.

EXTERNAL ROTATION—RECURVATUM TEST
With the patient supine, the examiner grasps one lower extremity under the heel. With his other hand he supports the calf. The knee is allowed to move from 10 degrees of flexion to full extension (Fig. 20-9). If the knee becomes hyperextended with external rotation of the tibia and tibial varus, the test is positive. This indicates injury to the ar-

Figure 20-8. Posterior draw test for posterior cruciate ligament dysfunction.

Figure 20-9. Recurvatum test.

cuate ligament, popliteus, and fibular collateral ligament.

MCMURRAY TEST
The McMurray test evaluates for meniscal tears. With the patient supine, the examiner grasps the foot with one hand and palpates the knee joint line with the other hand. The examiner acutely flexes the knee and rotates the tibia into medial and lateral rotation. With the tibia held in lateral rotation the examiner applies a valgus stress and extends the knee (Fig. 20-10). The maneuver is repeated with the knee held in medial rotation and a varus stress applied while extending the knee. A palpable or audible click within the joint is considered a sign of a meniscal tear.

APLEY'S COMPRESSION TEST
With the patient prone, the knee is flexed to 90 degrees. The examiner stabilizes the patient's thigh and leans on the heel, compressing the menisci between the femur and tibia, then rotates the tibia medially while maintaining this compression (Fig. 20-11). Medial joint pain produced by this maneuver suggests a medial meniscal tear, while lateral joint pain suggests a lateral meniscal tear.

APLEY'S DISTRACTION TEST
With the patient prone, the knee is flexed to 90 degrees. The examiner stabilizes the thigh by kneeling on it, then applies traction to the leg while rotating it medially and laterally (traction

Valgus

reduces meniscal pressure but increases ligamentous strain) (Fig. 20-12). Any pain elicited by this maneuver indicates medial or lateral ligamentous dysfunction.

KNEE JOINT EFFUSION TEST
The knee joint effusion test is performed in the same manner as the test for external rotation. Failure of the knee to extend fully indicates increased joint fluid.

PATELLA FEMORAL GRINDING TEST
The patient is supine with the knee extended and relaxed. The examiner pushes the patella caudad in the trochlear groove, then holds it in this position. The patient is instructed to tighten the quadriceps muscle against the examiner's resistance. Palpable crepitation of patellar motion is an indication of roughness of the articulating surfaces, potentially due to chondromalacia of the patella.

Figure 20-10. McMurray test for meniscal tears.

Figure 20-11. Apley's compression test for meniscal dysfunction.

Figure 20-12. Apley's distraction test for ligamentous dysfunction.

Common Musculoskeletal Knee Joint Disorders

MENISCAL TEARS
Common Findings
1. History of trauma.
2. Pain, swelling, and complaint of knee locking.
3. McMurray's test and the Apley compression test positive.
4. Arthroscopy necessary for confirmation.

CHONDROMALACIA OF THE PATELLA
Common Findings
1. First attack occurred prior to bony fusion.
2. Pain on sitting, climbing stairs, or prolonged walking.
3. Minor joint effusion present.
4. Recurrence with squatting.
5. Stiffness after sitting.
6. Patella femoral grinding test positive.
7. X-ray findings may be present.

PATELLAR TENDON TENDINITIS
Common Findings
1. Repeated stress applied to the insertion of the quadriceps tendon on the patella, producing tendinitis (stress may be at proximal, or more often, distal pole of the patella).
2. Pain worse after exercise.
3. Severe localized point tenderness.
4. No joint effusion.
5. Bone scan showing increased activity, as in stress fracture.

TRAUMATIC SYNOVITIS
Common Findings
1. Painful, swollen knee; difficulty with extension.
2. Suprapatellar pouch distended.
3. Patella is ballotable.
4. Knee only slightly warm.
5. History of trauma or chronic recurrence.

ANTERIOR FAT PAD LESION
Common Findings
1. Anterior knee pain of long duration.
2. Pain relieved by rest.
3. Pain relieved with knee in flexed position.
4. Tenderness anteriorly about the patellar tendon, usually of the fat pad itself on either side.
5. Joint line not involved

OSGOOD-SCHLATTER DISEASE
Common Findings
1. Point tenderness and swelling of the tibial tubercle.
2. Relieved with rest.
3. Localized traction tendonitis.
4. Heals with bone fusion.

PES ANSERINE BURSITIS
Common Findings
1. Located at insertion of pes anserine.
2. At medial aspect of knee but below joint space.
3. Severe point tenderness.
4. Worsens with contraction of the sartorius, gracilis, and semitendinous muscles.

INFRAPATELLAR BURSITIS (HOUSEMAID'S KNEE)
Common Findings
1. Localized swelling of bursa.
2. Usually not painful.
3. Caused by local trauma, usually recurrent.
4. Outside of joint capsule, does not interfere with function.

BAKER'S CYST (POPLITEAL CYST)
Common Findings
1. Usually arises from semimembranous tendon bursa.
2. May communicate with the joint.
3. Benign posterior joint space effusion.
4. Not painful unless size hinders joint motion.
5. Frequently related to rheumatoid arthritis.

THE FOOT AND ANKLE JOINTS
Stanley Schiowitz

The foot and ankle joints make up a complex unit of 28 bones. This unit must perform the functions of weight-bearing and adapting to terrain during walking or running, yet still remain sufficiently elastic to accommodate to additional stress. Some 40% of the entire population have foot abnormalities, which makes the study of this region extremely important.

Functional Anatomy
The ankle articulation consists of the distal end of the tibia and the medial and lateral malleoli, which together form a concave surface, the crural arch, into which is fitted the body of the talus. These bones are connected by the joint capsule and by the deltoid, anterior and posterior talofibular, and calcaneofibular ligaments. The tibial malleolus extends about one third of the way down the medial surface of the talus and is anterior to the lateral malleolus. The fibular malleolus extends down the entire lateral aspect of the talus. When viewed from above, the entire articulation is laterally angled, thus creating a toeing-out of 15 degrees (Fig. 20-13).

The body of the talus is wedge-shaped and wider in its anterior portion. Dorsiflexion creates a close-packed position of the talus in the crural arch. Further dorsiflexion induces separation of the tibiofibular articulation, with lateral and caudal displacement of the distal fibula and medial rotation around the tibia. This motion of the fibula can be a major source of fibular head dysfunction.

The major joint motions of the ankle are plantar flexion (to 50 degrees) and dorsiflexion (to 20 degrees) (Fig. 20-14). Accessory motions of side-to-side glide, rotation, abduction, and adduction are present if the joint is in plantar flexion.

The triangular deltoid ligament is located medially and is attached above to the medial malleolus and below to the tuberosity of the navicular, the sustentaculum tali of the calcaneus, and the medial tubercle of the talus. The deltoid ligament is so strong that trauma often causes fractures of its bony attachments rather than rupture of the ligament itself.

The anterior talofibular ligament goes from the anterior margin of the lateral malleolus forward and medially to attach to the lateral aspect of the neck and the lateral articular facet of the talus. The posterior talofibular ligament runs from the lower part of the lateral malleolus to the lateral tubercle of the posterior process of the talus. The calcaneofibular ligament runs from the apex of

Figure 20-13. Regional functional anatomy of the ankle joint.

Figure 20-14. Major motions of the ankle joint.

Figure 20-15. Ligamentous attachments at the ankle, posterior view.

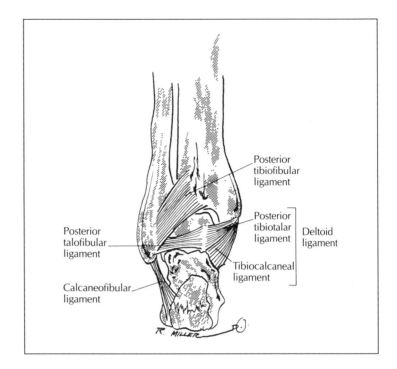

the lateral malleolus downward and backward to the tubercle on the lateral surface of the calcaneus (Fig. 20-15).

The shape of the crural concavity, the extent of the lateral malleous on the talus, and the strong ligamentous attachments deter joint dislocations unless accompanied by fracture of the malleoli.

The most common sprain represents an inversion and is usually caused by a combination of plantar flexion, internal rotation, and inversion. The lateral ankle ligaments sustain the initial impact. The type of ligamentous tear or fracture/dislocation will depend on the severity of the force.

The major muscle of ankle dorsiflexion is the tibialis anterior, assisted by the extensor digitorum longus, the extensor hallucis longus, and the peroneus tertius. The major muscles of ankle plantar flexion are the gastrocnemius and soleus, assisted by the plantaris, tibialis posterior, flexor hallucis longis, and flexor digitorum longus.

The subtalar articulation consists of the talus on the calcaneus. These bones have two separate concave-convex articulations. The major motions are calcaneal abduction (valgus) and calcaneal adduction (varus), in relationship to the fixed talus. The talus articulates with the navicular and the calcaneus articulates with the cuboid.

The combined motions of these joints create foot inversion and eversion (Fig. 20-16). Inversion is created by calcaneal adduction, navicular rotation, and glide on the talus. These motions raise the navicular and the medial border and depress the lateral border of the foot. Eversion is produced by an opposite series of motions. The muscles involved in the motion of inversion are the tibialis anterior and posterior. The muscles involved in the motion of eversion are the peroneus longus and brevis.

The cuboid motions on the calcaneus are glide with conjunct rotation. This usually accompanies the inversion/eversion motions of the combined articulations.

The forefoot consists of the metatarsals and phalanges. These bones have a combined motion of forefoot abduction and adduction (Fig. 20-17).

Pronation and supination of the foot are commonly described as a combination of various motions. Pronation consists of calcaneal abduction, subtalar-cuboid-navicular eversion, forefoot abduction, and ankle dorsiflexion. Supination consists of calcaneal adduction, subtalar-cuboid-navicular inversion, forefoot adduction, and ankle plantar flexion.

Figure 20-16. (**A**) Inversion of the ankle. (**B**) Eversion of the ankle.

Figure 20-17. (**A**) Abduction of the forefoot. (**B**) Adduction of the forefoot.

Figure 20-18. Transverse arches of the foot.

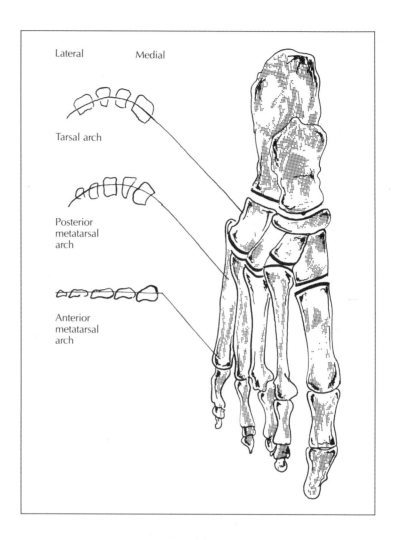

ARCHES OF THE FOOT

The longitudinal curve of the foot can be divided into medial and lateral longitudinal arches. The lateral arch is composed of the calcaneus, cuboid, and fourth and fifth metatarsal bones. This arch is low, with limited mobility; it is designed to transmit weight and thrust to the ground. Its major articulation is the calcaneocuboid, which has a limited range of motion. Stress through this arch can create a typical cuboid somatic dysfunction. Torsion through the anterior aspect of this arch will readily cause fracture of the fifth metatarsal.

The medial longitudinal arch is composed of the calcaneus, talus, navicular, cuneiforms, and the first three metatarsal bones. This arch is considerably higher and more mobile than its lateral counterpart. The plantar ligaments, plantar fascia, the tibialis posterior, flexor digitorum longus, flexor hallucis longus, and the intrinsic muscles of the foot assist in controlling the medial arch.

Evidently muscles contribute little to the maintenance of the arch, which instead is supported passively by the skeletal structure and ligaments. Muscles do play an active role in balance and gait.

Many authors describe a number of transverse arches (Fig. 20-18). With the exception of the metatarsal heads, these arches do not transmit forces to the ground. The anterior metatarsal transverse arch consists of the five metatarsals heads, with the second metatarsal as its highest point. With weight-bearing this arch is flattened. Depression of the anterior metatarsal transverse arch increases the weight-bearing burden of the metatarsal heads, creating dysfunction. A second, posterior metatarsal arch consists of the bases of the five metatarsals. A third, tarsal arch has been described, consisting of the navicular, cuneiforms, and cuboid bones. This arch assists in flexibility and the rotation motions of the foot. Diminution or absence of the tarsal arch is evident in pes planus (flat feet).

Common Musculoskeletal Disorders

PEDIATRIC CONGENITAL DEFORMITIES: ANATOMIC DEFINITIONS

Pes planus: Flattened longitudinal arches.
Equinus: Toes pointed down, foot in plantar flexion (Fig. 20-19A).
Calcaneus: Toes pointed up, foot in dorsiflexion (Fig. 20-19B).
Valgus: Toes pointed out, foot in abduction.
Varus: Toes pointed in, foot in adduction.
Eversion: Foot rotated externally on its longitudinal arch; sole faces laterally.
Inversion: Foot rotated internally on its longitudinal arch; sole faces medially.

COMMON CONGENITAL PEDIATRIC CONDITIONS

1. **Pes planus (dropped longitudinal arches).** Pes planus may be a normal finding in a child; however, it may also represent a congenital condition, either flexible calcaneal valgus or rigid vertical talus.
2. **Talipes equinovarus (clubfoot).** The foot is in the position of inversion, adduction of the forefoot, calcaneal varus, and equinus. The calf muscles are contracted.
3. **Metatarsus varus.** This condition is characterized by calcaneal valgus, the forefoot in adduction, and a convex lateral foot border.
4. **Tibial torsion.** In tibial torsion the tibia is twisted on its longitudinal axis and the relationship between the patella and the foot is abnormal. The condition can be secondary to femoral torsion. Bilateral torsion can create "pigeon toeing" or a Charlie Chaplin type of gait.

COMMON ADULT CONDITIONS

1. **Foot strains.** Foot strains are of several types, including (a) plantar fascia involvement of the medial longitudinal arch or at the calcaneal insertions, (b) medial and lateral ligament

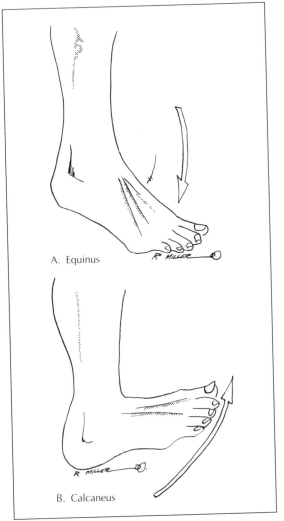

A. Equinus

B. Calcaneus

Figure 20-19. Pediatric congenital deformities.

involvement secondary to chronic or acute strains, and (c) metatarsalgia secondary to abnormal weight-bearing by the metatarsal heads.
2. **Morton's syndrome.** Morton's syndrome is a metatarsalgia caused by a short first metatarsal bone.
3. **Morton's neuroma.** Morton's neuroma is a fibroneuromatous reaction between the heads of the third and fourth metatarsals.
4. **March fracture.** March fracture is a stress fracture, usually involving the shaft of the second or third metatarsal.

5. **Hallux valgus.** Hallux valgus is a lateral deviation of the proximal phalanx of the first toe associated with soft tissue changes, pain, swelling, and inflammation at the medial aspect of the head of the first metatarsal, which is angled medially. This condition is also called a bunion.

6. **Hallux rigidus.** Hallux rigidus is an osteoarthrosis of the first metatarsophalangeal articulation. Joint motion is severely limited: there is no first toe push-off, and localized pain is present at that joint.

7. **Claw toe.** Claw toe is a fixed flexion deformity of the proximal interphalangeal joints associated with hyperextension of the metatarsophalangeal articulations.

8. **Hammer toe.** Hammer toe is similar to claw toe, but the distal interphalangeal articulation is in hyperextension. Usually only one toe is involved.

9. **Callus.** A callus is a hyperkeratotic response of the skin to excessive pressure.

10. **Corns.** Soft corns are hyperkeratotic lesions found between the toes, usually the fourth and fifth toes. They are extremely painful. Hard corns are usually found when hammer or claw toes cause abnormal shoe pressure on the hyperflexed or hyperextended joint.

The treatment and prevention of many of these adult dysfunctions require the proper fit of shoes and orthotic devices, as well as knowledge of osteopathic diagnostic and manipulative procedures.

References

Basmajian JV. 1978. Muscles Alive. Baltimore: Williams & Wilkins Co.

Cailliet R. 1968. Foot and Ankle Pain. Philadelphia: F.A. Davis Co.

D'Ambrosia RD. 1977. Musculoskeletal Disorders. Philadelphia: J.B. Lippincott Co.

Hoppenfeld S. 1986. Physical Examination of the Spine and Extremities. Norwalk, Conn: Appleton-Century-Crofts.

Jones L. 1955. The Postural Complex. St. Louis: Charles C Thomas, Publisher.

Kapandji IA. 1970. The Physiology of the Joints. Vol II. Edinburgh: Churchill Livingstone.

MacConaill MA, Basmajian JV. 1977. Muscles and Movements. New York: Robert E. Krieger Publishing Co.

O'Donoghue DH. 1970. Treatment of Injuries to Athletes. Philadelphia: W.B. Saunders Co.

Rasch PJ, Burke RK. 1978. Kinesiology and Applied Anatomy. Baltimore: Lea & Febiger.

Warwick RB, Williams PL. 1973. Gray's Anatomy, 35th British Ed. Philadelphia: W.B. Saunders Co.

Wells KF, Luttgens K. 1976. Kinesiology. Philadelphia: W.B. Saunders Co.

Wilson FC. 1983. The Musculoskeletal System, 2nd ed. Philadelphia: J.B. Lippincott Co.

21

Diagnosis and Treatment of the Lower Extremity

THE HIP
Stanley Schiowitz

This section describes the diagnosis and treatment of soft tissue dysfunctions of the hip joint. In most instances, these dysfunctions are evaluated by testing the range of anatomic or physiologic joint motion. The diagnosis of restrictive movements in the extremities can usually be simplified by comparing both sides. However, arthritic involvement of the hip joint can confuse the diagnosis, and it may be difficult to ascertain how much of the restriction is due to myofascial dysfunction and how much to joint lining disease. The techniques described here can be utilized when both conditions are present. After a few treatments the soft tissue components will improve, and any remaining restriction can be attributed to degenerative joint changes.

Most physicians treating musculoskeletal problems use the anatomic barriers to passive motion as their guide. The following discussion is presented with that in mind.

Screening Tests for Somatic Dysfunctions of the Hip

The following screening tests are performed to evaluate gross motions of the hip joint. Individual joint motions should be tested if any of the screening procedures are positive. Individual joint motions include abduction and adduction, internal and external rotation, flexion, and extension. Extending these procedures to their anatomic barriers of motion will result in full anatomic barrier motion measurements.

FABERE test. The FABERE test evaluates flexion, abduction, external rotation, and extension of one hip joint as compared with the other. The test is described in Chapter 20.

Squatting. The patient attempts to squat while holding onto support. Hip joint restriction will prevent this movement, as will knee joint dysfunction (Fig. 21-1).

Straight leg raising. The patient is supine with the legs together and extended. The physician stands on the side of the leg to be tested and grasps the patient's ankle with one hand while placing the other hand on the patient's opposite anterior superior iliac spine (Fig. 21-2). With the patient's knee extended, the physician lifts the patient's leg, flexing the hip, until motion is felt at the opposite anterior superior iliac spine. The angle of flexion from the table top is measured. The physician returns the leg to the table and repeats the maneuver from the other side of the table with the other leg. Any limitation of flexion is interpreted as being caused by contracted hamstring muscles.

Figure 21-1. Squatting test for hip joint restriction.

Figure 21-2. Straight leg raising test for limitation in flexion of the hip joint.

Thomas test for psoas contraction. In a supine position, the patient flattens the lumbar lordotic curve by flexing both hips and knees to the abdomen, then releases one leg to the table without creating lordosis. The clinician measures the extension of the leg. The maneuver is repeated with the other leg, and the two sides are compared. Inability to fully extend the leg may indicate iliopsoas contracture.

Treatment
MYOFASCIAL STRETCH—PASSIVE AND ACTIVE
1. Patient position: supine.
2. Physician position: standing on the side of dysfunction, facing the table.
3. **Technique:**
   a. The patient's hip and knee are flexed.
   b. The physician places his hands on the posterior aspect of the patient's thigh, near the popliteal region.
   c. The physician passively applies increasing force to the patient's thigh in the direction of limitation of motion, to the point of creating pain. This position is held for 3 seconds.
   d. The patient pushes his thigh against the physician's resisting hands, creating an isometric contraction in the direction opposite to the passive motion. This position is held for 3 seconds (Fig. 21-3).

e. The physician relaxes all force and returns the hip to the starting position.
f. The patient rests for 3 seconds, then the procedure is repeated.
   This maneuver should be performed three times, with each repetition allowing greater freedom of motion. The technique can be repeated in another direction of limitation of motion.

PASSIVE MYOFASCIAL RELEASE—COMBINED HIP AND KNEE
1. Patient position: supine.
2. Physician position: standing on the side of the dysfunction, facing the table.
3. **Technique:**
   a. The patient's hip and knee are flexed to 90 degrees, if possible.
   b. The patient's hip is placed into abduction and external rotation up to full pain-free motion.
   c. The physician places one hand on the medial aspect of the patient's knee, firmly holding that limb in its abduction–external rotation position.
   d. With his other hand, the physician grasps the patient's foot or shin and externally rotates the tibia to its maximum pain-free position (Fig. 21-4A).
   e. The physician holds this position for 3 seconds, increasing the motion pressure of both hands until the muscles relax.

Figure 21-3. Passive-active myofascial stretch of the hip.

A

B

Figure 21-4. (**A**) Passive myofascial release of the hip and knee, abduction–external rotation. (**B**) The hip and knee are returned to full extension.

f. Maintaining pressure with both hands, the physician slowly returns the patient's hip and knee to full extension on the table, releasing the pressure of both hands only at the last 5 degrees of full extension (Fig. 21-4B).

g. The patient rests, then the treatment is repeated.

This procedure can be performed with the patient's hip in adduction and internal rotation. The physician places one hand on the lateral aspect of the patient's knee and moves the tibia into internal rotation (Fig. 21-5).

Figure 21-5. (**A**) Active myofascial release of the hip and knee, adduction–internal rotation. (**B**) The hip and knee are returned to full extension.

A

B

Figure 21-6. Passive-active psoas adductor stretch.

Figure 21-7. Myofascial release with traction of the hip joint.

PSOAS ADDUCTOR STRETCH—PASSIVE AND ACTIVE

1. Patient position: supine.
2. Physician position: standing beside the table, on the side to be treated.
3. **Technique:**
   a. The patient flexes the dysfunctional hip and knee and places that foot on table beside the other knee, which is in full extension.
   b. The patient then abducts and externally rotates the flexed hip, so that the plantar aspect of the foot lies beside the medial aspect of the extended knee.
   c. The physician places one hand on the anterior superior iliac spine of the nondysfunctional side and the other hand on the medial aspect of the patient's flexed knee, holding it in its position of flexion, hip abduction–external rotation.
   d. The physician adds a gentle passive stretching force toward the table. This position is held for 3 seconds.
   e. The patient exerts a gentle force upward into adduction, internal rotation–flexion, against the physician's isometrically resisting right hand (Fig. 21-6). This position is held for 3 seconds.
   f. The patient relaxes. After 3 seconds the procedure is repeated.

MYOFASCIAL RELEASE WITH TRACTION OF THE HIP JOINT

1. Patient position: supine.
2. Physician position: sitting beside the table on the side of the dysfunction, facing toward the patient's head.
3. **Technique:**
   a. The patient's ankle and shin are placed in the physician's axilla and maintained in position by firm adduction of the arm.
   b. The physician grasps the patient's extended leg above the knee and rotates the hip internally and externally, testing for ease of motion.
   c. The hip is placed into its freedom of motion and firmly held there.
   d. The physician then applies traction to the entire leg by leaning back, creating a pull on the leg that is snugged in his axilla and gradually increasing rotation into the freedom of motion (Fig. 21-7). This position is held for 3 seconds, then the physician quickly rotates the hip fully in the opposite direction. This position is held for 3 seconds.
   e. The physician releases the leg and relaxes the position.
   f. The patient rests for 3 seconds, then the technique is repeated.

Figure 21-8. Passive-active hamstring stretch.

Figure 21-9. Locations of tender points of the hips. *PLT,* posterolateral trochanteric; *LT,* lateral trochanteric; *PMT,* posteromedial trochanteric.

HAMSTRING STRETCH — PASSIVE AND ACTIVE

1. Patient position: supine.
2. Physician position: sitting on the table on the side of the dysfunction, facing the patient.
3. **Technique:**
   a. The patient's ankle is placed on the physician's shoulder. The physician places both his hands on the anterior aspect of the patient's knee to maintain the leg in full extension.
   b. The physician stands up, raising the straightened leg higher into hip flexion. The hip is stretched to point of onset of pain and held at maximum painless stretch for 3 seconds.
   c. The patient presses that leg down onto the physician's shoulder for 3 seconds (Fig. 21-8).
   d. The leg is released, the patient relaxes for 3 seconds, and the technique is repeated.

Counterstrain Treatment

Three significant tender points are associated with the hip joint (Fig. 21-9). One might also consider the piriformis tender point when treating hip pain: the piriformis tender point is most closely associated with sacral dysfunctions and was discussed in Chapter 14.

POSTEROLATERAL TROCHANTERIC TENDER POINT

1. Tender point: on the posterolateral surface of the greater trochanter.
2. Patient position: prone.
3. Physician position: standing or seated beside the table.
4. **Technique:**
   a. The hip is extended and abducted (Fig. 21-10).
   b. External rotation may be needed.

LATERAL TROCHANTERIC TENDER POINT

1. Tender point: five to six inches below the trochanter on the lateral thigh.
2. Patient position: prone.
3. Physician position: standing or seated beside the table.

Figure 21-10. Counterstrain treatment of posterolateral trochanteric tender point.

Figure 21-11. Counterstrain treatment of lateral trochanteric tender point.

Figure 21-12. Counterstrain treatment of posteromedial trochanteric tender point.

4. **Technique:**
   a. The leg is abducted (Fig. 21-11).
   b. Some flexion may be introduced.

POSTEROMEDIAL TROCHANTERIC
TENDER POINTS
1. Tender point: two to three inches below the

trochanter along posterior shaft of femur over to the ischial tuberosity.
2. Patient position: prone.
3. Physician position: standing beside the table, opposite the tender point.
4. **Technique:**
   The thigh is extended, adducted and externally rotated (Fig. 21-12).

THE KNEE
Stanley Schiowitz

The knee joint is subject to numerous stresses in normal daily activities. Simply standing up from a sitting position can be difficult or painful if the knee joint is not fully functional. In addition, the resurgence of health consciousness has created a number of enthusiastic walkers, joggers, runners, and tennis players. Each of these activities can add greatly to knee joint dysfunction.

Before treating specific osteopathic articular somatic dysfunctions, the physician must evaluate and treat any soft tissue dysfunctions. The localized osteopathic joint motion dysfunctions discussed in this chapter involve minor or accessory motions.

Diagnosis of Somatic Dysfunctions of the Knee Joint
ABDUCTION — TIBIA ON FEMUR
This is a condition of varus stress of the tibia on the femur. It can be created by a blow to the medial knee joint or by a twisting motion that produces lateral ligamentous sprain. The lateral joint structures are lax, the medial knee joint approximates, and tibial motion on the femur is restricted in medial translatory slide.

1. Patient position: supine, with the knee fully extended.

Figure 21-13. Motion testing for medial-lateral translatory slide dysfunctions.

Figure 21-14. Motion testing for internal and external rotation of the tibia on the femur.

2. Physician position: standing on the side of the somatic dysfunction, facing the table.
3. **Technique:**
   a. The physician's cephalic hand grasps the patient's distal femur, holding it firmly and restricting its movement.
   b. With his other hand the physician grasps the patient's lower ankle and creates valgus/varus stress of the tibia on the femur. The varus motion should be greater than the valgus motion.
   c. The physician moves his hand up to the proximal tibia, then induces a straight medial-lateral translatory slide of the tibia upon the femur (Fig. 21-13). The lateral translatory motion should be greater than the medial translatory motion.

ADDUCTION — TIBIA ON FEMUR

This is a condition of valgus stress of the tibia on the femur. It can be created by a blow to the lateral knee joint or by a twisting motion that produces medial ligamentous sprain. The medial joint structures are lax, the lateral knee joint approximates, and tibial motion on the femur is restricted in lateral translatory slide.

1. Patient position: supine, with the knee fully extended.
2. Physician position: standing on the side of the dysfunction, facing the patient.
3. **Technique:**
   All positions are as described above for abduction; however, the findings are reversed: valgus motion is greater than varus, and

medial translatory motion is greater than lateral.

INTERNAL AND EXTERNAL ROTATION—TIBIA ON FEMUR

1. Patient position: supine. A pillow is placed under the knee to be examined to maintain slight flexion.
2. Physician position: standing on the side of the dysfunction, facing the table.
3. **Technique:**
   a. The physician's cephalic (with respect to the patient) hand grasps the patient's distal femur, holding it firmly and restricting its movement.
   b. With his other hand the physician grasps the patient's lower ankle and induces internal and external rotary motion of the tibia on the femur (Fig. 21-14).
4. **Interpretation:**
   Increased internal rotation with restricted external rotation signifies internal rotation dysfunction; increased external rotation with restricted internal rotation signifies external rotation dysfunction.

ANTEROPOSTERIOR SLIDE DYSFUNCTION—TIBIA ON FEMUR

In this condition the tibia is restricted in anterior or posterior slide. This motion is coupled to knee flexion-extension. Movement of the tibia on the femur into extension is coupled with anterior slide. Movement of the tibia on the femur into flexion is coupled with posterior slide. The initial complaints or findings are restrictions of flexion or extension movements. The physician must look for these dysfunctions.

The technique described below is a modified drawer test.

1. Patient position: supine, with the dysfunctional knee flexed and the foot flat on table.
2. Physician position: sitting on the patient's foot, anchoring it to the table.
3. **Technique:**
   a. The physician wraps both hands around the proximal tibia with his thumbs in front of the medial and lateral condyles and pressing on them. The physician's hand encircles the leg and grasps it firmly below the popliteal space.
   b. The physician creates a direct antero-posterior translatory slide of the tibia on the femur by first pulling the tibia forward with both hands and then pushing it backward with both thumbs (Fig. 21-15).

   Note: In performing this test, the physician is not evaluating for cruciate ligamentous tears. The anteroposterior force used must be greatly reduced.
4. **Interpretation:**
   a. Increased anterior slide with decreased posterior slide signifies anterior slide dysfunction; increased posterior slide with decreased anterior slide signifies posterior slide dysfunction.

Figure 21-15. Motion testing for anteroposterior slide dysfunctions of the tibia on the femur.

Figure 21-16. Motion testing for proximal fibular head dysfunctions.

PROXIMAL FIBULAR HEAD DYSFUNCTION— FIBULA ON TIBIA

These dysfunctions are not anatomically part of the knee joint. However, the proximity of the fibular head to the knee joint and the overlapping symptom complexes warrant inclusion of these dysfunctions here. When evaluating or treating a fibular head dysfunction, the physician should completely examine the distal articulation as well as the ankle joint.

1. Patient position: supine, with the dysfunctional knee flexed and the foot flat on the table.
2. Physician position: sitting on the patient's foot.
3. **Technique:**
   a. The initial steps are as in the modified drawer test (see anteroposterior slide dysfunction).
   b. The physician grasps the head of the fibula with his thumb and index finger (Fig. 21-16).
   c. A firm anteroposterior slide motion of the fibular head on the tibia is created.
4. **Interpretation:**
   a. Increased anterior slide with decreased posterior slide signifies anterior fibular head dysfunction; increased posterior slide with decreased anterior slide signifies posterior fibular head dysfunction.

Figure 21-17. Treatment of the knee using flexion-extension with anteroposterior translatory slide.

Treatment

Treatment of somatic dysfunctions of the knee begins with myofascial ligament-release techniques that encourage motion. The hip and ankle joints are included in the treatment. The somatic dysfunctions described in this chapter usually occur in combination. The techniques described below involve more than one joint or more than one dysfunction.

PASSIVE MYOFASCIAL RELEASE—COMBINED HIP AND KNEE

This treatment combines myofascial release of the hip joint with increasing internal and external rotation of the tibia on the femur (previously described under hip joint).

FLEXION-EXTENSION WITH
ANTEROPOSTERIOR TRANSLATORY SLIDE

1. Patient position: supine, the hip and knee on the side of the dysfunction flexed to 110 to 120 degrees.
2. Physician position: standing on the side of the dysfunction, facing the patient.
3. **Technique:**
   a. The patient's ankle is placed in the physician's axilla. The axillary grip must be firm enough that flexion-extension of the knee can be created by the to-and-fro rocking of the physician's body.

b. The physician grasps the proximal end of the tibia with his thumbs on the anterior tibia and his fingers clasped behind the leg, below the popliteal space.
c. The physician rocks forward, increasing knee flexion 5 to 10 degrees, and simultaneously pushes the tibia into posterior slide by the pressure of his thumbs (Fig. 21-17).
d. The physician rocks backward, decreasing the flexion, and simultaneously pulls the tibia into anterior slide with his fingers.
e. The to-and-fro rocking motion is repeated three to four times, increasing the anterior and posterior slide motions each time.

MYOFASCIAL RELEASE WITH TRACTION OF THE KNEE JOINT—INTERNAL AND EXTERNAL ROTATION

1. Patient position: supine. A pillow is placed under the knee to be treated, creating 10 to 15 degrees of flexion.
2. Physician position: sitting beside the table on the side of the dysfunction, facing the patient.
3. **Technique:**
   a. The patient's ankle and shin are placed in the physician's axilla and maintained in position by firm adduction of the physician's arm.
   b. The physician grasps that tibia at its proximal end, then translates the tibia on the femur anteriorly and applies traction by leaning back.
   c. The physician translates the tibia on the femur posteriorly and applies traction by leaning back.
   d. The physician rotates the tibia on the femur internally and applies traction by leaning back.
   e. The physician rotates the tibia on the femur externally and applies traction by leaning back (Fig. 21-18).
   f. The physician rests briefly, then repeats the set of maneuvers, increasing the rotation and slide motions but not the traction pull with each repetition.

KNEE AND ANKLE JOINT—
LONG-AXIS EXTENSION

1. Patient position: supine, with the hip and knee on the side of the dysfunction in 90 degrees of flexion.

Figure 21-18. Myofascial release with traction of the knee joint used for internal and external rotation, anterior and posterior translatory slide.

Figure 21-19. Treatment of the knee and ankle joints using long-axis extension.

2. Physician position: standing beside the table on the side of the dysfunction, facing the foot of the table.
3. **Technique:**
   a. The physician places his flexed elbow (closer to the table) in the patient's popliteal space and grasps the calcaneus with that hand.
   b. With his other hand the physician grasps the anterior aspect of the patient's ankle at the talus. A small towel or pillow can be inserted between the physician's elbow and patient's popliteal space for comfort, or if the patient's leg is longer than the physician's forearm.
   c. As the physician rocks backward, his elbow should separate the femur from the tibia, while his hands on the calcaneus and talus should separate the talus from the crural arch (Fig. 21-19).
   d. This position is held for 3 seconds, then the physician rocks forward to relax the traction force.
   e. Rest and repeat.
      Any of these techniques can be modified by introducing isometric resistance to create myofascial relaxation: for abduction, adduction, and internal or external rotation dysfunctions. The principle is the same in all cases. The joint is placed into its barrier to motion, then the patient actively attempts to reverse that motion against the isometric resistive force supplied by the physician.

Counterstrain Treatment

The locations of the tender points around the knee are shown in Figure 21-20.

ANTERIOR TENDER POINTS
The major anterior tender point is the patellar tender point, located just below the patella.

1. Patient position: supine.
2. Physician position: standing beside the table.
3. **Technique:**
   a. A rolled pillow is placed beneath the patient's calf.
   b. The knee is hyperextended by the physician pressing down on the anterior thigh just above the patella with a fair amount of force.
   c. The foot is internally rotated (Fig. 21-21).

POSTERIOR TENDER POINTS
A. Anterior cruciate tender point
   1. Patient position: supine
   2. Physician position: standing beside the table.
   3. **Technique:**
      a. A rolled pillow is placed under the thigh of the involved leg.
      b. The physician presses down on the lower leg just below the joint with a large amount of force (Fig. 21-22).
      c. This technique shortens the anterior cruciate ligaments.

Figure 21-20. Location of tender points around the knee. *PAT*, patellar; *LM*, lateral meniscus; *LH*, lateral hamstring; *MM*, medial meniscus; *MH*, medial hamstring; *EX*, gastrocnemius; *AC*, anterior cruciate; *PC*, posterior cruciate.

B. Posterior cruciate tender point
   1. Patient position: supine.
   2. Physician position: standing beside the table.
   3. **Technique:**
      a. A rolled pillow is placed behind the knee below the joint.
      b. The physician presses down on the dorsum of the ankle with a large amount of force.
      c. The foot is internally rotated (Fig. 21-23).
      d. This maneuver shortens the posterior cruciate ligament.
C. Gastrocnemius tender points
   1. Patient position: prone.
   2. Physician position: standing beside the table with his foot on the table.
   3. **Technique:**
      a. The foot is hyperextended over the physician's knee by a downward force on the posterior ankle (Fig. 21-24).
      b. This maneuver shortens the gastrocnemius muscle.

Figure 21-21. Counterstrain treatment of patellar tender point.

Figure 21-22. Counterstrain treatment for anterior cruciate tender point.

Figure 21-23. Counterstrain treatment for posterior cruciate tender point.

Figure 21-24. Counterstrain treatment for gastrocnemius tender point.

Figure 21-25. Counterstrain treatment for medial meniscus tender point.

MEDIAL TENDER POINTS

A. Medial meniscus tender point
1. Patient position: supine, involved leg off the table.
2. Physician position: seated beside the table.
3. **Technique:**
   a. The physician grasps the patient's foot and internally rotates the lower leg, keeping the knee slightly flexed.
   b. The knee is adducted slightly against the edge of the table (Fig. 21-25).

B. Medial hamstring tender point
1. Patient position: supine.
2. Physician position: standing beside the table.
3. **Technique:**
   a. The knee is flexed to about 60 degrees.
   b. The leg is externally rotated with a slight amount of adduction. This may be accomplished by grasping the patient's foot or ankle to use as a lever.

LATERAL TENDER POINTS

A. Lateral meniscus tender point
1. Patient position: supine, with the leg off the table.
2. Physician position: seated beside the table.
3. **Technique:**
   a. The leg is off the table with the knee slightly flexed.
   b. The physician grasps the patient's foot and internally rotates it (Fig. 21-26).
   c. The lower leg is slightly abducted.
   d. Occasionally external rotation may be needed.

B. Lateral hamstring tender point
1. Patient position: supine, with the leg off the table.
2. Physician position: seated next to the table.
3. **Technique:**
   a. The physician grasps the patient's foot and externally rotates it.
   b. The knee is flexed about 30 degrees and an abduction force is applied to the leg (Fig. 21-27).

Figure 21-26. Counterstrain treatment for lateral meniscus tender point.

Figure 21-27. Counterstrain treatment for lateral hamstring tender point.

Figure 21-28. High velocity, low amplitude thrusting technique for an anterior fibular head somatic dysfunction.

High Velocity, Low Amplitude Thrusting Techniques

A. Anterior fibular head somatic dysfunction
   1. Patient position: supine.
   2. Physician position: standing beside the table, on the same side as the dysfunction.
   3. **Technique:**
      a. The physician grasps the patient's foot on the side of the somatic dysfunction with his nonthrusting hand.
      b. The physician places the thenar eminence of his thrusting hand over the superolateral aspect of the fibular head.
      c. The patient's knee is placed in the close-packed position, then mildly flexed.
      d. The physician exerts a rapid knee extension while simultaneously introducing a downward and medial thrust through the fibular head (Fig. 21-28).
      e. Slight external rotation of the tibia facilitates the motion.
B. Posterior fibular head somatic dysfunction
   1. Patient position: supine.
   2. Physician position: standing beside the table, opposite the dysfunction.
   3. **Technique:**
      a. The physician grasps the patient's foot and ankle on the side of the dysfunction with his nonthrusting hand.
      b. The physician flexes the patient's hip and knee to 90 degrees.

   c. The physician places the index finger of his thrusting hand into the patient's popliteal crease, monitoring the dysfunctional fibular head.
   d. The physician locks the patient's foot on the side of the dysfunction in his armpit.
   e. The physician exerts a rapid downward thrust on the distal tibia and fibula while simultaneously pulling the fibular head anteriorly with his index finger (Fig. 21-29).
   f. Slight internal rotation of the tibia facilitates the motion.

Figure 21-29. High velocity, low amplitude thrusting technique for a posterior fibular head somatic dysfunction.

THE FOOT AND ANKLE
Stanley Schiowitz

The walking foot is constantly adapting to terrain. Beyond the calcaneus, the tarsal, metatarsal, and phalanges act as stabilizers, rising, falling, twisting, and turning to accommodate to every change in the road or our style of movement. These motions in turn are transmitted through the calcaneus, talus, and ankle mortice. This articulation is a secondary balancing mechanism, allowing dorsiflexion and plantar flexion, rotation, abduction, and adduction at the ankle.

Unexpected or uncompensated stresses or strains of the foot will create dysfunctions. These can occur at the articulations of the foot or at the ankle joint. A diagnosis is based on loss of joint mobility and tissue changes. Because the foot and ankle are attached to the body, the physician must always search out secondary dysfunctions.

Diagnosis of Somatic Dysfunctions of the Foot and Ankle Joint

The ankle joint is commonly involved in eversion and inversion strains or sprains, as well as in malleolar fractures. A thorough history, physical examination, and ancillary studies should be done before treatment is instituted. Dysfunction often follows immobilization treatment procedures. People with healed fractures may still have unresolved somatic dysfunctions.

The clinician should first examine a healthy extremity and test its motions. The findings in a healthy extremity provide a standard for comparison with a dysfunctional extremity.

MOTION TESTING
A. Dorsiflexion and plantar flexion
   1. Patient position: supine, with the knee slightly flexed and supported by a pillow.
   2. Physician position: standing at the foot of the table, facing the patient.
   3. **Technique:**
      a. With one hand the physician grasps the anterior ankle, locking both malleoli.
      b. With the other hand he grasps the forefoot, close to but not on the talus.
      c. The physician inverts the forefoot and, maintaining this position, places the foot into dorsiflexion and then plantar flexion (Fig. 21-30).
      d. Note degrees and freedom of motions as compared with the other foot.
B. Abduction-adduction (subtalar)
   1. Patient position: supine, with the knee slightly flexed and supported by a pillow.
   2. Physician position: standing at the foot of the table, facing the patient.
   3. **Technique:**
      a. The physician grasps the forefoot and

Figure 21-30. Motion testing for dorsiflexion and plantar flexion.

Figure 21-31. Motion testing for subtalar abduction-adduction.

Figure 21-32. Motion testing for calcaneal inversion-eversion.

Figure 21-33. Motion testing for a cuboid dysfunction.

places it into abduction and adduction (Fig. 21-31).

    b. Note degrees and freedom of motions as compared to the other foot.

C. Calcaneal inversion-eversion

  1. Patient position: supine, with the knee slightly flexed and supported by a pillow.

  2. Physician position: standing at the foot of the table, facing the patient.

  3. **Technique:**

    a. The physician grasps the calcaneus in one hand. His other hand is on the forefoot, locking the talus.

    b. The physician inverts and everts the calcaneus on the talus (Fig. 21-32).

    c. Note degrees and freedom of motions as compared to the other foot.

D. Cuboid dysfunction

  1. Patient position: prone.

  2. Physician position: standing beside the table, with one knee on the table.

  3. **Technique:**

    a. The patient's knee is flexed, with the foot resting on the physician's knee.

    b. The physician grasps calcaneus with one hand, locking it.

    c. With the thumb and index finger of the other hand, the physician grasps the cuboid and moves it dorsally and ventrally (Fig. 21-33).

    d. Note degrees and freedom of motion as compared to the other foot.

E. Fifth metatarsal dysfunction

  1. Patient position: prone.

  2. Physician position: standing beside the table, with one knee on the table.

  3. **Technique:**

    a. The physician grasps the cuboid with one hand, locking it.

    b. With his other hand he grasps the fifth metatarsal and moves it dorsally and ventrally (Fig. 21-34).

    c. To examine rotary motion of the metatarsal, the physician locks the fourth metatarsal and examines motion of the fifth. To examine motion of the fourth metatarsal, he locks the third metatarsal.

Figure 21-34. Motion testing for fifth metatarsal dysfunction.

d. Note degrees and freedom of motions as compared to the other foot.

F. Navicular dysfunction
  1. Patient position: supine.
  2. Physician position: seated at the foot of the table with his back to the patient. The foot to be examined lies on a pillow on his lap.
  3. **Technique:**
     a. The physician grasps the foot, including and locking the talus with one hand.
     b. With his other hand he grasps the navicular and moves it dorsally and ventrally (Fig. 21-35).
     c. Note degrees and freedom of motions as compared to the other foot.

G. Cuneiform dysfunction
  1. Patient position: supine.
  2. Physician position: seated at the foot of the table with his back to the patient. The foot to be examined lies on a pillow on his lap.
  3. **Technique:**
     a. The physician grasps and locks the navicular.
     b. The physician moves the cuneiform on the navicular.

H. First metatarsal dysfunction
  1. Patient position: supine.
  2. Physician position: seated at the foot of the table with his back to the patient. The foot to be examined lies on a pillow on his lap.

3. **Technique:**
   a. The physician grasps and locks the first cuneiform.
   b. He grasps the first metatarsal and moves it dorsally and ventrally.
   c. To examine for rotary motion of the metatarsals, the physician locks the second metatarsal to evaluate the first, and locks the third to evaluate the second.
   d. Note degrees and freedom of motions as compared to the other foot.

I. Phalangeal dysfunction
  1. Patient position: supine.
  2. Physician position: seated at the foot of the table with his back to the patient. The foot to be examined lies on a pillow on his lap.
  3. **Technique:**
     a. The physician grasps the metatarsal and locks it with one hand.
     b. With his other hand he grasps the first phalanx articulating with that metatarsal.
     c. After applying slight traction, the physician evaluates dorsal, ventral, abduction, adduction, and rotary motions (Fig. 21-36).
     d. Note degrees and freedom of motions as compared to the other foot.

Figure 21-35. Motion testing for navicular dysfunction.

Figure 21-36. Motion testing for phalangeal dysfunction.

Figure 21-37. Modified hand position for knee and ankle joint long-axis extension, utilized for treatment.

TREATMENT

A. Knee and ankle joint, long-axis extension
 1. Patient position: supine
 2. Physician position: standing with back to patient
 3. **Technique:**
   a. With the caudal (relative to the patient) hand the physician firmly grasps the forefoot and talus. With his other hand he holds the calcaneus.
   b. The physician's elbow maintains long-axis extension, with pressure at the popliteal region.
   c. The physician places the foot into corrective flexion-extension and abduction-adduction motions (Fig. 21-37).
   d. Maintaining the above position, the physician uses his cephalic hand to create calcaneal inversion and eversion.

B. Myofascial and joint motion—passive release
 1. Patient position: supine
 2. Physician position: standing at foot of table
 3. **Technique:**
   The physician applies mild traction force, then places the joint into the corrective motion direction.
   Note: This technique is applicable to all the joints examined as described in the first section of this chapter.

Counterstrain Treatment

The locations of the tender points on the lateral and medial aspects of the ankle and the dorsum of the foot are shown in Figure 21-38. There is also a tender point on the sole of the foot at the anterior end of the calcaneus.

Figure 21-38. Locations of foot and ankle tender points. *DM,* dorsal metatarsal; *MA,* medial ankle; *LA,* lateral ankle; *TAL,* talus; *DC,* dorsal cuboid; *NA,* navicular; *LC,* lateral calcaneal.

Figure 21-39. Counterstrain treatment of calcaneal tender point.

A. Calcaneal tender point
  1. Patient position: prone.
  2. Physician position: standing, with one foot on the table.
  3. **Technique:**
     a. The patient's foot rests on the physician's knee.
     b. The foot is plantar flexed against the physician's knee (Fig. 21-39).
     c. The physician grasps behind the heel and pushes toward the toes.
B. Dorsal metatarsal tender points
  1. Patient position: prone, with the knee flexed to 90 degrees.
  2. Physician position: standing beside the table.
  3. **Technique:**
     a. The physician strongly dorsiflexes the foot by placing a downward pressure on it (Fig. 21-40).
C. Medial ankle tender point
  1. Patient position: lying on his side, with the involved leg up.
  2. Physician position: seated beside the table.
  3. **Technique:**
     a. The patient's foot is brought off the table.
     b. A rolled towel is placed under the anterior ankle.
     c. The physician inverts the foot by pressing forcefully on the lateral side of the foot (Fig. 21-41).
D. Lateral ankle tender point
  This technique is the same as for the medial ankle tender point except that the ankle is forcefully everted (Fig. 21-42).

Figure 21-40. Counterstrain treatment for dorsal metatarsal tender point.

Figure 21-41. Counterstrain treatment for medial ankle tender point.

Figure 21-42. Counterstrain treatment for lateral ankle tender point.

Figure 21-43. Counterstrain treatment for talus tender point.

Figure 21-44. Counterstrain treatment of dorsal cuboid tender point.

E. Talar tender point
   This tender point is on the anteromedial ankle deep to the talus.
   1. Patient position: prone, with the foot up.
   2. Physician position: seated at the foot of the table.
   3. **Technique:**
      a. The foot is dorsiflexed, inverted, and internally rotated (Fig. 21-43).
F. Dorsal cuboid tender point
   1. Patient position: prone.
   2. Physician position: standing beside the table.
   3. **Technique:**
      a. The physician grasps the patient's foot and inverts it by applying pressure on the lateral side (Fig. 21-44).
G. Navicular tender point
   1. Patient position: prone.
   2. Physician position: seated or standing beside the table.
   3. **Technique:**
      a. The physician places his thumb or two fingers over the navicular bone to cause an inversion of the navicular.
      b. A slight amount of flexion is added (Fig. 21-45).

High Velocity, Low Amplitude Thrusting Techniques

A. Eversion/inversion somatic dysfunction of the ankle

Figure 21-45. Counterstrain treatment for navicular tender point.

   1. Patient position: supine.
   2. Physician position: standing at the foot of the table.
   3. **Technique:**
      a. The physician grasps the patient's foot on the side of dysfunction, placing one hand on the dorsal midtarsal region and using the other to grasp the calcaneus.
      b. The physician applies traction to the patient's leg (Fig. 21-46).
      c. If an inversion somatic dysfunction (i.e., eversion restriction) is present, the physician exerts rapid traction caudad through the calcaneus with simultaneous hypereversion of the ankle.
      d. If an eversion somatic dysfunction (i.e., inversion restriction) is present, the

Figure 21-46. High velocity, low amplitude thrusting technique for an eversion/inversion somatic dysfunction.

Figure 21-47. High velocity, low amplitude thrusting technique for tibiocalcaneal somatic dysfunction.

physician exerts traction caudad through the calcaneus while simultaneously hyperinverting the ankle.

B. Tibiocalcaneal somatic dysfunction
   1. Patient position: supine.
   2. Physician position: standing beside the table on the side of the somatic dysfunction.
   3. **Technique:**
      a. The physician cups the patient's tibia and fibula with one hand and places the thenar eminence of the other hand over the dorsum of the patient's forefoot.
      b. The physician applies traction cephalad on the patient's leg, through the tibia/fibula.
      c. The physician exerts a caudal and posterior thrust through the hand on the patient's forefoot. The physician's other hand stabilizes the ankle joint (Fig. 21-47).

C. Metatarsal somatic dysfunction
   1. Patient position: supine.
   2. Physician position: standing beside the table on the side of the somatic dysfunction.
   3. **Technique:**
      a. The physician grasps the patient's involved foot and places the pads of his thumbs, facing one another, over the junction of the metatarsal somatic dysfunction.

      b. The physician exerts a downward thrust through the thumbs, separating the joint articulation (Fig. 21-48).

D. Transtarsal somatic dysfunction
   1. Patient position: supine.
   2. Physician position: standing beside the table on the side of the somatic dysfunction.
   3. **Technique:**
      a. The physician places the patient's knee in flexion, abduction, and external rotation.
      b. The physician places the thenar eminence of one hand over the calcaneus; the other hand is placed over the first metatarsal and talus.
      c. The physician exerts a counterclockwise rotary thrust with the hand holding the talus while simultaneously exerting a downward thrust through the calcaneus with the other hand (Fig. 21-49).

E. Modified technique for transtarsal somatic dysfunction
   1. Patient position: supine and in FABERE position.
   2. Physician position: standing beside the table.

Figure 21-48. High velocity, low amplitude thrusting technique for metatarsal somatic dysfunction.

Figure 21-49. High velocity, low amplitude thrusting technique for transtarsal somatic dysfunction.

3. **Technique:**
   a. The physician exerts a simultaneous downward, lateral, and rotary thrust with the hand over the calcaneus. His other hand stabilizes the foot (Fig. 21-50).
F. Cuboid/navicular somatic dysfunction
  1. Patient position: prone.
  2. Physician position: standing beside the table on the side of the dysfunction.
  3. **Technique:**
   a. The physician flexes the patient's hip and knee on the dysfunctional side, then drops the leg off the side of the table.
   b. The physician grasps the patient's foot with both hands and places his thumbs in a V shape over the plantar surface of the cuboid or navicular.
   c. The physician exerts a downward thrust through his thumbs while simultaneously inducing a whiplike action at the patient's ankle and knee (Fig. 21-51).

Figure 21-50. Modified high velocity, low amplitude thrusting technique for transtarsal somatic dysfunction.

Figure 21-51. High velocity, low amplitude thrusting technique for a cuboid/navicular somatic dysfunction.

EXERCISE THERAPY FOR THE LOWER EXTREMITY
Stanley Schiowitz
Albert R. DeRubertis

The Hip
Related exercises are described in Chapter 11 (Treatment of the Lumbar Spine—Exercise Therapy). The clinician should review these exercises when prescribing exercise therapy for the hip.

MUSCLE STRETCH
A. Groin muscle stretch (Fig. 21-52)
  1. Patient position: standing, facing a firm support such as a table.
  2. **Instructions:**
    a. Place the sole of the foot of the leg to be treated on the edge of the table (the left foot is used as an example). The other foot remains on the floor, fully extended, with the toes pointing toward the table.
    b. Flex your left hip and knee as you lean your body toward the table. Continue leaning until you have achieved maximum painless stretch of the left groin muscles.
    c. Hold this position for 5 to 15 seconds.
    d. Straighten out the left leg. Relax, rest, and repeat.
    e. The stretch should affect the muscles of the medial, anterior, and posterior groin.

To stretch the right groin, repeat the exercise with your right foot on the table.
B. Groin muscle stretch (Fig. 21-53)
  1. Patient position: standing, facing a firm support such as a table.
  2. **Instructions:**
    a. Place the sole of the foot of the nondysfunctional leg on the edge of the table (the left leg is used as an example). The right leg is fully extended with the foot on floor and parallel to the table.
    b. Flex your left hip and knee as you lean your body toward the table. Continue leaning until you have achieved maximum painless stretch of the right medial groin muscles.
    c. Hold this position for 5 to 15 seconds.
    d. Straighten out the left leg. Relax, rest, and repeat.
    e. To stretch the left groin, repeat the exercise with your right foot on the table.
C. Bilateral groin muscle stretch (Fig. 21-54)
  1. Patient position: seated on the floor, with the hips and knees flexed and the soles of the feet resting against each other. The hands hold the toes or ankles.

Figure 21-52. Groin muscle stretch.

Figure 21-53. Groin muscle stretch.

Figure 21-54. Bilateral groin muscle stretch.

2. **Instructions:**
   a. Pull your body forward, bending from the hips, while keeping your back flat to avoid strain. Create a groin stretch.
   b. Place your elbows forward and resting on your legs. Lean on your elbows to push your thighs toward the floor.
   c. Hold a position of maximum painless stretch for 5 to 15 seconds.
   d. Relax, rest, and repeat.

MUSCLE STRENGTHENING

A. Hip flexors (Fig. 21-55)
   1. Patient position: standing, holding onto a firm support behind the patient; or seated with the legs dangling off a high table. A three- to five-pound weight is attached to the ankle of the leg to be exercised.
   2. **Instructions:**
      a. Slowly flex your knee and hip to 90 degrees.
      b. Hold this position for 5 to 15 seconds.
      c. Lower foot slowly to the floor.
      d. Relax, rest, and repeat.
B. Hip extensors (Fig. 21-56)
   1. Patient position: standing, holding onto a firm support with the hand opposite the leg to be exercised; or prone. A three- to five-pound weight is attached to the ankle.
   2. **Instructions:**
      a. Move your fully extended leg backward, keeping your low back flat.
      b. Hold this position for 5 to 15 seconds.
      c. Slowly return to the starting position.
      d. Relax, rest, and repeat.
C. Hip abductors (Fig. 21-57)
   1. Patient position: standing, holding onto a firm support with hand opposite the leg to be exercised; or lying on the side. A three- to five-pound weight is attached to the ankle.
   2. **Instructions:**
      a. Move the leg to be exercised directly sideways, fully extended, away from the midline of the body.
      b. Hold this position for 5 to 15 seconds.
      c. Slowly return to the starting position.
      d. Relax, rest, and repeat.

Figure 21-55. Hip flexor strengthening.

Figure 21-56. Hip extensor strengthening.

Figure 21-57. Hip abductor strengthening.

Figure 21-58. Hip adductor strengthening.

D. Hip adductors (Fig. 21-58)
  1. Patient position: standing, holding onto a firm support with the hand on the same side as the leg to be exercised. A three- to five-pound weight is attached to the ankle.
  2. **Instructions:**
     a. Extend the leg to be exercised and move it in front of the other leg and across the midline of the body.
     b. Hold this position for 5 to 15 seconds.
     c. Slowly return to the starting position.
     d. Relax, rest, and repeat.
E. Hip adductors (Fig. 21-59)
  1. Patient position: lying on the side to be exercised. The upper leg rests on a box or a chair, eight to ten inches above floor. A three- to five-pound weight is attached to the ankle.
  2. **Instructions:**
     a. Raise the leg to be exercised off the floor, toward the other leg. Keep the leg fully extended.
     b. Hold for 5 to 15 seconds.
     c. Slowly return to the starting position.
     d. Relax, rest, and repeat.

Figure 21-59. Hip adductor strengthening.

The Knee
MUSCLE STRETCH
A. Quadriceps (Fig. 21-60)
  1. Patient position: seated on a table with the hips and knees bent. The knee with contracted quadriceps will not fully flex to 90 degrees.
  2. **Instructions:**
     a. Place increasingly heavier weights on the ankle, forcing the knee into flexion and quadriceps stretch. Or,
     b. Have someone push down on your leg slowly, creating quadriceps stretch.
     c. Hold for 5 to 15 seconds. Return to the starting position.
     d. Relax, rest and repeat.

MUSCLE STRENGTHENING
A. Knee flexors (Fig. 21-61)
  1. Patient position: standing, holding onto a

Figure 21-60. Quadriceps stretch.

Figure 21-61. Knee flexor
strengthening.

support in front of the body. A three- to
five-pound weight is attached to the ankle.
  2. **Instructions:**
    a. Flex your knee as far as it will go. Keep
       your back straight.
    b. Lower your leg, slowly straightening out
       your knee. Count slowly to ten as you
       lower the foot to the floor.
    c. Relax, rest and repeat.
B. Knee flexors—prone position (Fig. 21-62)
  1. Patient position: prone, with a three- to
     five-pound weight attached to the ankle.
  2. **Instructions:**
    a. Bend your knee to 90 degrees.
    b. Very slowly lower that leg down into full
       extension.
    c. Relax, rest and repeat.

C. Terminal position of full knee extension (Fig.
   21-63)
  1. Patient position: seated on the floor or a
     table. A rolled towel or pillow is placed
     under knee to be exercised (about six
     inches high). A three- to five-pound weight
     is attached to the ankle.
  2. **Instructions:**
    a. Push your knee down against pillow,
       toward the floor, so that the weighted
       ankle comes off the table as the knee
       straightens out. Concentrate on pushing
       the knee down; do not try to extend the
       knee.
    b. Hold this position for 5 to 15 seconds.
    c. Slowly lower the weight to the table.
    d. Relax, rest, and repeat.

Figure 21-62. Knee flexor strengthening.

Figure 21-63. Terminal position of full knee
extension.

Figure 21-64. Isometric quadriceps contraction.

D. Isometric quadriceps contraction (Fig. 21-64)
  1. Patient position: seated, with one hand on the quadriceps muscle on the side to be treated.
  2. **Instructions:**
     a. Without moving your leg, try to contract the muscle you are touching so that the knee cap moves upward toward your hand.
     b. If the exercise is performed correctly, you will see the kneecap move and feel the muscle tighten.

The Foot and Ankle
STRETCH
A. Passive foot and ankle stretch (Fig. 21-65)
  1. Patient position: sitting, holding the foot to be stretched with one hand above the ankle and the other hand on the forefoot.
  2. **Instructions:**
     a. Push your forefoot down. Hold for 3 seconds. Relax.
     b. Push your forefoot up. Hold for 3 seconds. Relax.
     c. Push your forefoot in. Hold for 3 seconds. Relax.
     d. Push your forefoot out. Hold for 3 seconds. Relax.
     e. Rotate your forefoot in a clockwise and then counterclockwise direction, four times each way. Relax.
     f. Rest and repeat the entire exercise.

STRETCH–STRENGTHENING
A. Heel raising (Fig. 21-66)
  1. Patient position: standing with both feet flat on floor, six to eight inches apart.
  2. **Instructions:**
     a. Rise up on your toes. Hold onto something for balance, if necessary.
     b. Maintain this position for 5 to 15 seconds.
     c. Return to the starting position.
     d. Relax, rest, and repeat.

Figure 21-65. Passive foot and ankle stretch.

Figure 21-66. Heel raising to strengthen the gastrocnemius and stretch dorsiflexors.

Figure 21-67. Toe raising to strengthen dorsiflexors and stretch the gastrocnemius.

Figure 21-68. Toe stretch to stretch the arch and strengthen the peroneus longus.

B. Toe walking
   1. Toe walking is performed in the same position as the heel raising exercise. Walk forward on the toes for ten steps.
C. Toe raising (Fig. 21-67)
   1. Patient position: standing, with both feet flat on floor and six to eight inches apart.
   2. **Instructions:**
      a. Lean back on your heels.
      b. Maintain this position for 5 to 15 seconds.
      c. Return to the starting position.
      d. Relax, rest, and repeat.
D. Heel walking
   1. With the weight on the heels and the toes off the ground, walk backward on your heels for ten steps.
E. Picking up marbles (Fig. 21-68)
   1. Patient position: standing near support. Marbles are placed on the floor within reach of the foot to be exercised.
   2. **Instructions:**
      a. Pick up one marble with your toes.
      b. Lift this foot off the floor, cross it in front of the other leg, and release the marble into a container placed six to eight inches off the floor to the side of your stationary leg.
      c. In this manner pick up all the marbles on the floor, one at a time.

Figure 21-69. Toe stretch.

Figure 21-70. Toe curl.

F. Toe stretch (Fig. 21-69)
　1. Patient position: seated, with both feet resting flat on a book resting firmly on the floor.
　2. **Instructions:**
　　a. Lift up your toes only. Hold for 3 seconds. Relax.
　　b. Put your toes over the edge of the platform and push them down. Hold for 3 seconds. Relax.
　　c. Spread the toes far apart. Hold for 3 seconds. Bring them firmly together.
　　d. Curl your toes down as you bring your foot facing inward. Place your weight on the outer surface of your feet (Fig. 21-70). Hold for 3 seconds. Relax.
　　e. Place one foot forward and resting on its heel, with the foot and toes pointing up. Press down on that heel as you turn your foot in clockwise and counterclockwise circles. Your big toe should make complete circles. Repeat three times.
　　f. Relax, rest, and repeat the entire exercise.

22

The Temporo-mandibular Joint

ANATOMY AND BIOMECHANICS
Donald E. Phykitt

The temporomandibular joint (TMJ) is a synovial joint formed by the articulation of the condyle of the mandible with the mandibular (glenoid) fossa and the articular tubercle of the temporal bone. The joint is divided into superior and inferior compartments by a fibrocartilaginous disk. The major motions of the TMJ are depression of the mandible (opening the mouth) and elevation of the mandible (closing the mouth). These motions are achieved by rotation of the condyle in the mandibular fossa, accompanied by anterior or posterior glide on the articular tubercle, respectively. Furthermore, the joint allows protraction, retraction, and side-to-side glide of the mandible.

Anatomy
The mandibular fossa is an oval depression in the temporal bone just anterior to the external auditory meatus. It is bounded anteriorly by the articular tubercle, laterally by the zygomatic process, and posteriorly by the tympanic plate. The close proximity of the mandibular fossa to the external auditory meatus allows fingers placed in the meatus of each ear to palpate condylar motion as it rotates and glides in the fossa. Occasionally, a small ridge of bone (the postglenoid tubercle)

forms a prominence at the posterior border of the fossa.

The shape of the mandibular fossa does not exactly conform to the mandibular condyle. The articular disk molds the two surfaces together.

The mandibular condyle varies considerably in size and shape. The anteroposterior dimension of the condyle is approximately half the transverse dimension. The long axis of the condyle faces slightly posteriorly to the frontal plane and slightly medially.

The articular surfaces of the condyle are at its anterior and superior surfaces. These surfaces are convex. The posterior surface is broad and flat.

The articular disk is fibrous and is molded to the bony surfaces. It is variable in thickness, being thinnest centrally. Its margins merge with the joint capsule. The disk is more firmly attached to the mandible than to the temporal bone. Therefore, when the head of the mandible glides anteriorly on the articular tubercle (as when opening the mouth) the articular disk slides anteriorly against the tubercle.

The fibrous capsule of the TMJ is loose. It is attached to the margins of the articular area on the temporal bone and to the neck of the mandible. It is thickened laterally to form the temporomandibular ligament. This is a triangular ligament whose base attaches to the zygomatic process and the articular tubercle. Its apex is fixed to the lateral aspect of the neck of the mandible. The accessory ligaments of the TMJ are the stylomandibular, sphenomandibular, and pterygomandibular ligaments; none has any significant effect on joint movement.

The innervation of the joint is mainly supplied by the auriculotemporal branch of the mandibular division of the trigeminal nerve. Additional fibers are supplied by the masseteric branch of the mandibular nerve. The vascular supply is derived from the superficial artery and the deep auricular branch of the maxillary artery.

Movements of the TMJ result chiefly from the actions of the muscles of mastication—the temporalis, masseter, medial pterygoid, and lateral pterygoid muscles. The various movements of the TMJ result from the cooperative activity of several muscles, either bilaterally or unilaterally.

1. **Temporalis:** Extensive fan-shaped muscle covering the temporal region.
   Origin: Temporal fossa and temporal fascia.
   Insertion: Coronoid process and anterior border of the ramus of the mandible.
   Actions: Elevates the mandible (closes the mouth) and retracts the mandible after closure.
2. **Masseter:** A quadrangular muscle that covers the coronoid process and ramus of the mandible.
   It is easily palpated at the cheek when the teeth are clenched.
   Origin: Inferior margin and deep surface of the zygomatic arch.
   Insertion: Lateral surface of the ramus and corocoid process of the mandible.
   Actions: Elevates the mandible, clenches the teeth, and aids in protraction of the mandible.
3. **Lateral pterygoid:** A short, thick muscle with two heads of origin.
   Origin: Superior head—infratemporal surface of the greater wing of the sphenoid; inferior head—lateral surface of the lateral pterygoid plate.
   Insertion: Neck of mandible and the articular disk.
   Actions: When contracted bilaterally, the lateral pterygoid muscles protract and depress

the mandible. When contracted unilaterally they produce contralateral lateral glide of the mandible.
4. **Medial pterygoid:** A thick quadralateral muscle located deep to the ramus of the mandible; it embraces the inferior head of the lateral pterygoid muscle.
   Origin: Deep head—medial surface of lateral pterygoid plate; superficial head—tuberosity of the maxilla.
   Insertion: Medial surface of mandible, near its angle.
   Actions: Contracting bilaterally, it assists in elevating and protracting the mandible; contracting unilaterally, it produces contralateral lateral glide of the mandible.

Biomechanics

Mandibular movements may be classified as bilaterally symmetric or bilaterally asymmetric. Because the mandible is a single bone with two joints, movement through one joint cannot occur without a similar coordinating or dissimilar reactive movement in the other joint. Depression, elevation, protraction, and retraction of the mandible are bilaterally symmetric motions since they require similar motions in both joints. Lateral excursions (side-to-side movements) are bilaterally asymmetric, as there are dissimilar movements of the joints.

Depression. Hingelike rotation of the mandibular condyle is accompanied by simultaneous anterior glide of the condyles and articular disks on the articular tubercles. This is mainly produced by the lateral pterygoid muscles. Some assistance is gained from the suprahyoid and infrahyoid muscles. The axis of rotation is through the head of the mandible; the axis of glide is through the mandibular foramen.

Elevation. Elevation is the opposite of depression. The motion is achieved mainly through the actions of the temporalis and medial pterygoid muscles, with assistance from the anterior fibers of the masseter.

Protraction (protrusion). This motion involves anterior glide of both condyles and articular disks along the articular tubercles. It is achieved through bilateral contraction of the medial and lateral pterygoid muscles.

Retraction. This movement is opposite to that of protraction. It is produced by bilateral contraction of the horizontal fibers of the masseter muscles.

Lateral excursion. This movement involves lateral glide of the ipsilateral mandibular condyle, accompanied by slight medial rotation of the contralateral condyle about the medial, shifting axis. It is achieved by unilateral contraction of the contralateral medial and lateral pterygoid muscles.

EVALUATION AND TREATMENT OF TMJ DYSFUNCTION
Eileen L. DiGiovanna

Evaluation

A good history is the first step in evaluating a patient with temporomandibular joint (TMJ) dysfunction. The patient frequently reports pain in the jaw or temporal area of the head. Some report cracking or popping noises when they chew. Occasional patients experience pain in areas distant from the joint, such as headaches behind the eyes, neck pain, or low back pain. A few may report tinnitis or syncope.

Most symptoms outside the joint itself relate to involvement of the temporal bone with its intimate connections with the trigeminal nerve and with fascia and dura connected to other parts of the body. (The dura makes a significant connection between the bones of the cranium and the sacrum.)

HISTORY

The history should include questions regarding trauma to the face, in particular, the jaw. It is important to know if there has been recent dental work; poorly fitting appliances or prostheses are common causes of TMJ problems. Holding the mouth open for long periods of time, as during dental treatment, may cause problems. Frequent gum chewing, teeth grinding, and jaw clenching may contribute to TMJ dysfunction. Bruxism is one of the most frequent causes of TMJ dysfunction.

PHYSICAL EXAMINATION

Physical examination of the TMJ begins with observation. The examiner first notes any facial asymmetries or malocclusion of the teeth. Then, with the patient supine, the examiner sits at the head of the table and asks the patient to open and close the jaw slowly. The examiner looks for any deviation from the midline. The jaw may veer to one side or may travel on an S-shaped track back to the midline.

The examiner places one finger in the meatus of each ear and palpates the joint as the patient opens and closes the mouth, observing the quality of motion, any asymmetry, and the presence of clicking or grinding of the joint (palpable or audible) (Fig. 22-1). The muscles of mastication are evaluated for any tender areas or trigger points. Unusual tension of the pterygoids should be noted.

The cervical spine is evaluated next. It is fairly common to find dysfunctions of the occipitoatlantal joint, C2, C3. Finally, cranial motion, particularly of the temporal bones, is evaluated and any dysfunctions noted.

Treatment

The treatment of TMJ dysfunction has three components: (1) identifying and eliminating any treatable cause, (2) osteopathic manipulative treatment, and (3) prescribing an exercise regimen for the patient to use at home.

Figure 22-1. Evaluating TMJ function by observing tracking while palpating the joint through the auditory meatus.

ELIMINATING THE CAUSE

Since dental problems are a frequent cause of TMJ problems, the patient should be referred to a qualified dentist preferably one familiar with TMJ problems, for further evaluation of malocclusion, improperly fitted appliances or prostheses, or tooth grinding. Bruxism and jaw clenching may require psychologic counseling and help with stress management. Gum chewing may need to be eliminated. Balanced chewing habits may need to be taught to the patient.

OSTEOPATHIC MANIPULATIVE TREATMENT (OMT)

Persons with TMJ dysfunction may benefit greatly from one or more of the manipulative techniques described below.

Muscle Energy Techniques

Muscle energy techniques are designed to treat and relax the various muscles of mastication—those that open and close the jaw, and those that move it from side to side.

1. Patient position: supine.
2. Physician position: seated at the head of the table.
3. **Technique:**
   a. To treat the muscles that close the jaw, ask the patient to open her mouth. Place two fingers on the patient's chin. Ask her to attempt to close her mouth against your resistance (Fig. 22-2). Repeat three times.
   b. To treat the muscles that open the jaw, ask the patient to lightly close her jaw. Place two fingers under her chin and ask her to attempt to open her jaw against your resistance (Fig. 22-3). Repeat three times.
   c. To treat the muscles that move the jaw laterally, ask the patient to move her jaw away from the affected side. Place two fingers on the side of her jaw, and ask her to move her jaw back against your fingers as you provide a resistance (Fig. 22-4). Repeat three times, attempting to move the jaw further through its restriction.

Counterstrain Treatment

People with TMJ dysfunction frequently have a tender point in the masseter muscle of the affected side. This may be treated in the following manner:

Figure 22-2. Muscle energy treatment for muscles that close the jaw.

Figure 22-3. Muscle energy treatment for muscles that open the jaw.

1. Patient position: supine.
2. Physician position: seated at the head of the table.
3. **Technique:**
   a. One finger monitors the tender point in the muscle.
   b. The patient is asked to relax her jaw. With the other hand the physician moves the jaw toward the affected side until the point is no longer tender (Fig. 22-5).
   c. This position is held 90 seconds. The jaw is then returned to a neutral position.

Stretching Hypertonic Pterygoid Muscles

In some cases of TMJ dysfunction the pterygoid muscles are hypertonic. These muscles can be passively stretched by applying pressure with a gloved finger inside the mouth. The finger is gently slid along the muscle, massaging and stretching it.

Figure 22-4. Muscle energy treatment for muscles that move the jaw laterally.

Figure 22-5. Counterstrain treatment for tender point in the right masseter muscle.

Cervical Spine

Any somatic dysfunctions of the cervical spine should be treated to alleviate their contribution to the problem.

Craniosacral Concepts

Because the temporal bone is intimately involved in most TMJ dysfunctions, it must be evaluated and treated for any motion restriction found (see Chap. 25, Fundamentals of Craniosacral Osteopathy). Evaluation and treatment of the sacrum may provide important help as well.

EXERCISE PRESCRIPTION

An exercise program for home use should be prescribed for most patients with TMJ problems. The exercises are done in the same manner as the muscle energy treatments, with the patient providing her own resistance by placing her hand on the jaw as described. These exercises should be done two or three times daily, gradually building up to ten repetitions of each exercise during each session.

References

Berkowitz BKB, Moxham BJ. 1988. A Textbook of Head and Neck Anatomy. Chicago: Year Book Medical Publishers.

Jones LH. 1981. Strain and Counterstrain. Colorado Springs, Colorado: American Academy of Osteopathy.

Moore KL. 1985. Clinically Oriented Anatomy, 2nd ed. Baltimore: Williams & Wilkins.

23

Sinus Drainage Techniques

EILEEN L. DIGIOVANNA

Functional Anatomy

The nasal sinuses are a significant site of infection and a possible origin of headache. They include four pairs of aerated cells in the bones of the skull, named after the bones in which they are located: frontal, sphenoid, ethmoid, and maxillary.

Normally, secretions of the nasal sinuses drain into the nasal passages. The frontal sinuses drain primarily by gravity; the ethmoid, sphenoid, and maxillary sinuses rely heavily on the ciliated cells that line them to move mucus toward the nasal passages. The lining of the sinuses is similar to that of the upper respiratory tract and is affected by the same infectious processes and allergic responses.

Edema or tenacious mucus as well as slowing of ciliary movement may affect the discharge of secretions out of the sinuses. Secretory fluids build up, the passage of air is blocked, and unequal pressures result, leading to pain. This pain may be located over the sinuses or in the forehead, the orbits, or the cheeks, may be referred via reflexes to the occiput and neck, the teeth, the temples, or the ears.

Sympathetic innervation to the sinuses arises in the upper thoracic area and passes through the cervical ganglia. The upper thoracic and cervical areas should be evaluated for the presence of somatic dysfunction, and any dysfunction found should be treated. Probably the most consistent mechanical finding associated with sinusitis is occipitoatlantal dysfunction, which requires treatment for relief.

The osteopathic treatment of sinusitis has several goals: to relieve obstruction and pain; to improve venous and lymphatic flow from the area; effecting reflex changes; and to improve mucociliary clearance. Several manual techniques have been designed to aid in achieving these goals. Although only one set of sinuses may produce pain, the entire series of techniques should be performed, to assist drainage of all the sinus areas.

Treatment Techniques

The positions of patient and operator, described below, are identical for all the techniques:

1. Patient position: supine on the table, with her eyes closed, and relaxed.
2. Physician position: seated comfortably at the head of the table.

DIRECT PRESSURE AND "MILKING"
Pressure may be applied directly with the thumbs over the frontal sinuses. The pressure is gradually increased and released in a gentle, rhythmic motion, never hard enough to cause severe pain. The cycle is repeated several times (Fig. 23-1).

The thumbs are then placed side by side in the center of the forehead and, with gentle pressure downward, are moved laterally toward the temples. At the edge of the temporal fossae the thumbs are directed caudad to the zygoma. This cycle is repeated six or eight times.

Figure 23-1. Direct pressure applied over the frontal sinuses.

Figure 23-2. Gentle pressure applied over the supraorbital notch.

Figure 23-3. Pressure applied over the maxillary sinuses.

Figure 23-4. Direct pressure applied over the temporal areas.

Supraorbital notch. Gentle pressure may be applied over the supraorbital notch; then the thumbs swept along the eyebrow ridge bilaterally (Fig. 23-2).

Maxillary sinuses. The same technique can be applied to the maxillary sinuses. Pressure is applied over the sinuses with the thumbs. The nasal passages are "milked" by beginning with the thumb on each side of the nose and pressing down while sweeping the thumbs laterally along the maxilla (Fig. 23-3).

Temporal areas. Direct pressure may be applied over the temporal areas by gently placing the thenar eminences in the temporal fossae bilater-

ally and compressing these areas between the hands. Pressure is applied and released in gentle, rhythmic motions (Fig. 23-4).

INDIRECT PRESSURE

The fingers of the operator's hands are interlaced and laid palm up on the table under the patient's head. The thenar eminence of each hand is placed against the patient's head laterally on the occiput. Gentle, rhythmic pressure is applied to the head by pressing the hands together and releasing them. A counterstrain technique is applied in the same manner. The pressure is maintained for 90 seconds, then released very slowly. A similar

Figure 23-5. Sinus drainage technique for nasal congestion.

Figure 23-6. Counterstrain technique for the maxillary sinuses.

Figure 23-7. Counterstrain technique for supraorbital tender points.

technique involves cupping the occiput in one hand and placing the heel of the other hand in the center of the patient's forehead, compressing the head between the two hands in a gentle, rhythmic motion.

NASAL DECONGESTION

The nasal passages are milked by the examiner placing the thumb of the right hand on the left side of the patient's nose and the left thumb on the right side of the nose, the thumbs crossing above the bridge of the nose. Pressure is applied alternately by each thumb, moving down the length of the nose (Fig. 23-5). This is done several times, then the thumbs are reversed and a sweeping motion is made bilaterally down the sides of the nose and out over the maxillae.

COUNTERSTRAIN TECHNIQUES

Maxillary sinuses. The tender points are over the infraorbital nerves. An effective counterstrain technique for the maxillary sinuses is to interlace the fingers above the bridge of the nose with the thenar eminences resting on the lateral curve of the zygoma. Pressure through the thenar eminences, in a compressing and lifting motion, is maintained for 90 seconds, then released (Fig. 23-6).

Supraorbital tender points. The supraorbital tender points are located near the site of the supraorbital nerves. One arm rests on the patient's forehead, lightly pulling it superiorly, and, with fingers of the other hand pinching the bridge of the nose, the examiner distracts the nose caudad (Fig. 23-7).

24

Myofascial Release Concepts

PAULA D. SCARIATI

This chapter provides some basic rules and definitions, then outlines fascial anatomy and physiology and the properties of fascia that are of concern to the osteopathic physician. Finally, the principles of fascial release are explained and a few examples given. An understanding of myofascial release allows the clinician to create techniques appropriate to the clinical situation.

Rules

1. **Structure governs function (form governs function).** Structure that is not compromised at any level (i.e., anatomically, physiologically, biochemically, etc.) allows for proper function.
2. **Proper motion implies proper form.** This rule provides the basis for diagnosing somatic dysfunctions. Motion testing is used to determine the freedoms and restrictions of motion. A restriction of motion implies a problem with form, which is corrected with manipulative techniques.

Anatomy

Fascia is a sheet or band of fibrous tissue that lies deep to the skin and invests the muscles and the various organs of the body. It helps to form the strongest ligaments and tendons and is part of the structure of vessel and nerve sheaths.

Not only a sheath or aponeurosis, fascia is an extensive network that connects all the compartments of the body. Abnormal fascial tensions induced by trauma or stress may therefore cause problems distant from the actual site of dysfunction.

Anatomically, fascia can be divided into three types:

1. Superficial fascia
2. Deep fascia
3. Subserous fascia

The first two types occur everywhere in the body as complete ensheathments. Subserous fascia rests innermost on the deep fascia wherever there is a body cavity.

SUPERFICIAL FASCIA

Superficial fascia lies below and blends with the dermis of the skin. It is a loose, fatty, fibroelastic type of connective tissue with a distinct lower surface. Between the lower surface and the outer investing layer of deep fascia is a potential space where extravasating fluid can accumulate.

The superficial fascia serves an aesthetic purpose in that it helps to mold the skin. It also helps to insulate the body and invests the superficial muscles. Finally, the superficial fascia is considered to be the location of the deep pressure receptors (pacinian corpuscles).

DEEP FASCIA

Deep fascia is a tough, compacted, irregularly woven, fibroelastic tissue. It is reasonably pliant and has a feltlike consistency. It is modified in various areas of the body to form the perimysium, perineurium, peritendinium, and so forth. The deep fascia has discrete upper and lower surfaces, often widely separated, with septal layers lying intermediate between the two surfaces.

The deep fascia assists in motion. A classic example is the tensor fascia lata, which allows abduction and medial rotation of the thigh.

SUBSEROUS FASCIA

Subserous fascia is a loose fibroelastic type of connective tissue. It includes the pleura, pericardium, peritoneum, and tunica vaginalis. In general, it is the simple lining of the major body cavities, and thus most major organs are found within this fascial layer. Embryologically, the subserous fascia forms the substrate in which the visceral organs, blood, and blood vessels develop. This substrate also forms the attachments between organs.

Physiologic Characteristics

WOLFF'S LAW

According to J. Wolff, every change in the form and function of a bone, or any change in a bone's function alone, is followed by certain definite changes in its internal architecture, and secondarily by alterations in its external conformation. When stresses are applied to bone, the trabeculae within the bone adapt to accommodate the vector of stress. Thus, the bone develops the structure most suited to resist the forces acting on it. The same principle applies to fascia: it realigns itself to accommodate to changing stress patterns.

PIEZOELECTRIC FORCES

Piezoelectric forces are electrical charges produced in structures with changing lines of stress. Changing currents draw fibroblasts. The relationship of stress and the direction of fiber formation may involve fibroblast movement in patterns formed by piezoelectric currents. Thus, piezoelectric forces conceivably align the fibroblasts and determine the direction of reorganization of collagen in matrix.

GROUND SUBSTANCE

Ground substance is a colloidal suspension with high water content, mucopolysaccharides, and long chain carbohydrates. It serves to diffuse nutrients and acts as a mechanical barrier to bacteria. Colloids follow fluid mechanics generally in that they are not rigid, conform to the shape of their container, and respond to pressure even though they are not very compressible. They produce resistance to motion, internal molecular friction, called drag. The amount of resistive drag produced increases as the velocity of motion applied to the colloid increases.

These factors must be considered in the use of fascial release techniques. A light touch is imperative, not only to feel small motions but to avoid the colloidal response of viscous drag. The faster the clinician pushes, the more the ground substance resists. The goal of fascial release is to follow the wave in a fluid system within the connective tissue.

FASCIAL MOTION

Fascia responds to stress or traction in two phases. The first phase, or *immediate phase*, is abrupt and is presumed to represent the taking up of slack. The second phase, called *creep*, is a delayed but continual stretch over time in response to a constant load.

Inherent forces also come into play. These forces effect a change in the tissue (form), which, according to basic concepts, will change function. There is some question as to what these inherent forces are. Several hypotheses exist:

1. **Muscle spindle concept.** As in counterstrain therapy, shortening of the muscle results in a resetting of the muscle spindles to allow muscle relaxation.
2. **Central nervous system (CNS) adaptation.** When tissue is moved indirectly, the involuntary motion may cause a CNS response from feedback mechanisms.
3. **Cerebrospinal fluid (CSF) concept.** Upledger described a ball-and-valve mechanism in the arachnoid granulations that may turn the CSF flow on and off. This may explain the pulsations of the cranial mechanism (normally eight to ten pulsations per minute) and may be a source of force in fascial release. A Ciba monograph on trauma acknowledges CSF pulsations as a force causing dural herniations in cranial fractures, by forcing more fluid into the dura outside of the skull.
4. **Cytoskeletal changes.** Cytoskeletal changes may take place at the cellular level, with actin,

myosin, microtubules, and fibrils responding to new stresses.

STRESSORS

The stressors used by the clinician to challenge the fascia include the following:

1. Movement into the freedom of motion or the barriers to motion (indirect and direct stressors, respectively).
2. Traction or compression applied directly or via a lever arm (i.e., using the arm to release fascia in the cervical and thoracic regions).
3. Respiratory assist.

Fascial Properties and Functions

Contractility and elasticity are two important properties of fascia. Elasticity decreases during life, and this loss is an important contributor to the aging process. Contractility is not diminished with age and supercedes all other properties of fascia. With age or trauma, fascia undergoes changes such as thickening, shortening, calcification, and erosion, often losing its elastic properties and becoming painful. Many so-called trigger points correspond to points where the nerve pierces fascial investments.

These initial changes set off chain reactions that may compromise the vasculature, nervous system, and muscle, as well as change the movement of body fluids through the fascia.

Several other properties and functions of fascia are listed below.

1. It is provided with sensory and nerve endings.
2. It is extensively attached to muscles.
3. It helps regulate circulation, especially of the venous and lymphatic systems.
4. It assists in support and is a stabilizer, helping to maintain balance; the balance is suggestive of motion.
5. It assists in the production of motion, the control of motion, and the confluency of motion of related parts.
6. In many conditions resulting in chronic deformities, such as degenerative diseases or the aging process, fascial change precedes the bony and cartilaginous changes.
7. Fascial contraction and thickening predispose to chronic passive congestion. Chronic passive congestion precedes the abnormal production of fibrous tissue and is followed by an increase in the hydrogen ion concentration of articular and periarticular structures.
8. Many fascial specializations have special postural functions. In these, definite stress bands can be demonstrated.
9. Sudden stress on fascial membranes is often accompanied by a burning pain.
10. Inflammation and fluid often track along fascial planes.
11. The dura mater is a specialized connective tissue surrounding the CNS. In the skull, it is attached to bone. Changes in the tension and structure of the dura mater are important in the production of headaches and many disturbances of the brain.

Myofascial Release Techniques

INDIRECT VERSUS DIRECT TECHNIQUES

Conceptually, indirect fascial technique entails putting an area of restriction into its freedoms in an attempt to release it. This type of technique is analogous to pulling out a jammed drawer completely before pushing it back in. Direct fascial technique entails putting the area of dysfunction into its barriers to motion in an attempt to release it.

PRINCIPLES OF TECHNIQUE

Because fascial release is a concept, the clinician need only understand the principles, then apply them to any region of the body. The principles of fascial release technique are as follows:

1. **Indirect technique:** Carry the dysfunctional area into its freedoms of motion (where it moves most easily) in all planes. **Direct technique:** Move the area of dysfunction into its barriers to motion.
2. Hold the dysfunctional area in position.
3. Invite the patient's respiratory assistance, if feasible.
4. Wait for a sensation or thumping under your fingers that tells you the fascia is ready to move.
5. Follow the mechanism through its unwinding process until it is completed.
6. Reevaluate the ranges of the respective motions, which should now be more symmetric. If not, reengage the area to induce more fascial release.

Examples of Indirect Techniques

CERVICAL SPINE

1. Patient position: supine.
2. Physician position: seated at the head of the table.
3. **Technique:**
   a. The physician places the index finger of either hand on the transverse process of the vertebra that is to be released.
   b. The physician checks the range of motion of the vertebra in all planes—flexion/extension, rotation, and side bending.
   c. After determining which of the above are the freedoms of motion for this vertebra, the physician carries the vertebra into that position and holds it there.
   d. The physician asks the patient to take a deep breath in and out, waiting for a sensation in the tips of his index fingers that tells the physician that this vertebra is ready to unwind.
   e. The physician follows the vertebra with its associated fascia and muscle through the unwinding process until it is completed.
   f. The physician reevaluates the given dysfunction to determine if there is increased range of motion or decreased muscle tension.

   The above technique can be applied grossly to the entire cervical spine to unwind larger fascial planes. In this case the physician's hands would be placed on either side of the patient's cervical spine, supporting it, and the motions tested would be the gross motions of the cervical spine. The remaining steps would be the same.

THORACIC SPINE

The fascial restriction treated in the following technique is on the right side.

1. Patient position: sitting on the edge of the table.
2. Physician position: standing behind the patient, facing his right side.
3. **Technique:**
   a. The physician places his right arm across the patient's chest and holds the patient's left shoulder.
   b. With his left hand the physician monitors the area to be released.

Figure 24-1. Fascial release of the scapula.

   c. With his axilla over the patient's right shoulder, the physician evaluates the range of thoracic flexion/extension, rotation, and side bending for that thoracic segment.
   d. The physician moves the spinal segment into its freedoms of motion.
   e. The spinal segment is held in position.
   f. The patient's respiratory assistance is invited.
   g. The physician follows the region as it unwinds.
   h. Once the process has been completed, the physician reevaluates the dysfunctional segment to assess improvement.

SCAPULAE

1. Patient position: lying on his side. The scapula that is to be treated faces up.
2. Physician position: standing in front of the patient.
3. **Technique:**
   a. The physician's hand grasps the inferior angle of the patient's scapula. The physician's arm supports the patient's arm, which is completely relaxed.
   b. The physician's other hand grasps the medial border and angle of the patient's scapula (Fig. 24-1).
   c. Motions are tested for their freedoms: superior/inferior, medial/lateral, and clockwise/counterclockwise rotation.
   d. The scapula is placed in its freedoms of motion and held in position.
   e. The patient is asked to take a deep breath in and out, to assist fascial motion.

f. The physician waits for and follows the motion of the scapula as it unwinds.

g. The physician reevaluates scapular motion to assess its improvement.

SACRUM

During inhalation, the sacrum ascends and moves posteriorly at its base. During exhalation it moves caudad and anteriorly at the base.

1. Patient position: supine.
2. Physician position: sitting to one side of the patient, facing his head.
3. **Technique:**
   a. The physician introduces his palpating hand onto the sacrum by having the patient lift himself off of his back and sliding his hand between the patient's legs to cup the sacrum in his palm.
   b. The physician's fingertips should lie at the base of the sacrum.
   c. The patient lowers himself to the table again.
   d. The physician assesses the motion of the sacrum during inhalation and exhalation, noting any rotation or side bending deviation.
   e. The physician carries the sacrum into its freedoms of motion and holds it there.
   f. The patient's respiratory assistance is invited.
   g. The physician follows the motion of the sacrum as it unwinds.
   h. The physician reevaluates the motion of the sacrum to assess for improvement.

   Note: Many other positions can be used to release the sacrum.

Conclusion

The techniques described illustrate the principles of fascial release. Many other fascial release techniques are used by different osteopathic physicians; others can be devised to suit the clinical situation.

The point of complete unwinding, the goal of myofascial release, is not always ascertainable or achieved. At complete unwinding, a symmetric, respiratory-like motion should be palpable. During a release treatment, however, the area may fall into a repetitive figure 8 pattern that does not resolve. When this occurs, the physician must reengage the freedoms of motion or the barriers to motion in an attempt to release the fascia completely.

Myofascial release is a subtle technique that requires considerable concentration and experience. Novice clinicians are often frustrated by their inability to palpate and follow the fascial planes on their first few tries. Time and experience will lead to greater success.

References

American Academy of Osteopathy 1974 Yearbook. Colorado Springs, Colorado: American Academy of Osteopathy, 1974.

Becker RF. 1975. Meaning of fascia and fascial continuity. Osteopath Ann 3(7):35–47.

Cathie AG. 1974. Considerations of fascia and its relation to disease of the musculoskeletal system. 1974 Yearbook AAO, AAO.

———. 1974. The fascia of the body in relation to function and manipulative therapy. Yearbook AAO, AAO.

———. 1974. Osteopathic armamentarium: Seventh Annual Academy Lecture. 1974 Yearbook AAO, AAO, 1974.

Feltowitz J. 1986. Introduction to myofascial release. Westbury: New York College of Osteopathic Medicine Curriculum, December.

Greenfield GB. 1986. Radiology of Bone Diseases, 4th ed. Philadelphia: J.B. Lippincott Co.

Hubbard RP. 1983. Mechanical behavior of connective tissue. In Chila A, ed. Myofascial Release: The Integrator of Manipulative Procedures. Newark, Ohio: Tutorial.

Moore KL. 1980. Clinically Oriented Anatomy, 2nd ed. Baltimore: Williams & Wilkins Co.

Netter F. Summit, New Jersey: CIBA Pharmaceutical Co., vol. 24, 1972.

Truek SL. 1984. Orthopedics: Principles and Their Application. Philadelphia: J.B. Lippincott Co.

Warwick R, Williams PL. 1973. Gray's Anatomy, 35th British ed. Philadelphia: W.B. Saunders Co.

Wolff J. Das Gesetz der Transformation der Knochen, Berlin, Hirschwald, 1982.

Upledger, JE. 1983. Craniosacral Therapy, Seattle: Eastland Press.

25

Craniosacral Concepts

HUGH ETTLINGER
BONNIE GINTIS

The craniosacral concept was originally conceived by William Garner Sutherland as a direct extension of the theories of A. T. Still. This section introduces the basic principles of the craniosacral concept. It should be used as a stepping stone to the more complicated aspects of this field.

Principles of the Craniosacral Concept

Respiration and circulation are the processes by which cells exchange gases, nutrients, and wastes with their environment. Thoracoabdominal respiration and cardiovascular circulation are separate but interdependent processes. The craniosacral concept has to do with another aspect of these processes referred to as the *primary respiratory mechanism*. The primary respiratory mechanism is a palpable, cyclic, rhythmic wave of motion throughout the entire body. It is proposed to be a continuous flux of the extracellular fluid. The frequency of this wave is normally 8 to 12 cycles per minute.

The *cranial rhythmic impulse* is the primary respiratory mechanism as it exists in the central nervous system (CNS) and can be palpated via the cranium and the sacrum. There are five components of the cranial rhythmic impulse:

1. Inherent motility of the CNS.
2. Fluctuation of the cerebrospinal fluid (CSF).

3. Mobility of the intracranial and intraspinal membranes.
4. Articular mobility of the cranial bones.
5. Involuntary motion of the sacrum between the ilia.

Each of these is described below.

INHERENT MOTION OF THE CNS

It has been proposed that coordinated contraction of oligodendroglia causes inherent motion of the brain and spinal cord. Contractile elements have been identified in these cells. Whether or not rhythmic contractions occur, the brain and spinal cord would have to change shape slightly to accommodate to the changes in shape (not volume) of the cranium during the cranial rhythmic impulse.

FLUCTUATION OF THE CSF

Although usually considered a result of the primary respiratory mechanism, pressure gradients are produced by production and release of CSF into the cranial cavity by the choroid plexus in the ventricles, and drainage of CSF into the venous system. Its role in the cranial rhythmic impulse is probably limited to that of an enhancer rather than a prime mover. The pathways of CSF through the ventricles and beyond, shown in Figure 25-1, are as follows: lateral ventricles → foramen of Monroe → third ventricle → cerebral

Figure 25-1. Circulation of cerebrospinal fluid. (Adapted from Netter, Ciba collection.)

aqueduct → fourth ventricle → spinal cord-foramen of Magendie and foramen of Luschka → subarachnoid cisterns. There are four subarachnoid cisterns: (1) the cisterna basalis, at the base of the cerebrum; (2) the cisterna pontis, about the pons; (3) the cisterna superior, between the corpus callosum and the cerebellum; and (4) the cisterna magna, between the cerebellum and the medulla. CSF flows from cisterna magna to the other cisterns and finally to the arachnoid granulations (pacchionian bodies) and into the venous sinuses.

MOBILITY OF INTRACRANIAL AND INTRASPINAL MEMBRANES

The dural membrane system is central to the function of the cranial rhythmic impulse. Abnormal tensions in the dura may adversely affect neural function, either by causing direct pressure or by inducing local circulatory changes. The following discussion reviews the anatomy of the dural membranes, the venous system contained within it, and its motion.

The falx cerebri, falx cerebelli, and tentorium cerebelli form the dural membrane system. Magoun describes it as "three sickleshaped agencies, all of which arise from a common origin at the straight sinus, named the 'Sutherland fulcrum' in honor of its discoverer, and have their secondary insertion into the various bones of the cranium" (Fig. 25-2).

The falx cerebri arises from the straight sinus and extends upward along the sagittal ridge of the occiput, the sagittal suture, and the metopic suture. Both the free inferior edges and the attached superior edges insert onto the crista galli of the ethmoid. These attachments are called the anterior superior pole of the reciprocal tension membrane system (Fig. 25-3).

Each tentorium cerebelli makes up another sickle. Originating from the straight sinus, the tent is attached bilaterally to the occiput at the internal protuberance and along the transverse ridges. This is the posterior pole of the reciprocal tension membrane system. The very small attachment to the mastoid angle of the parietals is also considered part of the posterior pole. The tent then continues anteriorly, attached to the petrous ridge of the temporal bone on either side. These are the lateral poles of attachment. The lateral attached border of the tent attaches to the ipsilateral posterior clinoid process, and the medial free border attaches to the ipsilateral anterior clinoid process. These four attachments constitute the anterior inferior pole of attachment.

The diaphragma sella is part of the visceral dura. It completely encases the pituitary gland. Tension changes in this dura may alter the function of the hypothalamus-pituitary axis. The falx

Figure 25-2. Dural membranes, lateral view.

Figure 25-3. Reciprocal tension membrane system.

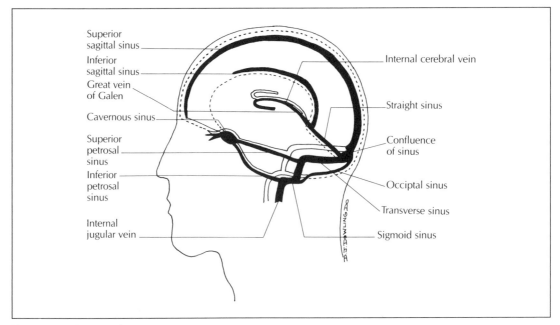

Figure 25-4. Venous sinus system.

cerebelli extends downward, attaches strongly to the foramen magnum, and continues as the dura surrounding the spinal cord, attaching inferiorly to the sacrum. This forms a separate pole of reciprocal tension and an important link between the cranium and the sacrum.

Before ossification, the tough, fibrous envelope of periosteum and dura maintains the shape and stability of the cartilaginous and membranous skull. After ossification, it guides and limits the motions in the cranium.

To ensure proper function, these sickles must operate from a suspended fulcrum that can shift and adjust to maintain balanced tension. This fulcrum exists somewhere along the straight sinus.

Dura invests all foramina leaving the skull. Any cranial nerve or vessel may be affected by changes in dural tension.

The venous sinuses lie between the two layers of dura. The superior and inferior sagittal sinuses lie within the falx cerebri. The transverse, sigmoid, superior, and inferior petrosal sinuses lie within the tentorium cerebelli. The straight sinus is at the junction of the falx and tentorium. The cavernous sinus and basilar plexus lie anterior and inferior to the tent (Fig. 25-4).

The drainage patterns of the venous sinuses are as follows:

Superior sagittal sinus → right transverse sinus → sigmoid sinus → internal jugular vein

Inferior sagittal sinus → great vein of Galen → straight sinus → left transverse sinus → sigmoid sinus → internal jugular vein

Occipital sinus → transverse sinus (ipsilateral) → sigmoid sinus → internal jugular vein

Cavernous sinus → superior and inferior petrosal sinuses → sigmoid sinus

These venous channels are void of the elastic and muscle tissue found in all other veins, eliminating elasticity and muscular contraction as enhancers of drainage.

Cranial nerves III and IV, the ophthalmic division of cranial nerves V and VI, and the internal carotid artery run through the cavernous sinus and may be affected by congestion of the sinus. Dural attachments around foramina investing nerves and vessels are continuous with cervical fascia. Thus, extracranial somatic dysfunction as well as cranial dysfunction can alter dural tension.

Figure 25-5. Types of sutures found in the skull.

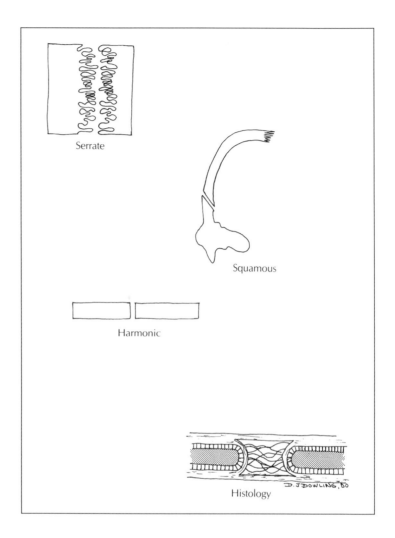

Serrate

Squamous

Harmonic

Histology

D. J. DOWLING, DO

ARTICULAR MOBILITY OF THE CRANIAL BONES

The cranial rhythmic impulse exists in the developing fetus, whose cranium begins as cartilage and membrane. As the skull ossifies, sutures form to accommodate this motion which is already present. The shape of the suture therefore reflects its motion. The basic suture types and their respective motions are shown in Figure 25-5 and listed below:

Serrate: Sawtoothed (e.g., the sagittal suture). Allows a rocking motion.
Squamous: Scalelike, or overlapping, such as the temporoparietal (squamoparietal) suture. Allows a gliding motion, determined by the bevel and groove direction of the two surfaces.
Harmonic: Edge to edge (e.g., the lacrimoethmoidal suture). Allows shearing.
Squamoserrate: A combination, found in the lambdoidal and coronal sutures.

INVOLUNTARY MOBILITY OF THE SACRUM BETWEEN THE ILIA

The sacrum rocks on a transverse axis through the articular pillar of the second sacral segment, posterior to the sacral canal (Fig. 25-6). This motion must be differentiated from respiratory sacral motion, which is caused by spinal motion and contraction of the pelvic diaphragm. The axis of

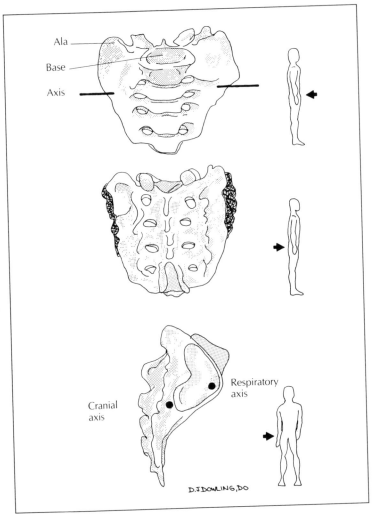

Figure 25-6. Axes of sacral motion.

involuntary sacral motion lies anterior to the sacral canal and passes through the body of S2 at the junction of the short and long arms of the L-shaped sacral articulation.

MECHANISM OF THE CRANIAL RHYTHMIC IMPULSE

The two phases of the cranial rhythmic impulse are flexion and extension (Fig. 25-7). Flexion is discussed in terms of the five basic components of the cranial rhythmic impulse. Flexion is an increase in the transverse diameter accompanied by a simultaneous decrease in the anteroposterior diameter of the cranium. The tentorium cerebelli is flattened and shifted anteriorly, allowing anterior rotation of the sphenoid by way of its attachment to the clinoid processes (Fig. 25-8). The falx cerebri moves centrally. The basiocciput moves anterosuperiorly. All paired bones externally rotate. The foramen magnum moves superiorly, drawing the sacral base posteriorly by its dural attachment on the anterior wall of the sacral canal, or on the posterior surface of the body of the second sacral segment. The brain and spinal cord change shape slightly with this motion.

In extension, these motions are exactly reversed (Fig. 25-9).

The cranial rhythmic impulse is a palpable wave of CSF. The driving force of this wave may be within or outside of the CNS. Coordinated con-

Figure 25-7. Extension and flexion phases of the cranial rhythmic impulse.

Figure 25-8. Cranial rhythmic impulse, flexion phase. (**A**) Relationship of sphenoid to occiput.
(**B**) Effects on reciprocal tension membrane system.
(**C**) Direction of force in flexion.

Figure 25-9. Cranial rhythmic impulse, extension phase. (**A**) Relationship of sphenoid to occiput.
(**B**) Effects on reciprocal tension membrane system.
(**C**) Direction of force in extension.

Extension   Flexion

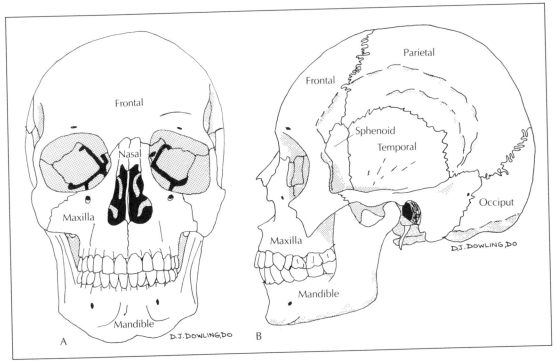

Figure 25-10. The skull (**A**) frontal view. (**B**) Lateral view.

traction of glial cells has been proposed as a mechanism. The heart and diaphragm must also be considered as significant fluid pumps in the body.

Osteology of the Skull

The skull consists of 22 bones, each articulating with several other bones. Some cranial bones articulate with up to 12 other bones. Sutures articulate these bones in such a way that no bone moves independently (Fig. 25-10). The motion of any one bone is greatly influenced by the motions or restrictions of the other cranial bones.

Sutures develop to accommodate motions which are present before the sutures exist. The motion of a bone may be deduced from the shape of its sutures. When an axis of motion crosses a suture line, the suture changes shape and develops a bevel, since motions on opposite sides of an axis are different. These points are called pivots (Fig. 25-11).

This section examines the bones of the cranial base and vault, their sutures, the pivots within them, and their motions. The facial bones are not considered, although they are affected by cranial mechanics.

THE SPHENOID

The motion of the sphenoid and occiput are considered the driving force of cranial articular motion. The sphenoid influences the ethmoid, frontal, and facial bones. The sphenoid primarily articulates with 12 bones (Fig. 25-12).

Parts

Structurally, the sphenoid consists of the body, the greater and lesser wings laterally, and the pterygoid plates inferiorly.

Articulations

1. **Occiput:** The sphenoids articulate with the basilar portion of the occiput (the sphenobasilar joint), a synchrondrosis that is cartilaginous until age 20 to 25 years, then converts to cancellous bone. It exhibits flexibility, not articular mobility.
2. **Temporals:** The sphenoid articulates at three places with the temporal bones. The most important articulation is the articulation of squamosal border of the greater wing of the sphenoid with the inferior border of the temporal squama. This articular surface must be divided into two portions, since there is an important change in bevel, called the

Figure 25-11. Bevel changes in skull sutures.

Figure 25-12. Sphenoid.

Figure 25-13. Sphenosquamous pivot.

sphenosquamous pivot (Fig. 25-13). This point represents an axis of motion between the sphenoid and the temporal bones. It is found directly behind the zygomatic arch. Above the sphenosquamous pivot, the articulation is mostly squamous and the sphenoid is externally beveled (the suture is on the external surface). The temporal bone is internally beveled (the suture is on the internal surface). More simply, the temporal bone overlaps the sphenoid here, and a primarily gliding motion exists. Below the sphenosquamous pivot, the articulation is more serrate (both are actually squamoserrate), less vertical, and more evenly beveled. The motion is more of a rocking motion.

3. **Parietals:** A small articulation exists at the pterion between the posterosuperior surface of the greater wing and the anterior inferior angle of the parietal bone. It is a squamous suture, allowing gliding motion. The sphenoid overlaps the parietal bone.

4. **Frontal bone:**
   a. An L-shaped articulation exists between the anterosuperior surface of the greater wings and the lateral inferior surfaces of the frontal bone. It is a serrate suture.
   b. Two other articulations, also serrate exist between the anterior border of the lesser wings laterally and the orbital surface of the frontal bone, and between the anterior superior surface of the body medially and the orbital surface of the frontal bone. Together, these two articulations allow the sphenoid to influence the lateral surfaces of the frontal bone laterally, anteriorly, and slightly superiorly as the sphenoid flexes.

5. **Ethmoid:**
   a. The anterior body of the sphenoid (ethmoid spine) articulates with the posterior border of the cribriform plate. This articulation is a gomphosis or peg-in-socket joint.
   b. Two other articulations, both harmonic, allow flexibility of motion in these areas of contact (laterally in the horizontal plane and midline in a vertical plane).
      Other articulations of the sphenoid indicate its area of direct influence (not discussed).

6. **Palatines** (2)

7. **Vomer**

8. **Zygomae** (2)

Motion
In flexion, the sphenoid rotates anteriorly about a transverse axis through its body at the level of the zygomatic arch. This motion is discussed in detail later.

THE OCCIPUT
The other driving force of the articular motion of the cranial rhythmic impulse, the occiput is as influential in the posterior of the cranium as the sphenoid is in the anterior part.

Parts
The structures of the occiput are shown in Figures 25-14 and 25-15.

1. **Basilar occiput (basiocciput):** anterior to and forming the anterior border of the foramen magnum.

2. **Condyles:** adjacent to and forming the lateral borders of the foramen magnum.

Figure 25-14. Occiput.

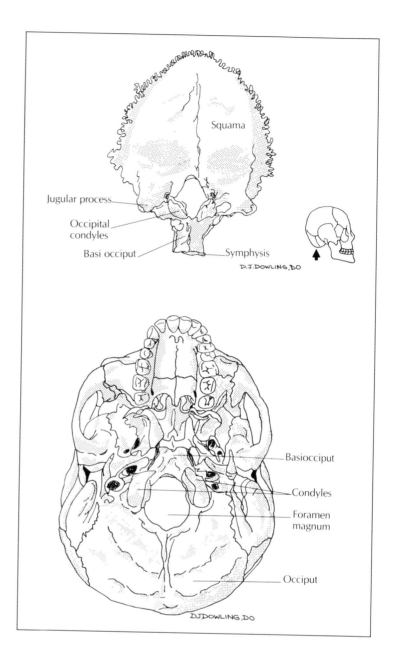

Figure 25-15. Base of skull—occiput.

3. **Squama:** body of the occiput, forming the posterior border of the foramen magnum.

Ossification of all parts is not complete until approximately 5 years.

Articulations
Articulating with six bones, the occiput is the primary mover of the temporals and parietals (Fig. 25-16).

1. **Sphenoid:** The articulation of the occiput with the sphenoid was discussed under the sphenoid bone.
2. **Parietals:** The lambdoidal suture between the superior surface of the occiput and the posteroinferior surface of the parietal bone is the site of articulation. The change in bevel along this articulation can be found by extending a superior temporal line from the parietal bone back to this suture (Fig. 25-17).

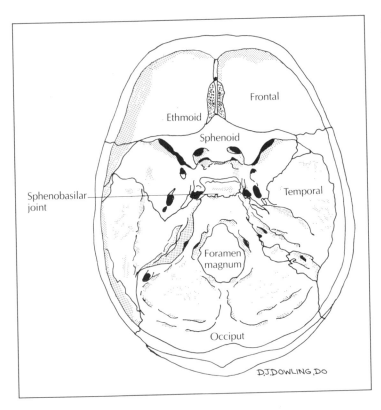

Figure 25-16. Superior view of skull with calvaria removed, showing articulations of the occiput.

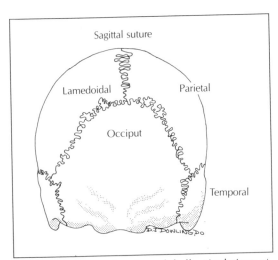

Figure 25-17. Posterior view of skull articulations of occiput.

The change in bevel occurs at the point at which the orientation of both bones changes from primarily the coronal plane (superior) to primarily the horizontal plane (inferior). From the midline to this point, the occiput is internally beveled (overlapping the parietal) and the suture is more serrate, although squamoserrate. Lateral to this point, the occiput is externally beveled (overlapped by the parietal bone) and the suture is less serrate, although still squamoserrate. The motion is primarily rocking, but there is some glide as the occiput slides anteriorly into flexion. The parietal motion is almost entirely lateral.

3. **Temporals:** There are three separate surfaces of contact of the occiput with the temporal bones (Fig. 25-18).

   a. The lateral posterior surface of the occiput articulates with the mastoid portion of temporal bone. The joint is convex on the temporal bone and concave on the occiput, almost describing an L shape. The point at

Figure 25-18. Articulations between the occiput and the temporal bone, superior aspect.

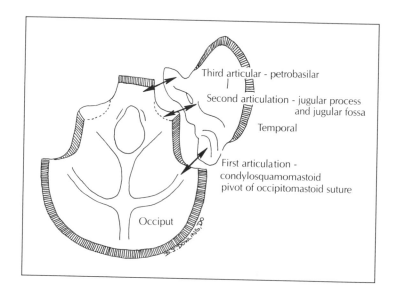

Third articular - petrobasilar

Second articulation - jugular process and jugular fossa

Temporal

First articulation - condylosquamomastoid pivot of occipitomastoid suture

Occiput

which the legs meet is a point of bevel change, called the condylosquamomastoid pivot. Superior and posterior to this point, the occiput is externally beveled (overlapped by the temporal bone); anterior to this point it is internally beveled (or flat). The joint is serrate, accommodating a rocking motion.

b. The jugular process of the occiput articulates with the jugular surface of the temporal bone. There are two parts to this articulation:

    i. The jugular notch of the occiput articulates with the jugular fossa of the temporal bone, forming a smooth, quadrangular articulation in the coronal plane.

    ii. An irregular, flat, rough surface posterior to the notch articulates with a surface on the temporal bone. It is in the horizontal plane. This is an extremely important articulation, for it is the means by which the occiput drives the temporal bones into external rotation. The temporal bone moves anteriorly and superiorly posterior to this point, anteriorly and inferiorly anterior to the point, laterally above this point, and medially below it.

    iii. The upper edge of the lateral border of the basiocciput articulates with the petrous portion of the temporal bone (inferior border). This is a tongue-and-

groove articulation, allowing a hinge and glide motion.

4. **Atlas:** The occipitoatlantal articulation is a synovial joint.

Motions
The primary motion of the occiput on the atlas is flexion-extension, with the occipital condyles convex and the superior articular facets of the atlas concave.

THE TEMPORAL BONE
Parts
The structure of the temporal bone is shown in Figure 25-19.

1. **Squama:** smooth body of the temporal bone.
2. **Mastoid portion:** posterior, including the mastoid process.
3. **Zygomatic arch:** anterior and lateral.
4. **Petrous portion:** medial, containing the auditory and vestibular apparatus. It is the surface for the attachment of the tentorium cerebelli.

Articulations
The temporal bone articulates with seven other bones.

1. **Sphenoid:** The articulation of the temporal bone with the sphenoid was discussed under the sphenoid bone.
2. **Occiput:** The articulation of the temporal bone

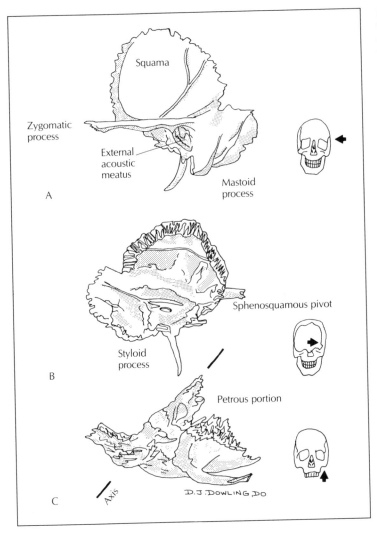

with the occiput was discussed under the occiput. This is the major influence on temporal motion.

3. **Zygoma:** The temporozygoma articulation forms the zygomatic arch, a serrate suture that allows rocking.

4. **Parietal:** The temporoparietal articulation can be considered as two separate articulations, or as one articulation with a change in bevel where the mastoid and squamous portions of the temporal bone meet. For present purposes it is considered as two separate articulations.

   a. The superior surface of the temporal bone, broadly beveled internally, articulates with the inferior anterior surface of the parietal bone, broadly beveled externally (the temporal bone overlaps the parietal bone). This suture is squamous, allowing medial and lateral glide of both bones as they rotate internally and externally.

   b. The superior surface of the mastoid portion of the temporal bone articulates with the posteroinferior surface of the parietal bone, forming an irregular, cobblestone articulation. There is a change in bevel at the center. This suture accommodates the rotary motion of the petrous portion of the temporal bone.

5. **Mandible:** The temporomandibular articulation is a synovial joint, found

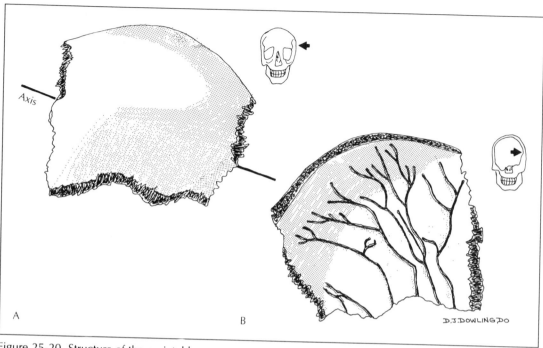

Figure 25-20. Structure of the parietal bone. (**A**) External view; (**B**) Internal view.

Figure 25-21. Sutures and articulations of the parietal bones of the skull, superior view.

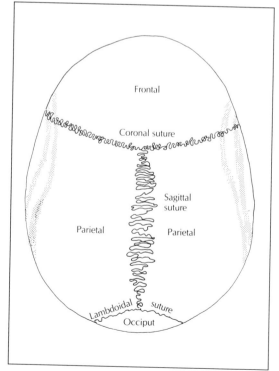

underneath the most posterior portion of the zygomatic arch.

THE PARIETAL BONES
Parts
The parietal bone has only one part (Fig. 25-20).

Articulations
The parietal bones articulate with five bones (Fig. 25-21).

1. **Parietal:** The interparietal (sagittal) suture is serrate, allowing a rocking motion as the parietal bones rotate internally and externally. It has fewer but wider serrations posteriorly to accommodate greater motion there.
2. **Frontal:** The coronal suture is squamoserrate with an external bevel medially and an internal bevel laterally on the parietal.
3. **Sphenoid**
4. **Occiput**
5. **Temporal**

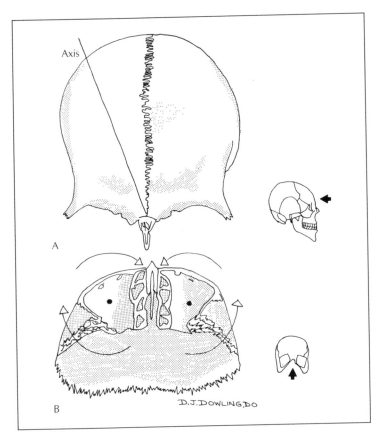

Figure 25-22. Frontal bone. (**A**) Anterior view; (**B**) inferior view.

FRONTAL BONE

Parts

1. **Nasal part:** inferior and midline, articulates with the ethmoid.
2. **Orbital parts:** lateral and inferior, forming the roof of the orbit.
3. **Squama:** forehead area, with frontal eminences laterally. A metopic suture exists in the midline in 10% of adults.

Articulations

The frontal bone articulates with 11 bones (Fig. 25-22).

1. **Parietal bones**
2. **Sphenoid**
3. **Ethmoid:** three sutures, two lateral, one in the midline anteriorly, all harmonic to accommodate gliding.
4. **Lacrimals**
5. **Maxillae**
6. **Nasal bones**
7. **Zygomae**

ETHMOID

Parts

1. **Horizontal cribriform plate:** where the falx cerebri attaches.
2. **Lateral masses** (2)
3. **Perpendicular plate**

Articulations

The ethmoid articulates with 12 bones (Fig. 25-23).

1. **Frontal bone**
2. **Sphenoid**
3. **Palatines** (2)
4. **Nasals** (2)
5. **Vomer**
6. **Inferior conchae**
7. **Maxillae** (2)
8. **Lacrimals** (2)

Figure 25-23. Structure and articulations of the ethmoid. (**A**) Superior view; (**B**) lateral view; (**C**) inferior view.

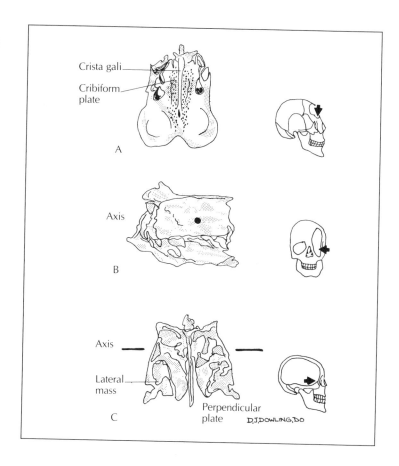

Cranial Articular Motions

No cranial bone moves independently. Restriction originating in any part of the cranium will cause changes in the motion patterns of the entire cranium.

Magoun has identified three factors essential for cranial articular motion.

1. **Plastic resiliency.** Every bone must be sufficiently resilient in itself and mobile in its sutures to move through its normal range without strain.
2. Resiliency of **contiguous bones.** The contiguous bones must be similarly resilient and mobile to accompany movement or compensate for it without strain.
3. **Unrestricted movement of dural membranes.** The dural membranes must be unrestricted in their arcs of reciprocal tension to allow such movement to occur within normal limits.

To this list one may add the influence of cervical fascia and muscles attaching to the cranial base, as well as sacral articular mobility.

Magoun emphasizes one further point referring to palpation of the cranial rhythmic impulse. "Do not look for movement as in the other joints of the body. This is merely a resiliency—a combination of slight yielding or suppleness in the articulation plus the flexibility of live and pliant bone."

Because the sphenoid and the occiput are considered to have the greatest influence on cranial articular motion, the sphenobasilar symphysis is the reference point for this section's discussion of physiologic and nonphysiologic cranial motion.

PHYSIOLOGIC MOTION—FLEXION
AND EXTENSION
Flexion of the sphenobasilar junction results in slight elevation of that articulation. The midline bones all rotate about a transverse axis into flex-

Figure 25-24. Flexion and extension at the sphenobasilar joint.

Figure 25-25. Transverse axes of cranial physiologic flexion and extension.

ion (Figs. 25-24 to 25-26). The compensatory response of the peripheral (paired) bones is external rotation. During extension, opposite motions occur (Fig. 25-27). All motions are subtle.

Occiput. In flexion, the occiput rotates about a transverse axis directly above the foramen magnum at the level of the confluence of sinuses. As it rotates, the basilar part and the condyles move anteriorly and superiorly, directly influencing the temporal bones, and the squama moves posteriorly and slightly laterally. The greatest lateral deviation occurs at the lateral angles.

Sphenoid. The sphenoid rotates on a transverse axis through the center of its body at the level of the floor of the sella turcica. The greater wings move forward, slightly laterally, and inferiorly, influencing the lateral edges of the frontal bone anteriorly and laterally. The pterygoid processes move posteriorly and slightly laterally.

Temporal bone. Influenced by the jugular process of the occiput, the temporal bone externally rotates around an axis running from the jugular surface to the petrous apex. This approximates a line running through the petrous portion along its

Figure 25-26. Flexion.

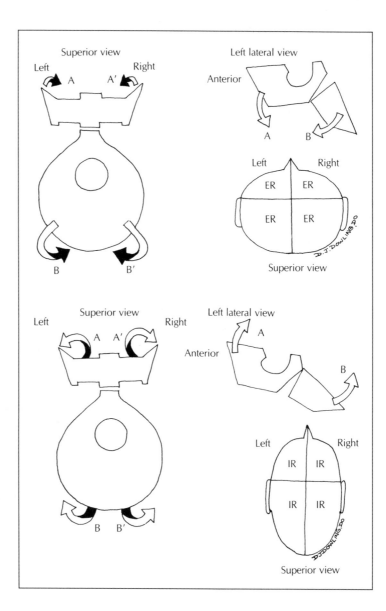

Figure 25-27. Extension.

long axis. The squamous portion and zygomatic arch move anteriorly, laterally, and inferiorly; the mastoid moves medially, superiorly, and slightly posteriorly; and the top of the petrous portion rotates laterally and slightly superiorly. The motion of the temporals has been likened to a wobbly wheel. Its motion influences the parietal bones and the occiput.

Parietal bones. The inferior surface of the parietal bone moves laterally around an axis connect-ing the anterior and posterior bevel changes (on the coronal and lambdoidal sutures). The posterior surface moves more laterally than the anterior surface.

Ethmoid. Influenced by the sphenoid and falx cerebri, the ethmoid rotates about a transverse axis through the middle of the bone, in the same direction as the occiput. The lateral masses move as paired bones into external rotation.

Frontal bone. The frontal bone acts as paired

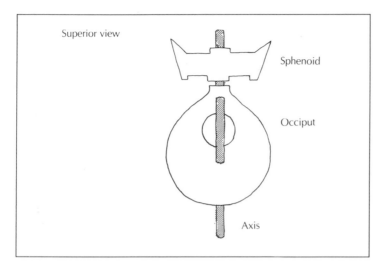

Figure 25-28. Torsional axis.

bones do, rotating externally under the influence of the sphenoid. The axis of rotation runs from the bevel change at the coronal suture through the center of the orbital plate. The inferior lateral angles move laterally and anteriorly. The glabella recedes slightly under the influence of the falx.

Sacrum. Pulled by dura, the sacral base moves posteriorly and the apex moves anteriorly about a transverse axis through the second sacral segment.

NONPHYSIOLOGIC MOTION
Torsion
Cranial torsion is a rotation of the sphenobasilar symphysis along an anteroposterior axis (Fig. 25-28). The sphenoid and occiput rotate in opposite directions. The axis runs from nasion to opisthion. The torsion is named for the side of the high wing of the sphenoid (Figs. 25-29, 25-30).

The following changes take place in the other bones and the membranes.

1. **Temporal bone:** relative external rotation on the side of the torsion.
2. **Parietal bone:** relative external rotation on the side of the torsion.
3. **Mandible:** shifted toward the side of the torsion.
4. **Orbit:** smaller on the side of the torsion.
5. **Membranes:**
   a. Falx cerebri: also torsioned, with the anterior end twisting in the same direction the sphenoid rotates, the posterior end

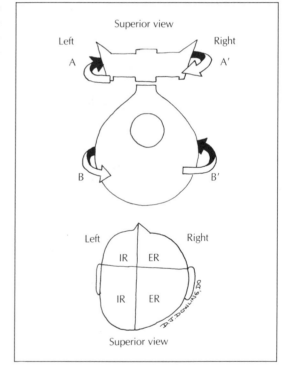

Figure 25-29. Right torsion.

twisting in the same direction the occiput rotates.

   b. Tentorium cerebelli: The tentorium is side bent in the same direction as the occiput rotates.

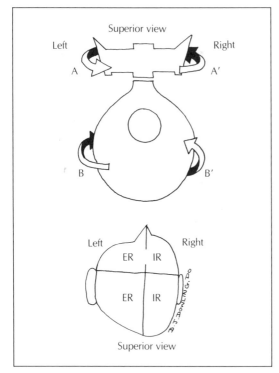

Figure 25-30. Left torsion.

c. Spinal dura: relaxed on the side of the low occiput, allowing the sacral base on that side to move inferiorly.

Side Bending and Rotation

Side bending and rotation are two separate motions of the sphenobasilar symphysis that occur simultaneously (Fig. 25-31). Side bending occurs by rotation around two vertical axes, one through the center of the body of the sphenoid and the other through the center of the foramen magnum (Figs. 25-32, 25-33). The sphenoid and occiput rotate in opposite directions on these axes, causing the side bending.

Rotation occurs on the same axis as torsion; however, the sphenoid and occiput rotate in the same direction. Rotation occurs toward the side of the convexity (convexity is lowered).

The following motions occur in the other bones and membranes:

1. **Temporal bones:** posterior on the convex side.
2. **Parietal bones:** posterior on the convex side.
3. **Mandible:** shifted to the convex side.
4. **Frontal bone:** anterior on convex side.
5. **Orbit:** anterior on convex side.
6. **Membranes:**
   a. Falx cerebri: side bent, following the convexity of the side bending of the sphenobasilar symphysis.
   b. Tent: follows occipital motion.
   c. Spinal dura: inferior on the side of the convexity (low occiput), dropping the sacral base on that side.

Figure 25-31. Side bending and rotation axes.

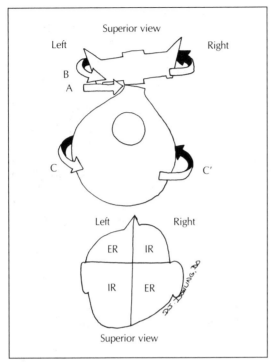

Figure 25-32. Right side bending and rotation.

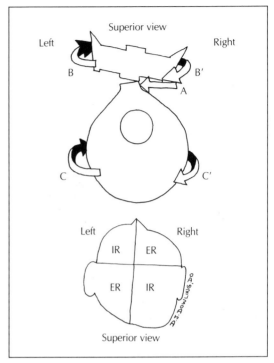

Figure 25-33. Left side bending and rotation.

Diagnosis and Treatment of Craniosacral Dysfunction

The cranial rhythmic impulse is a subtle mechanism consisting of small motions. Beginners commonly err by increasing their palpatory force in an effort to better sense these subtle motions. This inhibits the mechanism and makes more difficult palpation of the smaller motion restrictions so important to accurate diagnosis. As Magoun has stated, in palpation as in treatment, a light touch and gentle handling are essential. "To employ other than skillful and delicate sense perception is to lose the shades of physiological reaction so necessary for success. Living cells prefer persuasion to force, consideration to trauma, intelligence to ill-expended energy. *One must work with the tissues, not against them.*"

The primary respiratory mechanism is a fluid-based system. The pressures and motions come from the fluid. To work with this system, one must use certain basic principles of fluid dynamics. A common analogy is with a boat in water which, although solid, moves according to the mechanics of its fluid medium.

The clinician palpating the cranial rhythmic impulse is palpating the wave of fluid beneath the area contacted. Motion testing uses the momentum present in the system. Whenever possible, motion should be induced when the cranial rhythmic impulse is in the phase closest to that motion. This allows the system to supply most of the force necessary to carry out the motion test. When the motion being tested does not conform to motions already present, gentle continuous force is applied until the system begins to respond. This will create momentum in the desired direction. With rare exceptions, strong force is not used in the diagnosis or treatment of craniosacral dysfunction.

Treating craniosacral dysfunctions with indirect techniques allows the clinician to use the forces inherent in the mechanism. Indirect techniques are therefore preferred to direct techniques. Direct techniques are used primarily when treating small children and for sutural decompression. By their nature, direct techniques are more likely to cause adverse reactions and must always be applied with great care.

The cranial rhythmic impulse is the primary respiratory mechanism as it exists in the CNS. The CNS is extremely sensitive to changes in its internal environment (i.e., changes in hydrostatic or osmotic pressure, oxygen tension, glucose concentration, and so forth). Adverse reactions to craniosacral treatment are therefore more severe and easier to induce than with other manipulative treatment. The most common cause of an adverse reaction to cranial treatment is forceful, or heavy-handed manipulation.

DIAGNOSIS

History and observation are primary tools used in diagnosing craniosacral dysfunction. A history of trauma, especially to the head or buttocks (sacrum), is important. The direction and amount of force of the trauma should be noted. Any history of dental extraction or problems should be noted.

Observation will disclose general tendencies as well as asymmetries. Photographs of the individual taken before the traumatic incident are helpful for comparison with present conditions. Asymmetry may represent a functionally normal anatomic variant. Functional and dysfunctional asymmetries should be distinguished.

Some general tendencies found and certain skull types are described below:

1. Flexion: general appearance round. The transverse diameter of the skull is increased, the anteroposterior (AP) diameter is decreased. All quadrants are in external rotation (see Fig. 25-26).
2. Extension: General appearance long and narrow. The transverse diameter of the skull is decreased, the AP diameter is increased. All quadrants are in internal rotation (see Fig. 25-27). Extension is more common than flexion.
3. Torsion: named according to the side of the superior greater wing of sphenoid. The anterior and posterior quadrants on the side of the lesion are in external rotation. The relationships are reversed on the opposite side of the skull (see Figs. 25-29 and 25-30).
4. Side bending and rotation: named according to the side of convexity. The skull appears round on the side of the convexity and flat or slightly indented on the side of the concavity. The anterior quadrant on the convex side is in external rotation and the posterior quadrant is in internal rotation. These relationships are reversed on the opposite side of the skull (see Figs. 25-32 and 25-33).

Asymmetries in the following features should be noted:

1. Orbit: larger on the side of an externally rotated anterior quadrant.
2. Forehead: gradually sloping in flexion, a more vertical slope in extension. Reflects anterior quadrants.
3. Ears: reflect posterior quadrants. Flared and lowered in external rotation, close to the head in internal rotation.

Palpation

Palpation is the most important tool for cranial diagnosis. Before starting, the patient should be supine, relaxed, warm, and comfortable. The operator must also be comfortable and relaxed, with his arms resting on the table in minimal muscle contraction. The motions being palpated are minute, and operator tension or muscle contraction will send sensory impulses that may block or confuse signals coming from the fingers.

The operator places his hands on the patient's head to palpate motion. The hands are placed to contact very specific areas. Ordinarily the index fingers are placed over the greater wings of the sphenoid, the little fingers are placed on the occipital squama, and the two middle fingers are placed across the temporal and parietal bones, one on either side of the ear. When possible, the thumbs should touch each other and not the patient. The fingers and palm of the hand should contact the skull. The greater the area of contact, the easier it is to feel motion. One-half ounce of pressure is sufficient.

The cranial rhythmic impulse resembles a respiratory excursion; its rate should be approximately 8 to 12 cycles per minute, with small changes arising from metabolic activity or changes in respiration. Novice clinicians may have to concentrate for seconds to minutes before the rhythmic impulse is recognized. The palpated motion should be evaluated for rate, strength of excursion, and symmetry. These findings should be firmly established before any motion testing is initiated.

Passive motion is initiated slowly and gently. Once the motion is started, the operator simply follows the motion as the inherent forces (not the operator) carry it to its limit. In this way, both the physiologic and nonphysiologic motions may be tested for full range. Restrictions are noted accordingly.

TREATMENT

The goal of the treatment is to decrease or remove restrictions to motion in the cranial rhythmic impulse. Restrictions of motion may affect nerve function, circulation, and CSF fluctuation. Restrictions may be caused by membranous strains or articular dysfunctions. Whichever occurs first, both are always involved. This principle applies to the entire body.

Craniosacral dysfunction patterns involve the entire body. The primary dysfunction may occur in the spine or cranium. Treatment of both aspects is necessary for best results. Untreated musculoskeletal dysfunctions may prevent correction and induce recurrence of craniosacral dysfunctions. Areas of particular importance are the sacrum and upper cervical spine, to which the dura attaches directly.

Indirect technique utilizes the point of balanced membranous tension. This point is defined by Magoun as "that point in the range of motion of an articulation where the membranes are poised between the normal tension present throughout the free range of motion and the increased tension preceding the strain or fixation which occurs as a joint is carried beyond its normal physiology." Simply, it is the most neutral position within the range of motion, or the point of least tension or restriction. It is found by monitoring the mechanism gently through its entire range. The point of balanced tension is the point where the restriction in one direction ends, but before it begins in the opposite direction.

Three basic kinds of techniques are used to treat craniosacral dysfunctions: indirect techniques, direct techniques, and disengagement.

1. **Indirect techniques (exaggeration).** The mechanism is moved in the direction opposite the restriction (toward the freedom of motion). It is the direction in which the point of balanced membranous tension is almost always found. Indirect techniques are widely used in the treatment of craniosacral dysfunctions.
2. **Direct techniques.** The mechanism is moved through the barrier to motion in the direction of the restriction. Gentle encouragement is

maintained against the restrictive barrier until release occurs.
3. **Disengagement.** The joint is gapped. Traction or compression may be necessary for disengagement, according to the anatomy of the suture involved.

Two outside forces are used to enhance the effects of treatment:

1. **CSF fluctuation (or direction of fluid motion).** The operator places a finger at the spot on the skull at the greatest contralateral diameter from the restriction. This technique will be described in the next section.
2. **Respiratory assist.** Inhalation accentuates flexion and external rotation, exhalation accentuates extension and internal rotation. If treatment requires positioning in flexion, deep inhalation may aid in release. Treatment may utilize a series of deep breaths, or the operator may ask the patient to hold his breath in inhalation. Exhalation may be used for positioning in extension in the same manner.

Other factors to consider in treatment are described below.

Chronic or longstanding dysfunctions. Chronic dysfunctions usually require repeated treatments. Rarely are chronic dysfunctions correctable in one session, since the treatment may be traumatic and may increase the chance of a reaction, especially in the CNS, which is extremely sensitive to any change in its internal environment.

Sequence of correction. The sequence of correction will vary with the individual and the type of corrections needed.

Frequency. The frequency of treatment similarly varies with the individual case. Overtreatment can lead to problems if the body has not adjusted to the previous treatment. Too long an interval between treatments can diminish the effect of the previous treatment. The appropriate frequency of treatment will become apparent after several sessions with the patient.

Reactions. Reactions include headache, dizziness, nausea, and emotional or autonomic responses, sometimes quite severe. Heavy-handedness is a common cause of a treatment reaction; however, reactions may occur regardless of the operator's touch and experience. Reactions are quieted by relaxing the patient and keeping him warm. A fluid fluctuation technique may be used to quiet the cranial rhythmic impulse or to normalize its pattern. These techniques are described in the next section.

Contraindications. Increased intracranial pressure, intracranial hemorrhage, tumors, aneurysms, and skull fracture are absolute contraindications to craniosacral treatment.

Other variables. Nonsomatic factors may affect the disease process or the ability to treat the patient. Metabolic disease or disturbance and emotional factors are examples. These nonsomatic components are more difficult to diagnose and treat. Lack of response after several treatments may be a clue to the presence of nonsomatic factors. An incomplete or incorrect diagnosis may also contribute to lack of response.

Techniques to Alter the Pattern of Fluid Fluctuation

OCCIPITAL COMPRESSION (CV-4)

This technique is commonly called the CV-4 technique because its effects are postulated to be due to compression of the fourth ventricle, which lies anterior to the occipital squama. It is one of the most useful of all cranial techniques. Applications range from quieting an overactive cranial rhythmic impulse, to increasing the amplitude of the cranial rhythmic impulse, to moving fluids. The technique has been used successfully to relieve headaches, reduce fever, assist in difficult labor, relieve congested sinuses and lungs, and reduce edema. It can also be used to reduce trauma, such as a whiplash injury, or even the trauma of noncranial manipulative treatment.

To perform the CV-4 technique, the practitioner places her thenar eminences on the occipital squama, below the superior nuchal line. The hands must not be on the temporal bone or the occipitomastoid suture, as this will create dysfunctions. The O-M suture should be palpated before the hands are placed. Then the practitioner interlocks her fingers or overlaps her hands underneath. Once the hands are placed, the patient is instructed to lie still. The practitioner begins by monitoring the cranial rhythmic impulse through several cycles. Then the mechanism is followed into extension, with the practitioner resisting its attempt to flex. After a time the fluid flux will slow to a still point, during which no flux will be

palpable. At this point the practitioner may notice warmth in her palms or sweat on the patient's forehead, and the patient's breathing may change. To finish, the practitioner maintains her hand position, applying no pressure, until she feels the cranial rhythmic impulse return, slowly, to full force. This may take from 15 seconds to several minutes. This signifies the end of the treatment. In cases of acute head trauma or tenderness, this technique may be applied to the sacrum, with extension encouraged by directing the base anteriorly, resisting flexion.

VENOUS SINUS DRAINAGE

This nontraumatic technique may increase venous drainage. Before treatment is initiated, the thoracic outlet, cervical, and O-A dysfunctions must be mobilized to allow drainage into the thoracic cavity.

Step 1. The physician places four fingers across the superior nuchal line, pointed directly anteriorly toward the patient's face. This position is maintained with slight pressure (usually the weight of the head will suffice) until release or an apparent softening of the bone is felt beneath the fingers. This release is followed, to maintain balance of tension, until both sides release (this may take several minutes). This step promotes drainage of the transverse sinus.

Step 2. To drain the confluence of the sinuses, the same procedure is followed, except that one finger is placed on the inion.

Step 3. To drain the superior sagittal sinus, the physician begins at the inion and uses several fingers to V-spread the occipital squama (see below); the same release will be felt. Above lambda the sagittal suture may be spread with two crossed thumbs, disengaging the suture. The physician waits for release, then "climbs" up the suture one thumb at a time to bregma (coronal suture). Continue on the frontal bone in the same manner you did below lambda, separating with your fingers. This sequence is the reverse of the direction of sinus drainage. The end points must be drained before earlier sinuses can be drained.

V-SPREAD

V-spread is a combination of disengagement and direction of fluid. The physician places two fingers of one hand on either side of the suture to be released and exerts gentle traction to disengage the suture. Simultaneously, she places one or two fingers on the point of greatest distance from the suture on the contralateral side. Gentle pressure with these fingers will send a fluid wave toward that suture. This wave should be palpated by the V-spread fingers within a few seconds and will continue between the two hands. The physician adjusts the directing fingers until the pulse is palpated between the two V-spread fingers. Release or an apparent softening of the tissues will occur.

LATERAL FLUCTUATION/ROCKING

To perform this technique, the physician contacts the temporal bones bilaterally. One possible hand position entails placing the thumbs over the anterior aspect of the mastoid processes with the hands cupping the occipital squama. The physician gently encourages (rocks) one temporal bone into external rotation while simultaneously directing the other into internal rotation. When the limits of this phase are reached, the process is reversed by rocking each temporal bone in the opposite direction. The rocking is continued until a still point is reached. The physician continues monitoring until the cranial, rhythmic impulse returns, making sure the temporal bones are internally and externally rotating normally.

Somatic Dysfunction Diagnosis and Treatment

Dysfunctions of the sphenobasilar symphysis and the temporal, frontal, and parietal bones will be discussed. Dysfunctions of the facial bones, although relevant to complete cranial diagnosis and treatment, are beyond the scope of the chapter.

Sphenobasilar Symphysis

The sphenobasilar symphysis directs the motion of all the other bones of the skull. A peripheral (nonsphenobasilar) dysfunction (usually of the temporal bone, but sometimes of the parietal or frontal bone) will influence motion of the whole cranium and thus may mimic a sphenobasilar dysfunction. Therefore, the entire skull must be evaluated before deciding on any treatment plan. In addition, because a sacral dysfunction can prevent correction of a cranial dysfunction or induce its recurrence, sacral dysfunctions should also be diagnosed and treated as part of the treatment of cranial dysfunctions.

The clinician may use either the vault hold or the fronto-occipital hold; both holds are de-

scribed for each pattern. Always palpate gently for cranial motion as described earlier for general findings before undertaking specific motion testing.

1. Vault hold. The physician places his hands on either side of the head with the thumbs touching each other just behind the sagittal suture (they should not be touching the patient's head). The index fingers contact the greater wings of the sphenoid, the little fingers contact the occiput, and the middle two fingers contact the temporal and parietal bones (one on each side of the ear). The finger pads, not the tips are used. The entire finger and palm of the hand should contact the head.

2. Fronto-occipital hold. The physician places one hand under the patient's head, cupping the occipital squama. The other hand is placed across the forehead so that the thumb and index or middle finger of that hand contact the greater wings laterally. The entire hand, not just the finger pads, should contact the patient's head.

FLEXION/EXTENSION

Although flexion and extension are the normal physiologic motion present, they may be restricted in one direction. This dysfunction may occur without other associated nonphysiologic dysfunctions (see Figs. 25-26, 25-27).

General Findings and Observations

The general findings of a flexion or extension dysfunction are listed in Table 25-1.

Palpation for Motion

Do not encourage motion out of phase with the cranial rhythmic impulse.

1. Vault hold. The physician places his hands in the vault hold. Flexion is encouraged by directing both the greater wing of the sphenoid and the occipital squama inferiorly. Both hands move symmetrically caudad and expand laterally. Motion is started at the beginning of physiologic flexion and followed until resistance is met. This is the limit of flexion. Extension involves an opposite set of maneuvers: the hands (index finger and fifth finger) move cephalad and medially until resistance is met.

2. Fronto-occipital hold. The physician positions his hands in the fronto-occipital hold. To test

Table 25-1. Findings in a Flexion or Extension Dysfunction of the Sphenobasilar Symphysis

Parameter Evaluated	Flexion Dysfunction	Extension Dysfunction
Restricted motion	Extension	Flexion
Head diameter	Increased in transverse dimension	Increased in longitudinal dimension
Forehead	Wide and sloping	Vertical
Eyes	Prominent	Receded
Paired bones	Externally rotated	Internally rotated
Ears	Protruding	Close to head

flexion, he rotates the greater wings anteriorly and inferiorly and simultaneously rotates the occipital squama inferiorly and anteriorly. These motions are reversed to evaluate extension.

Dysfunction Correction
Indirect or exaggeration techniques are used to correct most cranial dysfunction patterns. The same holds and motions are used as were described for motion testing. Flexion is encouraged for a flexion dysfunction (extension restriction), extension is encouraged for an extension dysfunction (flexion restriction). However, instead of moving the joint to its limit of motion, the movement is stopped just as the beginning of restriction is encountered. This will place the mechanism in its most free state (the point of balanced membrane tension). The correction is then made by the inherent forces of the cranial rhythmic impulse. If this alone does not correct the dysfunction, two assistive forces may be used:

1. Direction of fluid. This force is called on by the physician placing a finger directly on the vertex. The technique is easiest with the vault hold, where the thumbs are over the point of contact. With the fronto-occipital hold, the index finger on the frontal side may be stretched to this point. Fluid is directed to the sphenobasilar symphysis.
2. Respiratory assist. For a flexion dysfunction, the patient is asked to inhale and hold her

breath for as long as possible. For an extension dysfunction, the patient is asked to exhale and hold for as long as possible.

TORSION
The reader should review the motion pattern described earlier. On one side the sphenoid wing is high and the occiput low, as rotation occurs about an anteroposterior axis (see Figs. 25-29 and 25-30).

General Findings and Observation
The side of the high sphenoid wing (and low occiput) are in relative external rotation. The side of the low sphenoid wing and high occiput are in relative internal rotation. Table 25-2 lists the important findings.

Palpation for Motion
1. Vault hold. Test motion by symmetrically rotating each hand in opposite directions around a horizontal axis.
2. Fronto-occipital hold. The frontal hand elevates one greater wing. The occipital hand lowers the occipital squama on the same side.

Dysfunction Correction
The sphenobasilar symphysis is moved into free motion until the first indication of resistance appears. The symphysis is then returned to the position of least resistance, or the point of balanced

Table 25-2. Findings in Torsion Dysfunction of the Sphenobasilar Symphysis

Parameter Evaluated	Side of High Sphenoid Wing	Side of Low Sphenoid Wing
Frontal lateral angle	Anterior	Posterior
Orbit	Wide	Narrow
Frontozygomatic angle	Increased	Lessened
Eyeball	Protruded	Retruded
Zygomatic orbital rim	Everted and externally rotated	Inverted and internally rotated
Symphysis menti	To this side	Away from this side
Mastoid tip	Posteromedial	Anterolateral
Ear	Protruding	Close to head

membrane tension. This position is held until release occurs. Directing fluid from the vertex to the symphysis may help. Having the patient inhale fully and holding for as long as possible may also encourage release. The range of motion is then rechecked.

SIDE BENDING/ROTATION

Side bending and rotation dysfunctions are named for the convexity of the side bending motion. The dysfunction was described previously (see Figs. 25-32 and 25-33).

General Findings and Observation

In side bending and rotation dysfunctions, one side of the head is relatively convex, the other relatively flat. The head may be imagistically divided into four quadrants—two anterior quadrants, influenced by the greater wing of the sphenoid on that side, and two posterior quadrants, influenced by the occiput on the side. In these dysfunctions, the anterior quadrant on the side of the convexity is in relative internal rotation, and the posterior quadrant on that side is in relative external rotation. Table 25-3 lists the important findings.

Palpation for Motion

1. Vault hold. The physician approximates the fingers of one hand while simultaneously lifting cephalad. The fingers on the opposite hand are spread and moved caudad.

Table 25-3. Findings in Side Bending/Rotation Dysfunctions of the Sphenobasilar Symphysis

Landmark	Convexity	Concavity
Lateral frontal angle	Posterior	Anterior
Orbit	Narrow	Wide
Frontozygomatic angle	Lessened	Increased
Eyeball	Retruded	Protruded
Zygomatic orbital rim	Prominent	Flat
Symphysis menti	To this side	Away from this side
Mastoid tip	Posteromedial	Anterolateral
Mastoid portion	Anterolateral	Posteromedial
Ear	Protruding	Close to head

2. Fronto-occipital hold. Side bending is induced first by approximating the fingers of both hands. Then rotation, which occurs automatically, can be assisted by rotating the fingers cephalad.

Dysfunction Correction

The motion is brought to its freest position, the point of balanced membrane tension. Directing fluid from vertex will assist, as will the patient's respiratory assistance.

STRAINS

Strains are serious dysfunctions and are almost always traumatically induced. There are two types of strains, vertical strains and lateral strains. Each is discussed separately.

Vertical Strains

Vertical strains are named according to the position of the basisphenoid. It can move superiorly or inferiorly, creating superior and inferior vertical strains (Figs. 25-34 and 25-35).

General findings and observation. A vertical strain is flexion of the sphenoid accompanied by extension of the occiput, or extension of the sphenoid with flexion of the occiput. Side-to-side findings are symmetrical. Evidence of the anterior quadrants in external rotation would indicate a superior vertical strain; if they are in internal rotation, there is inferior strain.

Palpation for motion.
1. Vault hold. To test for superior vertical strain, the physician rotates both hands forward, carrying the greater wings into flexion and the occiput into extension. These motions are reversed to test for inferior vertical strain.
2. Fronto-occipital hold. To test for superior vertical strain, the physician moves the frontal hand caudad, influencing the sphenoid toward flexion, and simultaneously moves the occipital hand cephalad, influencing the occiput toward extension. The directions of each hand are reversed to test for inferior vertical strain.

Dysfunction correction. This dysfunction is corrected in the same manner as other dysfunctions of the sphenobasilar symphysis. The physician finds the point of balanced membrane tension and holds it, directing fluid from the vertex.

Figure 25-34. Superior strain.

Figure 25-35. Inferior strain.

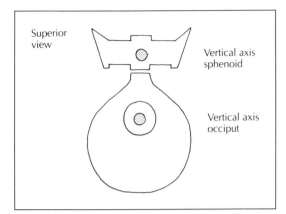

Figure 25-36. Lateral strain axes.

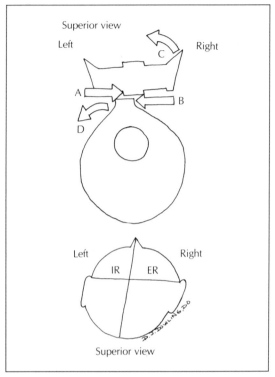

Figure 25-37. Right lateral strain.

Lateral Strain

A lateral strain is a side-to-side shearing of the sphenobasilar symphysis (Fig. 25-36). It is usually caused by trauma lateral to one side of the anterior cranium or the opposite posterior cranium (anterior or posterior to the sphenobasilar symphysis) (Figs. 25-37 and 25-38).

General findings and observation. Both bones rotate on a vertical axis in the same direction. The head may take on the appearance of a parallelogram (especially noticeable in infants). Regardless of age, side-to-side findings will not be symmetric.

Palpation for motion.
1. Vault hold. To test for lateral strain, the physician directs the sphenoid laterally in one direction with his index fingers while directing the occiput in the opposite direction with the fifth fingers.
2. Fronto-occipital hold. The physician directs the sphenoid laterally in one direction with the frontal hand and directs the occiput in the opposite direction with the occipital hand.

Dysfunction correction. The physician finds the point of balanced membrane tension (toward the freedom of motion), then assists by directing fluid from the vertex or by enrolling the patient's respiratory assistance.

COMPRESSION OF THE SPHENOBASILAR SYMPHYSIS

This dysfunction occurs as a result of pressure or trauma to the front of the head or face, to the back of the head, or to the entire periphery (i.e., compression of the infant cranium during a difficult birth) (Fig. 25-39).

General Findings and Observation

This dysfunction manifests as a restriction (mild, moderate, or severe) of all motions at the sphenobasilar symphysis. With severe compression, the cranium feels rigid.

Motion Testing

Any hold may be used. The dysfunction is recognized as the practitioner tests for all motion patterns and becomes aware of limited or absent motion in the sphenobasilar symphysis.

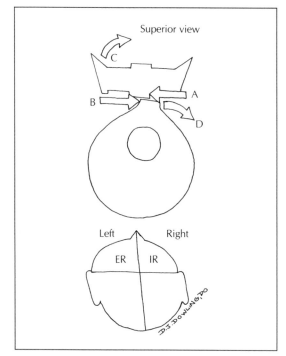

Figure 25-38. Left lateral strain.

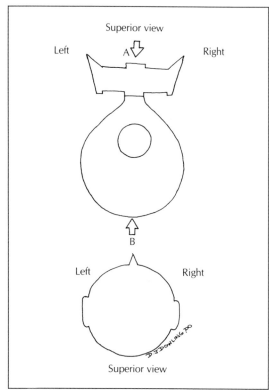

Figure 25-39. Compression.

Dysfunction Correction
Correction of this dysfunction is difficult, often requiring more than one practitioner. The technique will not be described here.

The Temporal Bone

The temporal bone is a common site of articular restrictions (specifically of the occipitomastoid suture). The motion of the temporal bone is very complex. The changes in bevel found on the temporal bone reflect at least two different axes of motion for the temporal bone. Four surfaces of the temporal bone can be evaluated separately. Internal and external rotation may also be tested.

DYSFUNCTIONS OF THE TEMPORAL BONE
General Findings and Observation
The general findings depend on whether the dysfunction is unilateral or bilateral. A temporal bone dysfunction may cause varied symptoms. The entire auditory and vestibular apparatus sits within the petrous portion of the temporal bone.

Cranial nerves IX, X, and XI exit from the jugular foramen along with approximately 90% of the venous drainage from the skull. Dysfunctions of the temporal bone can cause widespread and dramatic symptoms.

Palpation for Motion
Internal and external rotation are the physiologic motions of the temporal bones. To position the hands, the physician places the middle or index finger bilaterally inside the patient's ears, the middle or ring finger on the inferior surface of the mastoid tip, and the thumb on the superior surface of the zygomatic arch (temporal portion). The physician then encourages bilateral external rotation. Once the motion is felt it is allowed to continue until the limit of motion in that direction has been reached. The physician notes any restrictions or asymmetries. Then the physician's thumb and the finger are placed on the superior surface of the mastoid and the inferior surface of

the zygomatic arch, respectively, and internal rotation is encouraged.

There are four spring tests to evaluate the motion of four different portions of the temporal suture. These tests are different from the tests of physiologic motion and more like the spring tests used for evaluating any joint. Response (motion) should be immediate. Lack of response indicated a sutural restriction in that surface of the temporal suture.

1. **Occipitomastoid suture.** The occipitomastoid suture is a troublesome suture in the cranium and a common site of restriction. To test this suture, the physician uses the same hand position as for evaluating internal and external rotation, but on one side only. The other hand cups the occiput with the finger pads monitoring the occipitomastoid suture on that side. Then the physician springs the temporal bone into internal and external rotation (not through its full range) while stabilizing the occiput with the other hand, preventing it from moving. Motion should be felt at the occipitomastoid suture.
2. **Parietotemporal suture.** The physician finds the asterion, then palpates the posterior corner of the parietal bone. The parietals are sprung directly medially to diagnose a dysfunction.
3. **Sphenotemporal suture.** The physician palpates with his opposite hand at the pterion. The hand on the same side directs the mastoid posteriorly and medially, which should produce gapping at the pterion. A restriction could be temperosphenoid or sphenobasilar.
4. **Temporobasilar (petrobasilar) suture.** The physician positions the fingers of the opposite hand on the occiput in the same manner as in 1, then slides them deep into the occipital sulcus. The hand on the same side grips the temporal bone around the ear. Simultaneously the physician pulls the temporal anteromedially and the occiput posterolaterally, then reverses these directions, testing the glide of the petrous portion on the basilar part of the occiput.

These tests are not fluid motion tests. They are articular tests for specific joint motions of the temporal bone. Point tenderness on a suture may also indicate sutural restriction.

Dysfunction Correction

Internal rotation (external rotation restricted). The physician finds the point of balanced membrane tension and holds this position, aided by the patient holding his breath in exhalation. The hand placement is reversed for external rotation (internal rotation restricted), in which case the patient assists with a breath held in inhalation.

Specific joint mobilization. Regardless of where the articulation is, the physician uses V-spread and directs fluid as the appropriate treatment. The V-spread position is achieved by placing one finger on either side of the suture that is restricted. These fingers maintain constant, gentle traction. Simultaneously the physician directs fluid to the suture from the opposite pole, or from the place on the skull at the greatest contralateral distance. The position of this finger should be moved slightly until the pulse is felt directly between the two fingers.

Although tests for only four suture surfaces were described, Magoun lists eight areas for V-spread, as follows:

Restricted Suture	Directing Finger
Petrobasilar	Parietal eminence
Petrojugular	Lateral vertex
Occipitomastoid	Frontal eminence
Parietomastoid	Pterion
Parietosquamous	Parietosquamous
Pterion	Asterion
Sphenosquamous pivot	Parietal eminence
Sphenopetrous	Frontal eminence

FRONTAL BONE
Dysfunctions of the frontal bone are often secondary to sphenoid dysfunctions. Primary dysfunctions are either traumatic or secondary to sinus congestion in the ethmoid or frontal sinuses.

Palpation for Motion—Frontal Lift
In the frontal lift the physician uses one hand. The grip is the same as that of the frontal hand in the fronto-occipital hold, except that the fingers contact the lateral angles of the frontal bone, not the greater wing of the sphenoid. It is best to find a bump, usually detectable on the upper lateral

surface of the orbit. This will aid in gripping the frontal bone. The frontal bone is pulled superiorly, to separate it from the ethmoid and sphenoid bones (among others), and anteriorly, to gap the coronal suture. Restrictions should be noted.

Dysfunction Correction

The *frontal lift* is used to lift the frontal bone. The unrestricted side will move further before resistance is met. The physician follows this motion until resistance is equal on both sides, then maintains tension and waits for release of the restricted side. This is a direct technique and must be done carefully.

V-spread may be directed to any sutural restriction.

PARIETAL BONES

Dysfunctions of the parietal bones are often secondary to dysfunctions of the occiput or temporal bones. Primary dysfunctions are usually traumatic in origin.

Palpation for Motion—Parietal Lift

Palpation for motion of the parietal bones is a two-step diagnostic procedure. If the steps are not done in order, the procedure will not work.

1. With four fingers of each hand, the physician directs the entire parietal bone (both sides) medially. This will separate it from the temporal bone.
2. Once medial release of the parietals is felt, the physician lifts the parietals superiorly. Any restricted motions are noted.

Dysfunction Correction

The *parietal lift* is performed with the hands focused to either the front or back, depending on where restriction is felt. Lift is maintained until release occurs. Motion is then rechecked.

V-spread may be directed to any sutural restriction.

26

Facilitated Positional Release

STANLEY SCHIOWITZ

Facilitated positional release is performed using a modification of indirect myofascial release techniques. The advantages of facilitated positional release are the speed with which the dysfunction resolves and the improved results in managing difficult dysfunctions. The goal of manipulation is to restore normal tissue texture and joint motion. Should the applied technique fail in any instance, it can be repeated or another method can be used immediately.

A psssible explanation for the effectiveness of this treatment relates to the action of the muscle spindle gamma loop when the gain is suddenly decreased. According to Carew, with a sudden decrease in load, the spindles in the muscle become unloaded and the Ia fiber discharges from these spindles cease, thereby removing their excitation to motor neurons controlling the extrafusal muscle fiber. The muscle then begins to relax until it lengthens. This physiologic change may well account for the immediate effect felt when facilitating force is used in these techniques.

General Procedure

The physician modifies the patient's sagittal posture in the region to be treated, adding a facilitating force and placing the dysfunction into its freedoms of motion.

Joint motion and tissue texture influence each other reciprocally, and it may be difficult to ascertain which is the primary cause of the dysfunction. In doubtful cases, tissue changes should be treated first.

In general, hypertonic tissue found along the posterior aspect of the spine is shortened, with backward bending and side bending to the same side. If tissue hypertonicity is found anteriorly, forward bending is usually required. Some muscles have a contralateral side bending function or a rotary component; these muscles must be placed in their individual shortened positions. Careful localization of the component motions of facilitation, forward and backward bending, and side bending and rotation to the area of tissue texture change will produce more accurate results.

Specific Techniques

TECHNIQUES FOR MODIFYING TISSUE TEXTURE CHANGES

1. The patient assumes a relaxed position.
2. The physician flattens the anteroposterior spinal curve of the area to be treated.
3. The physician places the tissue into its ease of motion (i.e., shortened).
4. The physician applies a facilitating force (compression, traction, torsion, or a combination of these forces). Steps 3 and 4 may be applied in reverse order.
5. The position is held for 3 to 4 seconds.
6. The physician releases the position and reevaluates the dysfunction.

TECHNIQUES FOR TREATING INTERVERTEBRAL MOTION RESTRICTIONS

The procedures are the same as for treating tissue texture changes, except for step 3: the physician

Figure 26-1. Facilitated positional release for treatment of tissue texture changes of the cervical region: application of axial compression.

Figure 26-2. Facilitated positional release for treatment of tissue texture changes of the cervical region, with backward bending and left side bending added.

places the vertebra into its planes of freedom of motion. For example, a somatic dysfunction diagnosed as C5 F Sr Rr is treated by placing the fifth cervical vertebra into a position of flexion, right lateral flexion, and right rotation, with respect to the sixth cervical vertebra. Springing, exaggerating the freedoms of motion, may be added to completely release articular dysfunctions.

CERVICAL REGION TECHNIQUES
All techniques for treating cervical region dysfunctions are begun with a slight flattening of the region to be treated.

A. Tissue texture dysfunction, posterior right side, in region of C4 vertebra
  1. Patient position: supine.
  2. Physician position: seated at the head of the table.
  3. **Technique:**
    a. The patient moves up the table until his head and neck are off the table and supported by the physician.
    b. With the thumb, palm, and middle finger of the left hand, the physician cradles the patient's neck. His middle finger is on the tissue to be treated. The rest of the hand helps support the patient's neck.
    c. The patient's head is firmly supported in the palm of the physician's right hand, which will be used in the ensuing maneuvers.
    d. The physician gently bends the head and

neck forward to flatten the cervical lordosis.
    e. From this starting position the physician gently applies axial compression on the patient's occiput, with the vector of force directed through the patient's head toward his feet (Fig. 26-1). Less than 1 pound of force is sufficient—just enough to be felt at the physician's left index finger.
    f. Maintaining axial compression, the physician bends the patient's neck backward, then side bends it up to the physician's left index finger (Fig. 26-2). This maneuver causes shortening and relaxation of the tissue being treated.
    g. This position is held for 3 seconds, then released and the area of dysfunction reevaluated.
B. Somatic dysfunction (C4 E Sr Rr)
  1. Patient position: supine, as described in above technique.
  2. Physician position: seated at the head of the table, with hands placed as described in above technique.
  3. **Technique:**
    a. The physician places his finger at the articular facet of C4 on C5.
    b. After flattening the curve and adding a compressive force, the physician moves the patient's neck into extension and rotation.
    c. The physician then adds right lateral flexion of C4 on C5.

d. Immediate release of the articulation should be felt.

C. Somatic dysfunction (C4 F Sr Rr)

1. Patient position: supine as described in technique A.
2. Physician position: seated at the head of the table, with hands placed as in above techniques.
3. **Technique:**
   a. The physician gently bends the patient's neck forward to flatten the sagittal curve.
   b. From this starting position the physician applies compression.
   c. Maintaining compression, the physician gently increases the forward bending until flexion of C4 on C5 is felt by the monitoring finger. (With compression maintained, the degree of forward bending of the neck needed to achieve the necessary vertebral flexion is greatly reduced.)
   d. The physician adds right rotation and lateral flexion, up to monitoring finger (Fig. 26-3).
   e. After feeling an articular release, the physician holds the position for 3 seconds, then releases it and reevaluates the dysfunction.

THORACIC REGION TECHNIQUES

A. Tissue texture dysfunction, anterior left side, region of fourth costal cartilage

1. Patient position: seated.
2. Physician position: standing behind the patient.
3. **Technique:**
   a. The physician places his right hand around the front of the patient with the index finger on the dysfunction.
   b. The physician's left hand is on the patient's cervicothoracic junction, with the force arm resting on the superior aspect of the shoulder and the elbow over the acromiom process.
   c. The patient is instructed to sit up straight until the thoracic kyphosis flattens slightly.
   d. The physician applies compression at the cervicothoracic junction and left shoulder, directly toward the floor (Fig. 26-4). (Do not allow forward bending.)
   e. Maintaining the compressive force, the physician bends the patient's body forward up to the monitoring finger. (The patient may be told to drop his head forward.)
   f. The physician adds left side bending

Figure 26-3. Facilitated positional release treatment for C4 flexion dysfunction (C4 F Sr Rr).

Figure 26-4. Facilitated positional release treatment for anterior thoracic tissue texture changes: application of compression at the cervicothoracic junction.

Figure 26-5. Facilitated positional release treatment for anterior thoracic tissue texture changes, with forward bending, side bending, and rotation added.

Figure 26-6. Facilitated positional release treatment for posterior thoracic tissue texture changes: application of compression at the left cervicothoracic junction.

Figure 26-7. Facilitated positional release treatment for posterior thoracic tissue texture changes, with side bending and backward bending added.

until motion is felt at the monitoring finger. Rotation may have to be added (Fig. 26-5).

  g. The position is held for 3 seconds, then released and the dysfunction reevaluated.
     Note: Properly applied, this technique will also release many costochondral dysfunctions.

B. Tissue texture dysfunction, left posterior region of T7 vertebra
  1. Patient position: seated.
  2. Physician position: standing behind and to the left of the patient.
  3. **Technique:**
     a. The physician places his right index finger on the site of the dysfunction.
     b. The physician's left arm is placed on the patient's left shoulder with the elbow at the lateral aspect to allow direction and control of patient's motion.
     c. The patient is instructed to sit up straight until the thoracic kyphosis flattens slightly.
     d. The patient is told to push his chest out until backward bending is created up to the monitoring finger.
     e. The physician applies compression with his forearm near the patient's neck. The vector of force is aimed straight down (Fig. 26-6).
     f. Maintaining the backward bending and compression, the physician creates side bending up to the monitoring finger by

pressing down with his left elbow (Fig. 26-7).
     g. The position is held for 3 seconds, then released and the dysfunction reevaluated.

C. Somatic dysfunction (T7 E Sl Rl)
  1. Patient position: seated.
  2. Physician position: standing behind and to the left of the patient.
  3. **Technique:**
     a. The physician's monitoring finger is at the transverse process.
     b. All maneuvers as the same as for treatment of a tissue texture dysfunction, except that left rotation is added to the side bending.
  To treat a flexion dysfunction (T7 FS1 R1), flexion of spine is added after compressive force.

D. Thoracic dysfunction, patient prone (T3 E Sr Rr)
  1. Patient position: prone.
  2. Physician position: standing beside the table, opposite the side of the dysfunction.
  3. **Technique:**
     a. The physician places the index finger of his cephalic hand (with respect to the patient) at the transverse process. With the patient prone, mild flattening of the thoracic kyphosis is usually created. If not, a pillow is placed under the patient's head and neck.
     b. With his caudal hand the physician grasps the patient's acromial process.

Figure 26-8. Facilitated positional release treatment for T3 extension dysfunction (T3 E Sr Rr), patient prone. The physician applies a downward and parallel pull, creating compression and side bending.

Figure 26-9. A torsional motion is added, turning the shoulder upward and creating compression, extension, side bending, and rotation.

With his hand on the superior aspect of the shoulder girdle he pulls straight down, parallel to table and toward the patient's feet, until force is felt at the monitoring finger (Fig. 26-8).

c. Maintaining this force, the physician straightens up, thereby turning the patient's shoulder backward.

d. These combined motions create compression, extension, side bending, and rotation up to monitoring finger (Fig. 26-9). The physician should feel the tissue and/or the articular release.

e. The position is held for 3 seconds, then released and the dysfunction reevaluated.

E. First rib dysfunction

1. Patient position: supine.

2. Physician position: standing beside the table, on the side of the dysfunction.

3. **Technique:**

a. The physician places his caudal (with respect to the patient) hand over patient's rib with the fingers on the posterior aspect of the first rib (right hand on right rib). The hand placement may be modified laterally to treat tissue only, or at the costovertebral junction to obtain first thoracic articular release.

b. The physician bends the patient's elbow and places his left hand on the patient's flexed elbow.

c. The physician pushes down on the

Figure 26-10. Facilitated positional release treatment for first rib dysfunction: application of compression with internal rotation of shoulder.

patient's elbow directly into his monitoring fingers (Fig. 26-10).

d. Maintaining this compression, the physician adds internal rotation of the shoulder joint. This is accomplished by placing the patient's right forearm on the ventral aspect of physician's right forearm and turning the patient's forearm outwards by caudal motion of physician's forearm. This should create tissue release or articular motion.

e. The position is held for 3 seconds.

f. Maintaining the compressive torsional force, the physician brings the patient's arm toward midline (adducts it), then

Figure 26-11. Adduction followed by circumduction to release the arm.

Figure 26-12. Facilitated positional release treatment for lumbar tissue texture changes.

Figure 26-13. Facilitated positional release treatment for a lumbar extension somatic dysfunction.

circumducts the arm down to the tabletop (Fig. 26-11).

g. The position is released and the dysfunction reevaluated.

LUMBAR REGION TECHNIQUES

A. Tissue texture dysfunction, left low back

1. Patient position: prone, with a pillow under the abdomen. The pillow should be large enough to cause flattening of the lumbar lordosis.

2. Physician position: standing at the left side of the table. The physician's left index finger is placed on the site of tissue tension.

3. **Technique:**

   a. The physician places his left knee on the table beside the patient's left ilium.

   b. With his right hand the physician slides the patient's legs toward the left side of the table, producing side bending of the patient's lumbar spine over the physician's left knee. Side bending is continued until tissue motion is felt by the left (monitoring) index finger (Fig. 26-12).

   c. The physician releases the patient's legs, crosses patient's right leg over the left, and then places his right hand under the patient's right thigh. The physician grasps the patient's right thigh and extends and posteriorly rotates it until motion is felt by the left (monitoring) index finger in the area of tissue tenderness. A torsional motion is created up to the monitoring finger.

   d. This position is held for 3 seconds, then released and the dysfunction reevaluated.

B. Somatic dysfunction (L4 E Sl Rl)

1. Patient position: prone, with a pillow under the abdomen.

2. Physician position: standing at the left side of the table.

3. **Technique:**

   a. The physician monitors the left transverse process of the L4 vertebra with his left index finger.

   b. The physician grasps the patient's left lower leg or ankle with his right hand.

   c. The patient's left leg is brought into abduction until motion is felt at the monitoring finger, then internal rotation up to the monitoring finger is added.

Figure 26-14. Facilitated positional release treatment for a lumbar flexion somatic dysfunction.

Figure 26-15. Facilitated positional release treatment for lumbar diskogenic pain syndrome.

Figure 26-16. Facilitated positional release treatment for tissue texture dysfunctions in the gluteal region.

d. The patient's left leg is then pushed toward the floor until motion is felt by the physician's monitoring finger (Fig. 26-13). A small pillow is inserted between the patient's thigh and the table to avoid creating a painful pressure area. This pillow also assists in the creation of the desired fulcrum effect.

e. The position is held until the physician feels articular release. This usually occurs in 3 to 4 seconds.

f. The position is released and the patient is returned to neutral position. The dysfunction is reevaluated.

C. Somatic dysfunction (L4 F Sr Rr)

1. Patient position: prone, with a pillow placed under the abdomen.

2. Physician position: sitting at the right side of the table, facing the patient's head. The physician's left lateral thigh and knee are beside the table.

3. **Technique:**

a. The physician monitors the transverse process of L4 on the right side with one finger of the left hand.

b. The physician drops the patient's flexed right knee and thigh off the table over his left thigh.

c. The physician grasps the patient's knee with the right hand and flexes the patient's hip until motion is felt at the monitored transverse process.

d. The physician pushes the patient's right knee toward the table, into adduction, using his left knee and thigh as a fulcrum, until motion is felt at the monitored transverse process.

e. With his right hand the physician turns the patient's knee in a circular direction, creating internal rotation of the hip (Fig. 26-14).

f. This position is held until the physician feels articular release.

g. This position is held for 3 seconds, then released and the dysfunction reevaluated.

D. Lumbar diskogenic pain syndrome. This technique is useful for patients with radicular pain, post laminectomy, bulging disks, stenosis, or herniations. Treatment is described for a right-sided dysfunction.

1. Patient position: prone, with a pillow placed under the abdomen.

2. Physician position: seated at the right side of the table, facing the patient's head. The physician's thighs and knees are parallel to the table. The physician monitors the disk space to be treated with one finger of the left hand.

3. **Technique:**
   a. The patient's right hip and thigh are flexed and the thigh is placed over both of the physician's legs, allowing the knee to flex down toward the floor.
   b. The physician places his right hand on the patient's right shin or ankle.
   c. The physician raises his right foot off the floor, raising the patient's thigh, until motion is felt at the monitoring finger.
   d. The physician pushes his right knee laterally against the back of the patient's knee, creating a traction force, monitored by his finger.
   e. With his right hand the physician turns the patient's right leg down toward the floor, creating a rotary motion of the thigh and hip, with the knee acting as the fulcrum (Fig. 26-15).
   f. Mild tension is maintained at the monitoring finger until motion is felt. The physician will feel a release of tissue tension in 3 to 5 seconds.
   g. The physician releases the position, returns the leg to the table, and reevaluates the dysfunction.
      Note: This treatment may be applied to both sides for optimum results.

TISSUE TEXTURE DYSFUNCTIONS OF THE PIRIFORMIS AND GLUTEAL MUSCLES
1. Patient position: prone, with a pillow placed under the abdomen.
2. Physician position: sitting beside the table on the side of the dysfunction (right), facing toward the patient's head. The physician's left thigh and knee are beside the table.

3. **Technique:**
   a. The physician monitors the tissue to be treated with one finger of the left hand.
   b. The physician drops the patient's flexed right knee and thigh off the table over his left thigh.
   c. The physician holds the patient's knee with his right hand, gently flexing the patient's hip until motion is felt at the monitoring finger.
   d. The physician pushes the patient's right knee toward the table (adduction), using his left knee and thigh as a fulcrum, until motion is felt at the monitoring finger.
   e. With his right hand the physician turns the patient's knee in a circular direction, producing internal rotation of the hip, until motion is felt at the monitoring finger.
   f. With his right hand the physician pushes the patient's knee dorsally toward his monitoring finger, producing a mild compressive force (Fig. 26-16). There should be an immediate release of tissue tension.
   g. The position is held for 3 seconds, then released and the dysfunction reevaluated.

References

Carew, TJ., The Control of Reflex Action, in Kandel, ER., Schwartz, JH. (eds.). Principles of Neural Science, 2d ed., New York, N.Y.: Elsevier Science Publishing Co. Inc. 1985, p. 464.

Schiowitz, S., Facilitated positional release, JAOA, Vol. 901 no. 2, Feb. 1990, pp. 145–155.

27

Osteopathic Manipulative Treatment: Contraindications, Precautions, and Side Effects

EILEEN L. DIGIOVANNA

Although osteopathic manipulation is a highly effective treatment for many conditions and a useful adjunct in the treatment of others, certain precautions, contraindications, and side effects must be taken into consideration when formulating a treatment plan. Because of the wide variety of techniques available to osteopathic physicians, there is no absolute contraindication to at least some form of manipulation in any given patient or condition as long as the patient's condition is stable and motion permitted. It is important to make a careful diagnostic evaluation of the patient and to devise a treatment plan consistent with that patient's needs.

High Velocity, Low Amplitude Thrusting Techniques

Most of the severe iatrogenic complications reported as a result of manipulation are related to thrusting techniques. Most have resulted from chiropractic manipulation and have involved the upper cervical spine. Other complications included neurovascular accidents, aggravation of disk syndromes, and fractures. Missed diagnoses contributed significantly to complications.

Physician-related problems include diagnostic error, lack of skill, and the use of inappropriate force. Patient-related problems include abnormal bony structure, pathologic entities, intolerance of head motion leading to vertigo, and psychological intolerance of manipulation.

Perhaps the most significant complication reported is vertebrobasilar accident with rotary cervical manipulation, such as reported by Gittinger. In some persons, rotation and extension of the cervical spine causes narrowing of the vertebral artery on the side opposite the rotation. Occipital infarction may result, with various neurologic sequelae. Before initiating thrusting techniques for treatment of dysfunctions of the cervical spine, the physician may find it useful to extend and rotate the patient's head for 30 seconds while watching for nystagmus, nausea, or dizziness.

The most common side effect of cervical high velocity-low amplitude thrusting techniques appears to be vertigo. Although this may indicate impending vascular problems, in most cases it is of positional origin.

Hundreds of thousands of manipulative interventions are performed yearly by chiropractors, osteopathic physicians, and manual medicine practitioners in allopathic medicine. Perhaps half of these interventions are applied to the cervical spine, yet only a few hundred cases of significant patient injury have been reported.

Contraindications to thrusting techniques likely include the acute phase of arthritis, osteoporosis, bone cancer, fractures, atherosclerotic plaques, and cervical spondylosis with vertebral artery ischemia. Care should be exercised in treating patients with radicular pain from herniated disks, pregnant women, or patients with acute whiplash, Scheuermann's disease, and postsurgical conditions. Patients on anticoagulant therapy should be treated with great caution.

Muscle Energy Treatment

Muscle energy treatment is quite safe. Occasionally some muscle stiffness and soreness occur after the treatment. If the area being treated is not localized well or if too much contractive force is used, pain may be increased.

Sometimes the patient is in too much pain to contract a muscle, or for some reason is unable to cooperate with the physician's instructions or positioning. In such instances muscle energy treatment may be difficult to apply.

Counterstrain Techniques

Counterstrain is an atraumatic technique. Patients should be warned that they may feel sore several hours after the treatment. The soreness could last into the next day.

Craniosacral Treatment and Myofascial Release

These techniques are generally nontraumatic and, if applied properly, should cause no more than fatigue and lethargy after treatment. Emotional release, which may follow any type of manipulation, most commonly occurs after craniosacral or myofascial release. The physician must be prepared to deal with this situation. More rarely, nausea or vomiting, loss of appetite, dizziness, or headache may follow a cranial treatment.

Improperly applied craniosacral treatment may have more serious consequences. Because it has physiologic effects, certain untoward events could occur. Nerve injury is possible. One student developed hypopituitarism after force was applied intraorally to the sphenoid by an inept manipulator.

Eclectic Manipulation

Mastery of the multiple techniques of manipulative treatment will help the clinician determine and apply the most appropriate treatment in each patient. An analogy can be drawn with prescribing drugs: the more one knows about medications, their interactions, and their effects, the better treatment can be tailored to the individual case. Similarly, the more manipulative techniques the clinician knows, the more safely and effectively she can use them. Each patient and each physician are different. The manipulative procedures used should reflect these differences.

References

Bourdillon JF. 1982. Spinal Manipulation, 3rd ed. Norwalk, Conn: Appleton-Century-Crofts.

Brownson RJ, et al. 1986. Sudden sensori-neural hearing loss following manipulation of the cervical spine. Laryngoscope 96:166–170.

Gittinger JW. 1986. Occipital infarction following chiropractic cervical manipulation. J Clin Neuroophthalmol 6:11–13.

Grayson MF. 1987. Horner's syndrome after manipulation of the neck. Br Med J vol. 295, 6610:1381–1382.

Hoag JM, Cole WV, Bradford SG. 1969. Osteopathic Medicine. New York: McGraw-Hill Book Co.

Maitland GD. 1977. Vertebral Manipulation, 4th ed. Stoneham, Mass.: Butterworths.

28

The Hospitalized Patient

EILEEN L. DIGIOVANNA
BARRY ERNER
STANLEY SCHIOWITZ

The osteopathic physician is involved in the total care of the patient as well as the care of the total patient. The need for osteopathic evaluation and manipulative treatment does not cease when the patient is hospitalized. In fact, this may be the most crucial time for such management.

Upon admission all the health needs of the patient must be ascertained. This includes a careful history and a thorough physical examination, including a structural evaluation. A diagnostic plan must be developed, proper diet arranged, and a treatment plan set up. Structural evaluation may be a great help in formulating a diagnosis and is an important part of any physical examination.

Even when osteopathic manipulation is not the primary therapeutic modality, it still has a place as adjunctive treatment or, at the very least, as a means of making the patient more comfortable. All hospitalized patients can benefit from manipulative care; some patients need it more than others.

The Structural Examination

Each "history and physical" form in a patient's chart contains a section for the structural examination. It may include a body outline, with the various parts highlighted (Fig. 28-1). As for any other part of the physical exam, the notation "normal" or "within normal limits" is not helpful. Few people are "normal."

Whenever possible, the patient should be evaluated first standing, then seated, then supine and prone. Since many hospitalized patients are confined to bed, this paradigm may have to be altered.

The standing structural examination should include anteroposterior and lateral assessment, with any asymmetries or abnormal curves noted. To the extent possible, motion testing should be performed, including gross motion testing and evaluation at intersegmental levels of motion when indicated.

All patients may be palpated. Tissue textures should be evaluated, and any abnormal tension, bogginess, temperature changes, or fibrosis should be noted. This should be a layered palpation which evaluates skin, fascia, muscle, tendons, and ligaments.

If patients cannot be turned, the physician may gently slide her hand beneath them to assess tissues. If patients can be turned on their side this will facilitate the procedure. Asymmetric vertebral position should be noted, with any associated tissue changes. Abnormalities should be correlated with the patient's symptoms, since viscerosomatic reflexes may be of diagnostic importance.

With practice, the structural examination can be completed in a few minutes and can be integrated into the total physical examination. For example, while assessing the head and neck, the physician can evaluate the cervical spine.

All asymmetries and restrictions of motion

STRUCTURAL EXAMINATION

Examiner _____ Date _____

		Cervical	
		Thoracic	
		Lumbar	
		Sacral pelvis	

Spinal curves Sagittal plane	Increased	Decreased	Normal	Spinal scoliosis Frontal plane	Direction of convexity
Cervical lordosis				Cervical spine	
Thoracic kyphosis				Thoracic spine	
Lumbar lordosis				Lumbar spine	

Tissue diagnosis

Cervical region
Thoracic region
Lumbar region
Sacroiliac region

Summary of osteopathic structural diagnosis

_____

_____

Medical diagnosis

_____

_____

Suggested therapy

_____

_____

Reviewed by _____ Date _____

Figure 28-1. Structural examination.

should be noted in the proper places on the structural form. The body diagram may be used to pinpoint deviations of normal curves, to note areas of pain or tenderness, or to record sites of somatic dysfunctions. This will provide a quick overview of the examiner's findings.

A correlation of structural changes with findings on the physical examination is important in developing a differential diagnosis. In many cases such correlation may supply the diagnosis.

Items on the form for structural examination are discussed in sequence below.

Section 1: Sagittal and coronal plane diagrams of the human spine are shown in the chart in Figure 28-1. Each region of the spine should be palpated for somatic dysfunction, with findings recorded. An explanation of findings should be recorded in the space to the right of the spinal diagram.

Section 2: Any increase, decrease, or absence of changes in the normal patterns of kypholordosis in the frontal planes of the spine should be recorded.

Section 3: The presence or absence of spinal scoliosis should be recorded, along with the correct convexity of any curve observed.

Section 4: Tissue changes are commonly palpable in patients with somatic dysfunction. Indicate the tissue changes present under the proper spinal region.

Charting and Writing Orders for Osteopathic Manipulation

There must be proper chart documentation when ordering and delivering osteopathic manipulative treatments to a patient. It is recommended that the attending physician write the order for specific osteopathic manipulative treatments in accordance with the patient's condition. The physician can write the general order on the doctor's order sheet and provide a more detailed description in the progress notes. Some examples follow:

Date	Doctor's Orders
1/8/91	Osteopathic manipulative treatment: to be given by hospital medical staff as in progress note dated 1/8/91.

John Doe, D.O.

Date	Progress Note
1/8/91	OMT, myofascial-relaxing techniques with passive motion of the extremities to be performed daily.

John Doe, D.O.

The physician should record in the progress notes any manipulative treatment performed and an assessment of any benefits noted by the patient. If specific techniques have been ordered and the treating physician believes that other techniques may be needed, this information should be conveyed to the attending physician, who may change the prescription as she sees fit.

Osteopathic Manipulative Modalities

Following is a description of some available osteopathic manipulative modalities. These techniques may be used alone or in combination, depending on the needs of the patient.

MYOFASCIAL TREATMENT—RELAXING

This mode of treatment is used to relax contracted or contractured muscles. It should relieve pain, restore normal function, and increase arterial, venous, and lymphatic drainage. It is applied specifically and gently, as a gentle stretch, to the muscles. It should rarely elicit pain.

The progress note order should read as follows:

Myofascial treatment—relaxing to _____ area, _____ times daily.

MYOFASCIAL TREATMENT—STIMULATORY

Passive myofascial treatment can also be applied more rapidly with a minimum amount of force. It should never elicit pain. The goal is to increase muscle tone and to mildly increase circulation.

The progress note order should read as follows:

Passive myofascial treatment—stimulatory to _____ area, _____ times daily.

MYOFASCIAL RELEASE TREATMENT

This mode of treatment is used to release fascial tensions, to restore function, and to increase local circulation and lymphatic flow. Gentle force is applied in the direction of free motion, or the restrictions to motion are challenged, which affords release of tension and congestion in the tissues. This modality requires the operator to have special training in its techniques.

The progress note order should read as follows:

Myofascial release treatment to _____ area, _____ times weekly.

MUSCLE ENERGY TREATMENT

Muscle energy treatment is used for restrictions of motion between individual vertebrae. The technique utilizes the Golgi tendon reflex, reciprocal inhibition, or direct muscle pull on a specific bony attachment to restore the normal physiologic range of motion at the joints. Treatment should be applied gently and should rarely elicit pain. It requires patient cooperation.

The progress note order should read as follows:

Muscle energy treatment to somatic dysfunctions in _____ area [or specific somatic dysfunctions can be listed, e.g., C4 E Rr Sr].

HIGH VELOCITY, LOW AMPLITUDE THRUSTING TECHNIQUES

This mode of treatment is applied to restricted joint motions that result in abnormalities of position of the bones at a given articulation. This modality focuses a specific localized force into the given segment. After the segment is localized, a very gentle thrust is needed to move the segment. Myofascial relaxation should always be used prior to the thrust to remove tensions from the surrounding tissues. This technique should rarely elicit pain.

The progress note order should read as follows:

High velocity, low amplitude therapy to somatic dysfunctions in the _____ area, [or specific somatic dysfunctions can be listed, e.g., T6 F Sl Rl].

RANGE OF MOTION THERAPY

This mode of therapy is used in the treatment and prevention of restrictions in joint motions due to the development of fibrous adhesions or loss of mechanoreceptors in joint articulations. The joint is put through the full range of normal physiologic motion. After passive range of motion, active range of motion therapy may be used, which entails the use of isometric contraction to treat motion barriers. This modality is applied without

force by the operator, except when acting as the resisting force in the active variant. It should rarely elicit pain. Examples are the Spencer techniques for the shoulder girdle, and sacral rocking.

The progress note order should read as follows:

Passive/passive and active range of motion therapy to _____ joint(s), _____ times daily.

COUNTERSTRAIN TECHNIQUE

This mode of treatment is used for discrete tender points in muscles, ligaments, and fascia. The patient is placed in the position of greatest comfort to relieve tenderness at these points. With the aid of patient relaxation, the operator maintains the position until the tenderness and tension are gone. This modality is applied slowly and gently and should rarely elicit pain. It may be used safely even in patients who are quite ill. It may be utilized one to three times weekly. This modality requires the operator to have special training in its techniques.

The progress note order should read as follows:

Counterstrain techniques to the _____ area.

CRANIAL THERAPY (CV-4)

This cranial technique is designed to normalize fluctuations of the cerebrospinal fluid. There is also a relaxation of secondary dysfunctions in the spine. The result is a feeling of calm and well-being in the patient. This modality requires the operator to have special training in its techniques.

The progress note order should read as follows:

CV-4, _____ times weekly.

LYMPHATIC PUMP TECHNIQUES

This mode of treatment assists the normal physiologic pumping of the lymph through its channels. The operator applies a gentle rhythmic force to the chest or extremities for 30 seconds to 3 minutes. Lymphatic drainage may also be applied to the anterior cervical area to encourage lymph drainage from the head and neck into the thoracic area. Thoracic methods or arm methods are used to encourage lymph drainage from the thorax and its associated viscera into the lower extremity, with foot rocking used to promote drainage.

Each of these methods affects the lymphatic flow throughout the body. This is especially true for the thoracic, sacral, and foot rocking methods. They can be used when the structures in the area to be treated are too tender to allow forceful motions. For example, the foot rocking method may be substituted for the thoracic method, and vice versa.

This treatment is applied gently and should not cause pain or discomfort. This modality is useful in the treatment of edema, enlarged and painful lymph nodes, lymph stasis, and bronchial congestion (e.g., pneumonia or fever). Treatment should be provided at least twice a day and may be provided as often as every two hours every day until congestion is relieved.

The progress note order should read as follows:

Lymphatic pump treatment, _____ method to be applied, _____ times daily.

RIB RAISING

This mode of treatment is used to free restrictions in rib cage motion. These restrictions decrease the normal respiratory effort and increase the flow of venous blood and lymph. The technique consists of gentle mobilization of the ribs within their normal physiologic range of motion. One technique allows the patient to remain supine in bed; another is done with the patient seated. Either technique may be modified to have the patient on his side.

The progress note order should read as follows:

Rib raising treatment, _____ times daily.

SINUS DRAINAGE

This treatment is designed to alleviate the pain and discomfort resulting when the nasal sinuses fail to drain properly into the nasal passage. Several manual techniques are involved, including both direct and indirect pressure on the sinuses, counterstrain, and anterior cervical lymphatic drainage. This modality is utilized to relax the patient and to relieve discomfort. It should never be painful.

The progress note order should read as follows:

Sinus drainage techniques, _____ times daily.

Examples of Indications for Osteopathic Manipulation

BEDRIDDEN PATIENTS

1. Hypotonicity of muscles and decreased circulation. Treatment: myofascial/stimulatory.
2. Decreased function of mechanoreceptors, leading to loss of normal gait. Treatment: range of motion exercises for extremities, active and passive.
3. To prevent the development of phlebitis and emboli from circulatory stasis. Treatment: range of motion exercises, active and passive; lymphatic pump.
4. Muscle contracture. Treatment: myofascial, relaxing, stretching, and range of motion techniques.

The first two orders should be written for all bedridden geriatric patients. The orders must be written immediately upon the patient's admission, because it is impossible to remedy the massive loss of muscle tone and the loss of mechanoreceptors once they have occurred.

CARDIOVASCULAR DISORDERS

1. Myocardial insufficiency or following myocardial infarction. Treatment: muscle energy techniques to treat rib somatic dysfunctions, especially of the upper thoracic ribs on the left; myofascial relaxation of T1–T5, especially T4 and T5, to decrease autonomic nervous system output and to prevent development of shoulder-hand syndrome; myofascial relaxation of the occipitoatlantal and atlantoaxial joints.
2. Congestive heart failure. Treatment: lymphatic pump/pedal and thoracic areas, and rib raising to increase circulation; myofascial relaxation of T1–T4.
3. Hypertension. Treatment: counterstrain treatment or myofascial relaxation treatment of upper cervical and midthoracic areas.

EENT DISORDERS

1. Sinusitis. Treatment: sinus drainage; myofascial relaxation techniques (active and passive) for the cervical area; muscle energy techniques and high velocity, low amplitude, thrusting techniques.
2. Tonsillitis. Treatment: myofascial techniques for occipitoatlantal joint; muscle energy or

thrusting techniques to occipitoatlantal joint; anterior cervical drainage and lymphatic pump.

3. Otitis media. Treatment: sinus drainage and lymphatic pump to the anterior cervical area; myofascial release of the cervical area; jaw lift to stretch eustachian tubes. Jaw lift entails protracting the jaw, with gentle stretching traction applied anteromedially to the posterior border of the mandibular ramus ipsilateral to the infected ear. This traction is maintained for 30 to 60 seconds.

4. TMJ somatic dysfunctions. Counterstrain or muscle energy techniques.

GASTROINTESTINAL DISORDERS

1. Adynamic ileus, postoperative or posttraumatic. Treatment: myofascial treatment of the lumbar area; direct pressure over the lower thoracic and lumbar areas; muscle energy techniques or high velocity, low amplitude thrusting techniques to treat somatic dysfunctions in the lower thoracic and upper lumbar regions if not contraindicated; abdominal myofascial release.

2. Constipation. Treatment: myofascial, muscle energy, or thrusting techniques applied to the lumbar area; abdominal myofascial release.

3. Gallbladder disease and post-GB surgery. Treatment: myofascial treatment of T6–T10 and lower ribs on the right; muscle energy techniques or high velocity, low amplitude thrusting techniques for somatic dysfunctions.

4. Abdominal muscle spasm. Treatment: fascial release and counterstrain techniques.

5. Peptic ulcer. Treatment: myofascial, muscle energy, and counterstrain techniques applied to left midthoracic region (especially T5–T6) on the left and the sacroiliac and occipitoatlantal areas; abdominal myofascial release.

6. Subtotal gastrectomy. Treatment: myofascial, muscle energy, and counterstrain treatment for acute changes in the T5–T7 area.

7. Functional diseases of the colon. Treatment: myofascial, muscle energy, and counterstrain techniques applied to mid and lower thoracic area and upper lumbar area.

GENITOURINARY DISORDERS

1. Bladder problems. Treatment: muscle energy treatment of the sacral and pubic areas; sacral rocking.

2. Initiation of urination postoperatively. Muscle

energy treatment of the sacral and pubic areas, sacral rocking for somatic dysfunctions; myofascial relaxation to the thoracolumbar area.

3. Dysmenorrhea. Treatment: sacral rocking; myofascial treatment of the lumbar area; muscle energy techniques for sacral and lumbar somatic dysfunctions; counterstrain treatment for anterior and posterior pelvic and lumbar tender points especially the midpole sacral tender point and iliacus tender point.

4. Urinary tract infection. Treatment: myofascial release and counterstrain techniques applied to the lower thoracic, lumbar, psoas, and quadratus lumborum muscles; muscle energy techniques for pubic somatic dysfunction.

OBSTETRIC CARE

1. During labor. *First phase:* myofascial and muscle energy techniques applied to the lumbar area to relieve spasm and pain and to decrease the duration of this phase. *Second phase:* sacral rocking to release the sacral motion necessary for nutation of sacrum in second phase. *Third phase:* remove mother's legs from stirrups, one at a time, putting the hips through adduction, internal rotation, and extension, in sequence; then place the legs flat on the table. This prevents sacroiliac dysfunction due to increased elasticity of pelvic ligaments.

2. Prenatal and postnatal muscle spasm and somatic dysfunction. Treatment: myofascial, muscle energy, thrusting, myofascial release, and counterstrain treatment of the lower thoracic and lumbar areas secondary to baby's position, and to the midthoracic area secondary to milk production.

3. Dilation and curettage. Treatment: same as in the third phase of labor, removing the woman's leg from the stirrups, as described above.

RESPIRATORY DISORDERS

1. Bronchitis and pneumonia. Treatment: rib raising, and lymphatic pump; myofascial techniques for cervical and upper thoracic (T1–T5) areas.

2. Asthma and chronic obstructive pulmonary disease. Treatment: rib raising and lymphatic pump; myofascial treatment of the upper thoracic (T1–T5) spine and of the thoracolumbar junction (diaphragmatic attachments).

SURGICAL PATIENTS

1. Muscle spasm and somatic dysfunctions in areas of spine segmentally related to the viscera or body part on which surgery is performed. Treatment: myofascial treatment of the area; muscle energy techniques or high velocity low amplitude thrusting techniques if indicated for somatic dysfunctions.
2. Muscle contraction and somatic dysfunction resulting from position during surgery. Treatment: myofascial treatment of the area; muscle energy techniques or thrusting techniques for somatic dysfunctions.
3. Pneumonia or atelectasis. Treatment: prophylaxis to enhance respiration, ventilation, and circulation.
4. Edema (noninfectious). Treatment: lymphatic pump.
5. Restriction of motion due to adhesions, and to prevent the development of phlebitis and emboli. Treatment: passive range of motion exercises; rib raising; lymphatic pump.

HEADACHES

1. Migraines and other headaches (frequently associated with upper cervical muscle tension or somatic dysfunction, especially in the occipitoatlantal area). Treatment: myofascial treatment of the cervical area; muscle energy techniques, high velocity, low amplitude thrusting techniques, or counterstrain treatment for somatic dysfunctions.

29

Practical Applications of Osteopathic Manipulative Treatment

WHIPLASH INJURIES
Donald E. Phykitt

"Whiplash" is commonly used to describe an injury caused by acute hyperextension-hyperflexion of the cervical spine. Motor vehicle accidents account for a significant proportion of such injuries. The victims commonly are passengers in a stationary or slowly moving vehicle that is struck from behind, or passengers in a moving vehicle that strikes an immovable object (deceleration injury). Tissue damage and injury can occur when the offending vehicle is moving as slowly as 7 miles per hour.

Whiplash injuries are more accurately described as inertial injuries, since they result from a discrepancy between the inertia (resistance to movement) of the head and the momentum (tendency to keep moving) of the trunk. Inertia and momentum meet in the highly mobile cervical spine; for this reason, considerable research has focused on cervical injury.

Osteopathic medicine, however, regards whiplash as an insult to the entire body, including the pelvis, spine, and cranium and their connecting soft tissues (fascia, tendons, ligaments, muscles). This insult results in both local and distant re-flexes that affect every organ system in the body. Heilig in 1963 aptly summarized the situation:

"Whiplash" describes the *mechanism* of a whole series of vertebral and paravertebral injuries. It is not a typical syndrome, nor any particular injury. It is characterized only by the fact that damage has occurred to tissues as a result of forces of inertia and their effect on contiguous or connecting tissues and not because of external contact of the injured area.

Evaluation of the whiplash patient includes a complete history and physical examination. Special attention should be given to neurologic deficits, structural deviations, primary and compensatory somatic dysfunctions (cervical, thoracic, lumbar, sacral, cranial), and areas of sympathetic hyperactivity. The clinician should attempt to reconstruct the events of the accident and to uncover any predisposing structural or medical conditions.

Treatment is individualized for each patient. It will include osteopathic manipulative treatment, exercise, thermal and physical modalities, pharmacologic therapy, and emotional support.

Mechanism of Injury

Three theories are commonly proposed to explain the mechanism of injury in whiplash. All three recognize that the impact producing whiplash propels the body in a linear horizontal direction. Because of inertia, the head momentarily remains in its original position. It then abruptly moves in the direction opposite the impact force vector. Cessation of the impact, along with an acute stretch reflex of the neck muscles, causes the head to recoil in the same direction as the initial impact force vector.

For example, if a stopped car is struck from behind, the driver's body is propelled forward. After a brief pause the head moves backward into hyperextension, damaging the soft tissues on the anterior aspect of the neck. The head then recoils forward into hyperflexion, damaging the soft tissues in the posterior cervical region. Both motions can cause vertebral injuries as well.

The three theories on causation differ, however, with respect to the exact paths followed by the head and neck during the hyperextension and hyperflexion, and with respect to the forces that result in vertebral injury. According to the most widely held theory, the head follows an arc above the shoulders, and damage results from rapid tissue stretch secondary to traction, hyperflexion, and hyperextension.

A second theory, proposed by McKeever, contends that the injurious force results from horizontal translation of the body with respect to the head. McKeever postulates that the head remains at the same horizontal level throughout the injury (i.e., it does not follow an arc). Thus there is shortening of the neck with resultant severe compression when the head is directly above the shoulders. These compressive forces result in avulsion injuries of vertebral structures.

A third theory agrees that the cervical vertebrae are compressed. However, it postulates the concomitant presence of torques at the level of C1 and C7. It proposes that horizontal translation of the body is accompanied by an extension torque of the head at C1 and a flexion torque of the trunk at C7. Accordingly, the most severe injury is thought to occur in the midcervical region.

It is most likely that the actual mechanism of injury combines elements of all three theories. Most investigators believe that hyperextension causes greater injury than hyperflexion, for the following reasons:

1. The original force (usually directed from behind) most often comes as a surprise, giving the victim less chance to prepare by tightening his muscles.
2. Flexion is restricted by the impact of the chin on the chest. This motion is within the physiologic and anatomic limits of cervical motion.
3. However, nothing restricts extension until the occiput strikes the back of the seat. This motion is well beyond the anatomic barriers to motion, and soft tissue and osseous injury can occur.

Pathophysiology

Regardless of the mechanism of injury in whiplash, the damage caused to the cervical tissues remains the same. Tissue and structural injury in the cervical spine will be discussed in reference to the superficial soft tissues, the vertebral complex (vertebrae, ligaments, tendons), the peripheral and sympathetic nervous systems, the vascular system, and the cerebrum.

SUPERFICIAL SOFT TISSUE
Hyperextension

Abrupt elongation of relaxed, unprepared muscles initiates an acute stretch reflex. Rear-end acceleration accidents result in hyperextension of the cervical spine with concomitant stretching of the neck flexors. Similarly, hyperflexion during deceleration accidents is accompanied by stretching of the extensor muscles.

When a muscle is stretched acutely, most of the stretch is sustained by the intrafusal muscle fibers of the muscle spindles, which normally monitor muscle length. Abrupt, forceful elongation of the muscle initiates a neural reflex and results in a proportionately stronger contraction of that muscle. The reflex does not cause the subsequent spasm directly but contributes strongly to the recoil of the neck after the initial hyperflexion or hyperextension.

If the degree of stretch is sufficient, the fibrils of the extrafusal fibers (contractile elements of the muscle) will tear. The gross muscle is not injured, so there is usually no gross hemorrhage or edema. And because major nerves are not initially involved, there may be no immediate pain, paresthesia, or paresis. Severe injury, however, can cause nerve damage and gross bleeding.

Edema and microhemorrhage can serve as foci of muscle irritability, resulting in painful muscle spasm. Sustained contraction inhibits motion and impedes circulation, resulting in the buildup of metabolites, notably lactic acid. This compounds the muscle hyperirritability. The final result is fibrous contracture, trigger point formation, and chronic pain and immobility.

Hyperextension results in damage to the anterior cervical muscles. Minor injury may only traumatize the sternocleidomastoid muscle. However, this can lead to pain and trigger point formation along the whole muscle, especially at the origin, and can result in the head tilt and painful torticollis experienced by many patients.

More severe hyperextension damages the deeper neck flexors, notably the scalenes and longissimus colli. Severe hyperextension is often accompanied by stretching and subsequent edema of the pharynx and esophagus. Retropharyngeal hematoma can develop, causing dysphagia and pain on swallowing soon after an accident.

The prevertebral fascia of the anterior neck is continuous with the fascia of the mediastinum, which in turn is continuous with the crura of the diaphragm and the fascia surrounding the psoas major muscles. Thus, hyperextension can set up fascial strain patterns that can contribute to dysfunction in the thorax, abdomen, pelvis, and even the lower extremities.

Hyperflexion

Hyperflexion injuries cause less severe damage than hyperextension injuries but still contribute greatly to a patient's symptoms and incapacitation, for the following reasons:

1. The musculature of the posterior neck is both intricate and widespread. It includes the intrinsic muscles (e.g., the multifid and rotator muscles) as well as the extensive paravertebral muscles and the muscles of the shoulder girdle (the levator scapulae, rhomboid, and trapezius muscles). Moreover, numerous muscles attach to the occipital and suboccipital joints. These joints are highly mobile and consequently highly susceptible to injury. From these anatomic relationships, it can be understood why patients often complain of cervical pain radiating up to the occiput and down to both shoulders and the midthoracic region.

2. The posterior neck is richly innervated by afferent fibers. Not only do these fibers travel to the muscles, they also pierce the muscles on their way to innervating the skin of the posterior neck and scalp. Muscle spasm and waste buildup irritate the nerves. Such irritation of the occipital nerves (sensory for the scalp) causes much of the cephalgia reported.

VERTEBRAL COMPLEX

When muscles are elongated beyond their physiologic limits, tendons, ligaments, and articular capsules are stretched or torn. Vertebral subluxations or fractures can result.

Hyperextension is accompanied by posterior translation of a vertebra on the one below it. It may also involve traction on the anterior portion of the vertebral body and compression of the posterior articulation, with these consequences:

1. Anterior traction can result in strain or even tearing of the anterior longitudinal ligament and annulus fibrosis, with hemorrhage and edema.
2. Posterior compression can lead to fractures of the vertebral body or the spinous process.
3. Posterior glide causes facet encroachment onto the intervertebral foramen, with possible impingement on the nerve root.
4. Posterior translation accompanied by posterior compression can lead to acute facet impingement.

Hyperflexion is accompanied by anterior translation of a vertebra on the one below it. It may also include anterior compression and posterior traction, with the following consequences.

1. Anterior compression can cause fracture of the vertebral body.
2. Posterior traction can result in sprain or tearing of the supraspinal ligaments, interspinal ligaments, or posterior longitudinal ligaments.
3. Anterior glide can cause capsular tears of the articulation with or without facet subluxation or dislocation. This translation is also associated with foraminal narrowing and possible nerve root impingement.
4. Rarely, hyperflexion can cause posterior disk herniation. This injury is most often associated with rotational forces or horizontal shear forces at the time of impact.

Strains, sprains, and tears of the muscles, ligaments, tendons and capsules can all contribute to myofascial pain reflexes. They cause alterations in the function of bony articulations. They also lead to gross, usually palpable restrictions of vertebral motion.

After the acute injury, scar tissue forms in the overstretched tissues. Chronic pain and joint disability ensue as a result of osteophyte formation, traumatic arthritis, bony overgrowth, and synovitis at intervertebral joints. Delayed disk degeneration is often observed.

PERIPHERAL NERVES

Peripheral nerves can be injured anywhere along their course. Impingement on the nerve roots as they exit the vertebral foramina occurs during subluxation, dislocation, and facet synovitis. Other nerve injuries can occur:

1. Acutely, when the nerve is irritated as it pierces contracted or inflamed musculature or fascia
2. Chronically, as perineural scar tissue forms
3. As part of a neurovascular compression syndrome (usually scalenius anticus, hyperabduction, or costoclavicular).

A significant example of peripheral nerve irritation is seen in the occipital region. The intricate musculature in the suboccipital region and the torque forces sustained during impact make this area especially vulnerable to extensive muscle strain. The greater and lesser occipital nerves as well as the suboccipital nerve (C1–C2) pierce these tissues. Irritation of these nerves causes much of the cephalgia and neck pain experienced by whiplash victims.

Conversely, injury to the deep anterior structures of the neck is likely to cause brachial plexus damage. The plexus passes laterally between the anterior and middle scalene muscles. Plexus injury can result from stretching (extension, contralateral lateral flexion) during impact or from hypertonicity and inflammation of the scalenes.

SYMPATHETIC NERVOUS SYSTEM

Sympathetic nervous system symptoms are common after whiplash injuries. No sympathetic fibers are found in the intermediolateral cell column of the cervical spine. The cervical nerves are connected to the sympathetic nervous system via preganglionic fibers that arise in the lateral horn cells from T1 to T6. These fibers proceed up the sympathetic chain to enter the cervical ganglia and synapse with postganglionic fibers.

The inferior cervical ganglion is usually fused with the superior thoracic ganglion, in which case it is referred to as the cervicothoracic or stellate ganglion. It lies at the level of the superior border of the first rib, just anterior to C7. Some postganglionic fibers join the seventh and eighth cervical nerves to supply the blood vessels, sweat glands, and piloerector muscles of the upper extremity. The inferior cervical ganglion also sends branches to the heart.

The middle cervical ganglion lies anterior to the vertebral artery at about the level of the transverse process of C6. Postganglionic fibers pass to the fifth and sixth cervical nerves. Some fibers are also sent to the heart and thyroid gland.

The superior cervical ganglion lies at the level of the atlantoaxial joint. Some postganglionic fibers accompany the internal carotid and ophthalmic arteries into the orbit, where they supply the dilator muscles and smooth muscle of the upper lid. Other fibers accompany the external carotid artery to supply glands of the head and face. The superior cervical ganglion also contributes fibers to the first four cervical nerves.

A final path the sympathetic fibers in the cervical region can take is in the form of the vertebral nerve. Postganglionic fibers accompany the vertebral arteries and enter the skull to supply the vestibular portion of the ear, certain cranial nerves, and the pharynx.

Sympathetic symptoms can occur as a result of stimulation of peripheral nerves (containing sympathetic nerves) as they pierce inflamed soft tissue, stimulation of sensory elements of C1 and C2, simultaneous sympathetic irritation during nerve root compression in its foraminal passage, and compression of the vertebral artery. Sympathetic symptoms can be aural (tinnitus, deafness, postural dizziness), ocular (blurred vision, retrobulbar pain, and a pupil that dilates when the head is turned and returns to normal in the neutral position), vestibular (vertigo), and others, such as miosis, rhinorrhea, sweating, lacrimation, photophobia.

VASCULAR

Vascular compromise often occurs as a result of vertebral artery compression or spasm. The vertebral artery can be compressed anywhere along its course as it passes through the foramina in the transverse processes of the cervical spine. However, compression most often occurs at the levels of C1 and C2. The prevalence of compression here is due to the susceptibility of the region to injury and to the acute turn the artery makes as it enters the skull. Vertigo, syncope, near syncope, or nystagmus on rotation of the head are highly suggestive of vertebral artery compromise.

CEREBRAL

Patients with inertial injuries may also sustain cerebral concussion. This is most likely the result of the impact of the brain against the vault during rapid flexion and extension of the neck. Although head trauma is not necessary for concussion to occur, its presence makes the diagnosis more likely. The patient usually describes a "blinding" or "exploding" sensation in the head at the time of impact, followed immediately by headache, restlessness, insomnia, or mood change.

Factors Affecting Degree of Injury

Individuals subjected to identical forces may sustain different injuries or have different courses of recovery. A number of variables, including both the mechanics of the impact and the individual's condition at the time of the accident, determine the type and degree of injury sustained. Among these factors are the following.

1. **Force of impact:** The severity of injury is directly related to the force of impact. The force of impact is determined by the size of the offending vehicle and the speed at the time of impact.
2. **Position of the head:** Quite often, at the time of impact the victim has his head turned, to speak to someone or to look in the mirror. Head rotation at the time of impact increases the severity of the injury sustained and predisposes to greater injury on the side of the neck toward which the head is turned, for the following reasons:
   a. Rotation of the spine results in narrowing of the intervertebral foramen on the side to which the head is turned. This increases the likelihood of unilateral nerve root compression on that side.
   b. Rotation of the head greatly reduces the physiologic range of extension in the cervical spine. This increases the chance that the physiologic range of extension will be exceeded at impact, producing tissue damage.
   c. Many authorities believe that vertebral fracture and intervertebral disk herniation are more likely to occur when rotation accompanies flexion and extension at the time of impact.
3. **Position of the hands:** Bracing the hands against the steering wheel reduces anterior translation of the body, thereby reducing cervical injury but increasing the probability of injury to the shoulders, ribs, and thoracic region.
4. **Awareness of impending accident:** When the victim is aware that impact is about to occur, he may tense his muscles, in this manner reducing the pendular action of the head and the subsequent tissue damage.
5. **Head rests:** Properly adjusted head rests at the level of the occiput reduce hyperextension and the recoil into flexion by reducing the stretch reflex. This greatly decreases the severity of injury.
6. **Preexisting conditions:** Preexisting medical conditions (e.g., degenerative joint disease, osteoporosis) and previous trauma increase the likelihood of injuries such as fractures or nerve root impingement.

The Scope of Whiplash Injury

From an osteopathic viewpoint, the body is a unit mechanism, and all parts are deranged in a whiplash injury. This discussion considers the widespread effects of whiplash injury.

SACRAL INJURY

Injury to the sacrum occurs simultaneously with injury to the cervical and thoracic regions. These sacral dysfunctions apparently serve to maintain disability in cases that fail to respond to therapy (Becker, 1961).

The anterior longitudinal ligament fastens to the basiocciput, runs anterior to the bodies of the cervical vertebrae, and then attaches to the anterior vertebral bodies from T2 to the second sacral segment. The posterior longitudinal ligament extends from the occiput to the coccyx. Posteriorly, the supraspinal and interspinal ligaments and the ligamentum nuchae connect the spinous process. The dura is firmly attached at the basiocciput and the first two cervical vertebrae, then continues down the spinal canal without attachments until it reaches the anterior aspect of the second sacral segment, where it is again attached.

During cervical hyperflexion and hyperextension, the continuity of the various muscular, ligamentous, and dural attachments causes the sacrum to be forcibly lifted and dislodged from its floating position between the ilia. On rebound the sacrum lodges at varying degrees between the ilia. Locking invariably results in restriction of the involuntary flexion-extension movements of the sacrum in relation to the craniosacral mechanism. Craniosacral restriction may be accompanied by gross lumbosacral and sacroiliac dysfunctions (e.g., unilateral sacral flexion, sacral torsion).

The diagnostic and therapeutic consequences are several:

1. Freedom of voluntary sacral motion depends on freedom of craniosacral motion. Thus, the unilateral sacral flexion or sacral torsion cannot be successfully treated until the craniosacral mechanism has been restored.
2. Restriction of sacral motion locks the entire craniosacral mechanism, preventing it from carrying out its healing and life-sustaining functions. Restriction of craniosacral function can result in pain, fatigue, and disability of the whole body.
3. Loss of sacral motion places greater stress on the already injured tissues of the cervical and thoracic regions, hindering the self-reparative process. In essence, sacral dysfunction disturbs the body's balance and homeostatic mechanism, which hinders the healing process.

PELVIC INJURY

Iliosacral lesions are common after motor vehicle accidents. They are most frequently associated with having one foot planted, as when the driver sharply depresses the brake pedal at the time of impact. Both iliac rotations and superior pubic shears are observed. The paravertebral muscles of the spine and the latissimus dorsi attach to the iliac crests. Therefore, movements of the spine and shoulder girdle operate against the resistance of the locked ilium.

THORACIC AND LUMBAR INJURY

Many anatomic factors promote thoracic and lumbar dysfunction after whiplash injury. First, the continuity of the cervical, thoracic, and lumbar spine that is provided by the ligamentous attachments and paravertebral musculature transmits the acute strain to the thoracic and lumbar region. Second, lateral and rotary forces are experienced in the thoracic and lumbar region, which results in alteration of the normal anteroposterior and lateral curves, narrowing of the intervertebral foramina, and establishment of somatic dysfunctions. Third, the thoracic spine's proximity to the cervical spine and its intimate relationship with the muscles of the shoulder girdle make it especially susceptible to dysfunction. Special attention should be given to the upper thoracic region and the upper ribs.

CRANIAL INJURY

Dysfunctions of the cranium are almost invariably present after whiplash injuries. As a rule, the occiput and sacrum exhibit the same restriction (e.g., flexion or extension, to the right or left). The same forces that act on the cervical spine act on the cranium. Asymmetric traction by muscles that attach to the cranium can result in torsions and side bending or rotary dysfunctions. The temporal bones are especially vulnerable to these forces. Strain patterns are usually present if the victim's head has struck any object.

UPPER EXTREMITY INJURY

Injury to the upper extremity usually results from having the hand braced against an immovable object, such as the steering wheel or dashboard. Injuries usually involve the soft tissues of the shoulder—the glenohumeral capsule, the acromioclavicular and coracoclavicular ligaments, the rotator cuff muscles, and the trapezius. Tender points and fascial strains are common in the supraspinatus, trapezius, and latissimus dorsi muscles.

Pain radiating down the arm, with or without weakness or parethesias, does not necessarily indicate foraminal nerve root compression. It can be secondary to peripheral nerve irritation, neurovascular compression of the brachial plexus, or sympathetic nervous system irritation (referred pain). A careful neurologic and structural examination should be performed to uncover the cause.

Localized dysfunctions of the hands, wrists, and elbows may also occur.

LOWER EXTREMITY INJURY

The lower extremity can be involved in whiplash injury, exhibiting pain and decreased range of motion of various articulations secondary to sacral and ilial dysfunction, iliopsoas strains, and strain or sprain of the hip, knee, foot, and ankle. Hip and pelvic fractures are quite common if the victim's foot was firmly planted at the time of impact.

THORACIC, ABDOMINAL, AND PELVIC CAVITY INJURY

Fascial connections with the deep cervical fascia make the mediastinum and abdominal diaphragm susceptible to fascial strain. Fascial strain can limit thoracic visceral function and weaken the structures supporting the abdominal viscera. Sacral and ilial restrictions can weaken the support of the pelvic viscera and cause strains in the pelvic diaphragm. Contractures of the abdominal and pelvic diaphragms impede lymphatic and venous return, creating visceral congestion.

Symptoms

The whiplash patient often has no immediate pain and refuses medical treatment at the scene of the accident. A few hours later she may experience minor pain and stiffness in the neck and back. By the following day, sufficient edema and inflammation have accumulated to increase the severity of the pain and stiffness. Pain may be felt in the anterior or posterior aspect of the neck and radiating to the occiput, one or both shoulders, and the midthoracic region. The pain may radiate down either or both arms and may or may not be accompanied by numbness, weakness, and paresthesias.

Headaches are usually occipital but may radiate to the frontal region. Occasionally they are frontal or retrobulbar; rarely, they are bitemporal.

Other symptoms may not be evident for a few days to two or three weeks. These may include symptoms caused by involvement of the sympathetic nervous system, vascular impairment, dysphagia, nausea, vomiting, fatigue, low back pain, temporomandibular joint dysfunction, and severe emotional and psychological symptoms.

The multiple areas of body involvement, the

potential severity, and the variety of symptom complexes that may develop mandate a comprehensive history and physical examination in the patient with whiplash injury, even if the original complaints seem minor.

Treatment

Treatment of whiplash injuries is individualized for each patient, by stage of recovery and with consideration for the patient's total health needs. Common pitfalls in treatment are treating only the cervical and upper thoracic regions, and overtreating injured tissues. It must be remembered that the body has sustained tissue injury and the physician only aids the body's own reparative mechanisms. Extensive therapy may exceed the point of restoration of health and add to the injury.

This section presents guidelines and suggestions for a treatment regimen based on the severity and time of the patient's injury. The stages are not well demarcated, and the time frames are only guidelines. A patient's course of recovery will vary according to the severity of the injury, preexisting conditions, and the individual patient's physiology. Furthermore, many patients are first seen long after the onset of the injury. Delay before initiation of treatment greatly alters recovery time. The most accurate way to assess the patient's condition is with a comprehensive history and physical examination.

The treatments described below fit into the following three classifications: (1) osteopathic manipulative treatment, (2) adjunctive therapy (thermal, physical, and pharmacologic modalities), and (3) physical activities. Each category is reviewed separately for acute, early chronic, and late chronic stages of injury.

ACUTE STAGE (THREE TO FIVE DAYS)

The acute phase of whiplash injury is characterized by acute muscle contraction and moderate to severe limitation of motion. Tissues often are warm and edematous. Occasionally ecchymosis is present. Pain is usually confined to the neck and upper thoracic area, with or without radiation to the skull, shoulders, and upper extremities. Low back pain, dysphagia, and sympathetic nervous system symptoms may be present.

A patient seen immediately after injury may exhibit no signs or symptoms. This is not a reason to withhold therapy. On the contrary, proper treatment initiated early may greatly reduce the edema and resultant incapacitation.

Osteopathic Manipulative Treatment
Osteopathic manipulation should be instituted as soon as possible after the patient has been stabilized. The goals are to minimize edema and tissue reaction. The treatment is gentle, indirect, and perilesional, i.e., it addresses areas adjacent to the injured tissues.

A useful approach is to restore respiratory motion in both the cranium and the sacrum, followed by treatment of the pelvis and voluntary sacral motion. Myofascial release or muscle energy therapy is commonly employed. If the patient cannot cooperate or cannot be positioned for muscle energy therapy, the pelvis can be treated positionally either with fascial release (using the lower extremities) or with counterstrain techniques. Sacral motion in the incapacitated patient may be induced by sacral rocking, similar to the method described for the obstetric patient later in this chapter. This is followed by treatment of the lumbar and thoracic regions. Treatment should be restricted to soft tissue techniques. If the patient is bedridden, the physician may treat the spinal areas by placing her hands under the patient and applying steady pressure with her fingertips against the paravertebral muscles. Specific techniques are described in Chapters 9, 11, 14, and 17.

A major purpose of manipulation is to restore circulation. Many experienced clinicians avoid vigorous manipulation of acutely inflamed areas, believing that the increased blood flow may increase hemorrhage and fluid leak, thus causing more damage. Perilesional treatment may divert blood flow from the injured tissues to those in adjacent areas. This, combined with gentle lymphatic drainage of injured areas, may reduce the edema.

Manipulation of acutely injured areas should be both gentle and brief. It entails (1) indirect treatment of soft tissues in the cervical and upper thoracic region, (2) passive range of motion exercises, and (3) lymphatic drainage. Gentle occipital traction is useful and well tolerated. Tender points in the occipital region, sternocleidomastoid, levator scapulae, and rhomboids should be sought and treated.

The anterior neck is best treated by counter-strain techniques applied to the anterior tender points and by fascial release of the hyoid bone. Passive range of motion therapy should be instituted without creating pain.

Adjunctive Therapy
1. **Thermal.** Ice packs or ice massage (seven minutes each hour) should be instituted for the first 18 hours after injury, followed by heat therapy, dry or moist. Moist heat may be used at home. Ultrasound or diathermy have also been recommended any time after the initial 48 hours of injury.
2. **Immobilization.** The whiplash injury is a sprain/strain injury. For this reason, many clinicians recommend using a cervical collar, with the following stipulations:
   a. It is used only when acute inflammation is evident.
   b. It must be properly applied, usually with the spine in slight flexion.
   c. Its use should be limited to the acute period. Prolonged use results in muscle atrophy and disability. As the patient improves, the hours of wear should be reduced. First the patient wears the collar only while sleeping and driving, then only while sleeping.
3. **Traction.** Mechanical or manual traction should be used only if the patient obtains relief with its use. Mechanical traction is begun with a light weight (6 to 8 lb) that is slowly increased as the patient improves.
4. **Pharmacologic therapy.** Nonsteroidal anti-inflammatory drugs may be useful during the acute inflammatory stage. A lower analgesic dose can be prescribed once the inflammation has been controlled.

Physical Activity
Severely injured patients should be placed on bed rest for at least two to three days. If they feel better after this period, they may begin limited activity. If they have not improved, they should stay in bed for the remainder of the week. Passive exercises may be started in bed to avoid tissue atrophy.

Patients not confined to bed should be encouraged to begin limited activities immediately as tolerated. Passive range of motion exercises can be performed daily. Patients should also be instructed in which activities to avoid (e.g., rapid turning of the head).

EARLY CHRONIC PHASE
(ONE WEEK TO ONE MONTH)

Acute inflammation has subsided but increased tissue tension remains. Range of motion has improved. Pain is usually still present but is not as acute. Radiation of pain may still be present. Sympathetic nervous system symptoms may have begun or persist.

Osteopathic Manipulative Treatment

More aggressive treatment may now be employed. It is useful to treat in the same order as during the acute phase, but direct techniques may be added. Muscle energy techniques as well as high velocity, low amplitude thrusting techniques directed toward the lumbar and thoracic region may be tolerated. The cervical spine should be treated with muscle energy techniques and more vigorous lymphatic drainage techniques, in addition to occipital release, counterstrain therapy, and fascial release. Direct thrusting techniques to the cervical region should be avoided. Careful attention is paid to the cranium, sacrum, and anterior neck. Active myofascial treatment for range of motion may be instituted.

Adjunctive Therapy

1. **Thermal.** Moist heat, ultrasound, and diathermy may be continued.
2. **Immobilization.** A cervical collar should be minimal if at all.
3. **Pharmacologic therapy.** Nonsteroidal anti-inflammatory agents may be continued in analgesic dosage if necessary.
4. **Physical modalities.** Electrical muscle stimulation is often useful to induce muscle relaxation.

Physical Activity

The patient should be walking and at close to or full activity. The patient should be encouraged to increase his cervical range of motion exercises. Both active and passive isometric resistance can be added if tolerated. He should also begin range of motion exercises as needed for other spinal regions. Weight lifting is to be avoided.

LATE CHRONIC PHASE (ONE TO THREE MONTHS OR LONGER)

Mild pain with or without radiation is all that remains. There may be residual limitation in range of motion, especially in the neck or upper extremities. Tissue changes are usually chronic in nature.

Osteopathic Manipulative Treatment

Treatment includes the whole body. High velocity, low amplitude thrusting techniques may now be employed in the cervical region. A good practice is to begin with soft tissue techniques, then position the neck and spring it a few times. If this does not cause pain, the thrust may be performed. If springing causes pain, thrusting should not be performed. Vigorous, active range of motion therapy should be employed.

Adjunctive Therapy

Adjunctive therapy is similar to that in the early chronic phase, with the following differences:

1. Electrical stimulation should be adjusted to stimulate the muscle and thus decrease atrophy.
2. Trigger point therapy may be employed, using either vapocoolant sprays, deep pressure, or injection of a local anesthetic.
3. Physical therapy is begun to strengthen the extremities and improve aerobic capacity.

Physical Activity

The patient should be encouraged to work toward full activity. He participates in physical therapy, as previously described.

Emotional Support

Throughout the recovery process, the patient should be given strong emotional support. The following are guidelines for the physician.

1. Explain the injury and describe the plan of treatment.
2. Empathize with the patient's incapacity.
3. Encourage the patient and point out progress.
4. Describe the prognosis fully, in language that the patient understands. Do not guarantee results.
5. Set goals that are realistic. Review these goals with the patient as the treatment progresses.

HEADACHES
Donald Hankinson

Headache is commonly seen by physicians in general practice. According to the *Cecil Textbook of Medicine,* headache is the ninth most common reason for visiting a physician. In a New York Hospital study, 46% of patients in the hospital complained of headache.

The causes of headache are many and varied and include muscle tension, migraine, sinus congestion, trauma, hypertension, premenstrual syndrome, tumors, and meningitis. The vast majority of headaches are due to muscle tension or migraine. A 28-year study at the Headache Unit of Montefiore Hospital found that 90% of patients had either migraine, tension headaches, or a combination of the two. Even head pain usually attributed to other causes, most notably sinus congestion and mild hypertension, are thought by some clinicians to be misdiagnosed tension or migraine headaches. Although standard textbooks of medicine agree on a musculoskeletal pathologic basis for cephalgia, this factor is rarely considered in the diagnosis or treatment of headache.

This section explores the role of the musculoskeletal system in the pathogenesis, diagnosis, and treatment of migraine and tension headaches.

Pathogenesis

The brain itself is almost totally insensitive to pain. Extracranially, the pain-sensitive structures are the scalp, arteries, muscles, mucous membranes of the sinuses, external and middle ear, and the teeth. The musculoskeletal pathogensis of tension headaches is fairly straightforward. According to Cecil's *Textbook of Medicine,* "The contracting muscles or nerves supplying them may release vasoactive substances such as lactate, serotonin, bradykinin and prostaglandins which lower the pain threshold." The crucial area here is the suboccipital and upper cervical area. In the upper two cervical segments the sensory fibers of the first three cervical segments are joined by the descending tracts of cranial nerves V, IX, and X. These three cranial nerves, along with the second cervical nerve, mediate the referral of excessive connective tissue tension in the cervical area, as pain in the cranial vault, or cephalgia.

Intracranially, only the dura and large arteries at the base of the skull, the dural arteries, and the venous sinuses are sensitive to pain. Guyton states that the pain of migraines is secondary either to stretching of the dura at the cranial base, tugging on the venous sinuses, or damage to the tentorium. This prolonged tension causes a reflex vasospasm. The ischemia that develops results in loss of vascular tone for as long as 48 hours. The subsequent excessive stretching of the arteries causes the actual pain of a migraine. Biochemical substances, specifically norepinephrine (increased) and serotonin (decreased), are postulated to mediate the vasodilatory and vasoconstrictive phases, but their role remains speculative. What is known is that connective tissue stresses that cause tension or drag on dural structures create an environment for the development of migraines. Thus, headache is part of an evolving process, not an isolated event. In both migraine and tension headache, excessive tonus of connective tissue structures is a primary etiologic factor.

Evaluation

How should the osteopathic physician approach the patient with headache? A complete history is essential to determine whether a tension or migraine headache is present or whether further diagnostic workup is necessary to evaluate the possibility of a less common, potentially more ominous etiology. These two types of headaches have rather characteristic presentations, which, in allopathic medical practice, form the basis of diagnosis.

Tension headaches are bilateral, are usually preceded by emotionally stressful situations, and worsen as the day progresses. The pain is described as a constant tight pressure encircling the head like a hat band. The pain may last for weeks, months, or years. It remits with alcohol ingestion but is often unchanged with rest. Migraine is often preceded by an aura consisting of sensory, motor, and mood changes. The pain is usually mechanisms. One study in animals found an increase in type I oxidative fibers on the convex side of scoliotic curves. However, it is unclear whether this finding is part of the neuromuscular dysfunction or a secondary development. The results of many other studies in animals and humans indicate that the etiology is probably multifactorial, and the condition is partially hereditary.

Denslow and Korr state that "[t]he osteopathic lesion represents a hyperexcitable segment of the spinal cord through which impulses are channelled into muscles receiving innervation from that segment." If these segments persist, proprioceptive nerve endings in the peripheral muscles and joints could be maintained under continuous bombardment. This continuous stimulation could lead to increased muscle tension, and the segment would eventually be less able to withstand the stresses of daily living. Such persistent lesions could be a factor in the etiology of scoliosis.

Clinical Findings

Scoliosis can be divided into *structural* and *functional* groups; some curves have features of both. A structural curve does not correct on lateral bending of the trunk. This type of curve is relatively fixed and inflexible. There are changes in bone symmetry, with shortened ligaments and muscles on the concave side of the curve. Structural curves can occur due to fracture of the vertebrae, congenital anomalies, or soft tissue trauma such as burns or irradiation.

Functional curves can be partially or completely straightened by lateral bending in the opposite direction. Functional curves may be either *postural* or *compensatory*. Postural curves are slight deviations in a normal spine that correct voluntarily and disappear with movement. Compensatory curves are a manifestation of an underlying dysfunction that produces a lateral curve. A short leg produces a compensatory spinal curve. Uncorrected functional curves eventually develop a structural component.

Some 80% of all structural scoliotic curves are idiopathic. This condition is thought to be inherited in autosomal dominant fashion with incomplete penetrance. Idiopathic scoliosis is commonly divided into infantile, juvenile, and adolescent kinds. *Infantile idiopathic scoliosis* occurs from birth to three years of age. It is more

common in boys and in Europeans. Potential causes include molding in utero, injury to the skull during birth, or cranial asymmetry caused by laying babies in cribs on their sides. However, none of these causes has been demonstrated experimentally. Infantile idiopathic scoliosis usually resolves spontaneously.

Juvenile scoliosis occurs from four to ten years of age. It may represent a late infantile form of scoliosis that resolves or a more serious form that persists into adolescence.

Adolescent idiopathic scoliosis occurs from age ten until skeletal maturity. It is often present at an earlier age but remains unnoticed until the adolescent growth spurt occurs. This form of idiopathic scoliosis is the most significant and prevalent form and can become progressively worse during the growth spurt.

Idiopathic curves can occur at any area in the spine. Five of the most common curves are listed below:

1. Right thoracic curve
2. Right thoracolumbar curve
3. Double major curve—usually right thoracic, left lumbar
4. Lumbar curve
5. Cervicothoracic curve

The right thoracic curve is usually highly structural and the ribs can have increased angles on the convex side. This curve can develop quickly and requires early intervention to achieve a functional and cosmetic outcome. When a thoracic curve reaches 70 degrees, there can be significant cardiopulmonary dysfunction. The right thoracolumbar curve is usually less disruptive and cosmetically deforming but can cause severe rib and flank distortion due to rotation. The lumbar major curve can be very rigid, causing severe pain and dysfunction during childbirth and leading to arthritic changes later in life.

The remaining 20% of structural scolioses (nonidiopathic) occur secondary to congenital anomalies, neuromuscular diseases, tumors, trauma, infections, and iatrogenic causes. Congenital scoliosis occurs due to malformation of spinal elements or the development of bony bridges over growth areas. There are open and closed vertebral forms. Meningomyelocoele and spina bifida are two examples of the open form. In these closed parts of vertebrae are unfused or missing altogether. The closed vertebral forms are various, some bizarre. There can be failure of vertebral formation, in which hemivertebrae form, or failure of segmentation, in which unilateral and bilateral bars form. Hemivertebrae cause severe curves because they tend to grow. Unilateral bars and hemivertebrae are the worst combination; they progress rapidly until spinal fusion is needed.

Neuromuscular scoliosis occurs secondary to muscle weakness and imbalance caused by central or peripheral nervous system disease. These scolioses can be divided into neuropathic and myopathic forms. The neuropathic form is due to central nervous system dysfunction and damage. Some examples are poliomyelitis, cerebral palsy, and syringomyelia. The myopathic form includes muscular dystrophy, amyotonia congenita, and Friedreich's ataxia.

The neuromuscular scolioses are generally relentlessly progressive. Victims have decreased respiratory function due to the scoliosis and respiratory muscle weakness. Their scolioses are difficult to manage because of multiple anomalies and medical problems.

Traumatic scoliosis can occur secondary to fracture in which the epiphyseal growth plate is injured, causing asymmetric growth of the vertebrae. Irradiation of the thorax or abdomen can cause similar damage to the growth plate. Wedge fractures in older persons can also cause slight curve formation.

Scoliosis capitis is probably caused by persistent malfunction of the occiput secondary to the stress of labor and delivery. The occipital dysfunction causes cranial obliquity with flattening on one side of the face and increased roundness on the opposite side. The sacrum and pelvis assume the same obliquity and increase the scoliotic tendency.

OSTEOPATHIC NOTES
The body always tries to keep the eyes level. If for whatever reason there is a curve in the spine, the compensatory curves will form to keep the body balanced.

Scoliosis is not just pure lateral flexion, there is also a significant rotational component. The vertebrae involved follow Fryette's first law of vertebral motion. That is, in the neutral position, adjacent vertebrae rotate and side bend in opposite directions. The ribs follow the vertebral motion. The ribs on the convex side separate and

move posteriorly, producing the rib hump noted in scoliosis. The ribs on the concave side move closer together and anterior. Rotational stresses in scoliosis occur with enough force to deform the vertebral body. Disk spaces are narrowed on the concave side of the curve. The vertebral body tends to be wedged and thickened on the concave side of the curve. The vertebral canal may also be narrowed on the convex side of the curve.

The body changes follow Wolf's law, according to which the bony shapes and internal structures reflect the habitual stresses that have acted on the plastic osseous tissue. The changes that occur in a scoliotic patient with growth follow the Hueter-Volkman principle. The three basic parts of this principle are:

1. Increased pressure on a vertebral growth plate retards growth.
2. The less pressured side of the plate grows more.
3. This unequal growth influences the endochondral ossification and causes wedging.

The change from a functional to a structural scoliosis also follows this principle. There are progressive soft tissue shortening, body changes, and disk degeneration. The ligaments and fascia become more fibrotic, and there is decreased active and passive range of motion.

Diagnosis and Evaluation
Certain clues in the history may help establish the diagnosis. Although back pain is a rare symptom in children, 40% to 80% of adults with scoliosis may present with back pain. The pain is usually mild to moderate and worse at the end of the work day or after strenuous activity. The area of pain is variable but is often at the apex or junction of a curve. In a child, the parents may have noticed a round back or shoulders, or prominence of one hip. The patient may complain of difficulty in fitting a hem or sleeve lengths.

The physical examination begins with observation of the patient's gait. Observe for patterns indicating asymmetric pelvic rotation or drop which may indicate a short leg. Examine the patient from the back, sides, and front. Any asymmetry of the neck musculature or unequal scapular angle level is noted. Decide if the trunk seems to be balanced over the pelvis. If a plumb line dropped from the inion does not divide the body in half, the scoliosis is probably more severe. Look for a rib hump, unilateral muscle prominence, an asymmetric waist crease, or an unequal distance between the arms and trunk.

Ask the patient to bend forward from the hips with the knees extended. Observe the patient's back at eye level from in back and in front. A rib hump will become more prominent in this position. The rib hump represents posterior rotation of the spine and ribs on the side of the convexity of the curve. A curve with 10 degrees of angulation can be detected visually.

Assess the flexibility of the curve by having the patient side bend without flexing forward. Mark how far down the lateral leg the patient can reach. Functional curves are more flexible, but it is not uncommon for a structural curve to have a functional component.

The degree of chest wall flexibility should also be examined. Place both hands over the ribs and note any asymmetry of inspiration or expiration. A cardiopulmonary assessment should be considered in severe scoliosis or in any patient with signs of cor pulmonale, dyspnea on exertion, or repeated bouts of respiratory illness. This should include an electrocardiogram to look for right ventricular hypertrophy, and baseline pulmonary function studies.

Radiographic studies are used to determine the type and magnitude of the spinal curve. Scoliosis patients tend to receive a large amount of radiation in the course of a lifetime, so each study should yield maximum information with minimum radiation. Standing PA films on 30 × 90 cm cassettes have been suggested. The initial study can also include a lateral radiograph to determine the degree of kyphosis and lordosis of the spine.

The magnitude of the curve is generally measured by the Cobb method:

1. Locate the vertebral bodies at the extreme ends of the curve. The top of the superior vertebrae and the bottom of the inferior vertebrae tilt toward each other more than the other vertebrae.
2. Draw horizontal lines from the top of the superior vertebrae and the bottom of the inferior vertebrae into the concavity of the curve.
3. Drop intersecting perpendicular lines from the horizontal lines and measure the acute angles.

There is a great deal of controversy as to how often a curve should be reassessed. Curves of less than 10 degrees should be reevaluated in six months to a year. Curves of more than 10 degrees should be reexamined in four to six months. Curves of more than 20 degrees should be examined at four-month intervals.

Progression of 5 degrees or more is an indication for treatment. Curves of more than 30 degrees should be treated. A curve of less than 20 degrees in a skeletally mature adult usually will not progress, but the patient should be followed if she is symptomatic because she is at greater risk for degenerative disk disease and back strain. Skeletally mature adults with curves of 20 degrees or more should ideally be followed up at one- to two-year intervals.

Progression of a scoliotic curve is defined as an increase of greater than 5 degrees of curve magnitude between two visits. Bracing with either the Milwaukee brace or the Boston brace (molded orthosis) effectively prevents progression in about 90% of cases.

Treatment

Transcutaneous electrical nerve stimulation is used at night to involuntarily contract the paraspinal musculature on the convex side. The effectiveness of this treatment is inconclusive; some studies show improvement and some failure.

Nonoperative treatment consists of braces, active and passive stimulation, and exercise. There is a great deal of controversy as to whether exercise is beneficial in conjunction with other treatment modalities such as bracing to preserve muscle tone and keep the correction. The exercises should stress pelvic tilt, trunk shifting, and flexibility. Noncontact sports such as swimming are also beneficial.

Surgery is considered if bracing does not prevent progression or if the curve is greater than 50 degrees on initial evaluation. The most common reason for surgical correction is to prevent the cardiopulmonary complications of severe scoliosis. The most commonly used device is the Harrington rod.

Osteopathic manipulation should be aimed at increasing the intrinsic sustaining forces of the musculoskeletal system. This can be done by using active and passive techniques to increase muscle balance on both sides of the curve. The technique used depends on the physician's expertise and experience. Muscle energy and fascial release will increase muscle balance and relieve stress caused by muscle spasm and contracture. High velocity, low amplitude techniques can be used to correct specific acute somatic dysfunctions that occur in the curve. Craniosacral techniques can be used to alleviate strain patterns that occur in the cranium and sacrum secondary to the scoliosis or primary patterns that may have precipitated formation of the scoliosis.

The prognosis of untreated scolioses depends on many factors such as age, sex, skeletal maturity, and curve magnitude. About 75% percent of all scolioses progress, so the likelihood of spontaneous remission is low. Girls generally progress more often than boys. The larger the curve at ini-

tial diagnosis, the more progression is to be expected. Curves may also progress after skeletal maturity is achieved (Duiez, 1967). Certain patients who have had a compensated scoliosis throughout life may start to progress as they grow older.

The goals of the primary care physician in treating scoliosis are twofold. The first goal is to prevent severe scoliosis, which causes deformity and cardiopulmonary crowding, through early screening of children for scoliosis, with periodic rechecks. The second goal is to coordinate the treatment of the patient with scoliosis by making sure the patient gets thorough and adequate follow-up with timely referral to a specialist in the treatment of scoliosis where needed.

THORACIC OUTLET SYNDROME
Eileen L. DiGiovanna

Thoracic outlet syndrome is an umbrella term for a complex of signs and symptoms of various causes. The common denominator is compression of nerves or vascular structures as they pass through the thoracic inlet, traverse the shoulder girdle and axilla, and begin their descent into the arm. The axillary artery or components of the brachial plexus may be compressed.

Symptoms of nerve compression are pain or dysesthesia of the upper extremity. Arterial compression results in typical ischemic signs and symptoms whose severity depends on the degree of compression. These manifestations may include coldness, pallor, cyanosis, and occasionally Raynaud's phenomenon. The anatomic location of the veins in this area protects them from the forces acting on the nerves and arteries, so venous compression is rarely a problem.

Etiology
The anatomy of the area may contribute to the development of thoracic outlet syndrome. The neurovascular structures must pass through several narrow passageways. Three passageways are of particular concern. One is the triangle formed by

the anterior and medial scalene muscles and the first rib, which provides a passageway for the subclavian artery and nerve plexus. The second is where the neurovascular bundle passes between the clavicle and the first rib. The third is along the border of the pectoralis minor near its attachment to the coracoid process as the neurovascular bundle passes between it and the rib cage. As the arm is hyperabducted, the pectoralis minor is pulled taut and may compress the neurovascular bundle against the rib cage.

There are numerous causes for narrowing of these areas. Some require orthopedic or neurosurgical treatment, such as cervical ribs (which may be asymptomatic), improperly healed clavicle or first rib fractures, aberrant muscle slips, and the like. However, many other causes of thoracic outlet syndrome are amenable to osteopathic manipulation. Tension in muscles and fascia may compromise the free passage of nerves and arteries. Restricted motion of joints in the area, particularly at the junction of the clavicle and first rib, may be a source of chronic pressure on these structures. Edema as a result of somatic dysfunction is another source of pressure. All of these causes respond to osteopathic manipulation.

Figure 29-1. Adson test.

Evaluation

Before treatment is initiated, a thorough assessment is necessary. The clinician must identify conditions that should be referred for specialist care and rule out conditions that produce referred pain, numbness, or parasthesia of the arm and hand. A differential diagnosis would include cervical root compression or radiculitis, Pancoast tumor, Sudek's dystrophy or shoulder-hand syndrome, and carpal tunnel syndrome. The patient should be examined for joint motion of the upper ribs, clavicles, and cervical and thoracic spine. Tissue tension should be assessed in the area of the thoracic inlet.

Depending on which structures are involved, impingement may occur in any of several patient positions. Several special tests have been designed to better localize the area of impingement.

1. **Adson test.** The patient's affected arm is abducted and the physician palpates the radial pulse. The patient is instructed to turn her head toward the affected side and extend the neck,

then take a deep breath (Fig. 29-1). The test is positive if the pulse disappears or diminishes or if the patient's symptoms are elicited. If nothing happens with this maneuver, the patient is asked to turn her head away from the affected arm.

2. **Spurling maneuver.** The Spurling maneuver is done with the patient seated. The physician applies a compressive force to the top of the patient's head (Fig. 29-2). Pain down the arm indicates that the problem is probably not thoracic outlet syndrome but rather a nerve root compression.

3. **Hyperabduction test.** As in the Adson test, the radial pulse is monitored. The patient's arm is elevated 180 degrees (Fig. 29-3). The test is positive if the pulse diminishes or if symptoms are elicited.

4. **Costoclavicular test.** The patient is asked to assume a "military" posture—chest out, shoulders back and down (Fig. 29-4). Again, the radial pulse is monitored. The test is positive if the pulse diminishes or if symptoms are elicited.

If the Adson test is positive but cervical rib radiographs are normal, the area of the scalenes should be examined. The osteopathic physician may be able to relieve the symptoms by gentle stretching and relaxation of the scalenes if they exhibit increased tension or fibrosis. Fibrous bands may also be stretched sufficiently to relieve some of the symptoms. The patient should be placed on an exercise program for use at home.

Figure 29-2. Spurling maneuver.

Figure 29-3. Hyperabduction test.

Figure 29-4. Costoclavicular test.

Stretching exercises rather than isometric exercises should be used if there is any evidence of muscle hypertrophy.

If hyperabduction of the arm is the problem, any abnormal tensions of the pectoralis muscles should be addressed. However, the patient will likely have to avoid holding the arm in this position for extended periods of time, as in painting ceilings or trimming trees.

If the patient sleeps with her arm over her head, awareness of the problem is usually sufficient to correct it. Some patients find it helpful to tie their wrist with a piece of gauze or nylon stocking that is long enough to allow motion but not long enough for the arm to be placed over the head.

Restrictions of the clavicle and first rib are commonly seen and quite responsive to manipulation. Any somatic dysfunction involving the clavicle, the first rib, the seventh cervical, vertebra, or the first thoracic vertebrae seems capable of producing thoracic outlet syndrome symptoms. Frequently such dysfunctions occur in combinations.

Structural motion in addition to tissue changes in the area should be assessed. The second thoracic vertebra and the second rib are commonly involved. Somatic dysfunctions must be diagnosed and corrected if the problem is to be solved.

Three motions should be restored to the clavicle: motion in abduction-adduction, flexion-extension, and longitudinal rotation. Both sternoclavicular joints should be examined. Articulation of these joints may be sufficient, or muscle energy techniques may be used.

The first rib may be examined by the clinician sitting at the head of the supine patient and placing his thumbs on the flat posterosuperior portion of the rib, then springing it gently. It may also be assessed by following its motion during inhalation and exhalation. Motion may be improved utilizing muscle energy techniques or high velocity, low amplitude thrusting techniques.

Any somatic dysfunctions involving the upper

thoracic area should be treated. The cervical spine should be assessed and treated to restore motion to all vertebrae.

After motion is restored to all ribs and vertebrae, it may be helpful to reevaluate the area for any fascial tensions or tender points which remain. These should be treated with fascial release or counterstrain. The removal of tender points seems to decrease proprioceptive overactivity which may recreate the former dysfunctions.

Stretching of any tight muscles or fibrous bands is helpful. The patient should be placed on an exercise program at home to continue stretching the muscles of the cervical and upper thoracic spine, pectorals, and shoulder girdle.

The patient's posture needs to be evaluated and corrected, since drooping shoulders, forward carriage of the head, and rounded thoracic spine may contribute to the problem.

LUMBAR RADICULOPATHIES
Barbara Polstein

The term *radiculopathy* refers to a disease process involving one or more spinal nerve roots. There are three common causes of lumbar radicular syndromes: herniated nucleus pulposus, central spinal stenosis, and lateral spinal stenosis. In addition, three pseudoradicular syndromes are frequently responsible for low back pain radiating to the buttock and lower extremity: posterior facet joint syndrome, sacroiliac joint syndrome, and piriformis and other myofascial syndromes. These pseudoradicular syndromes do not compress the spinal nerves. Their manifestations are often similar to those of true radiculopathies, they may occur alone or in combination with disk herniation or spinal stenosis, and they respond favorably to manipulative treatment.

Functional Anatomy
The basic functional unit of the spine is a three-joint complex—an intervertebral disk set between two vertebral bodies anteriorly, and two posterior facet joints. In the absence of pathology, this three-joint complex serves to house and protect the spinal cord, offers unhindered passage of the spinal nerve roots to the periphery, helps to disperse external forces during normal weight-bearing and more vigorous activity, and facilitates spinal motion. When the balance in this complex is lost, as it may be in degenerative diseases, its functions are compromised, often resulting in compression of one or more spinal nerve roots.

INTERVERTEBRAL DISKS
The intervertebral disks act as hydrolic shock absorbers. Each is composed of strong, concentrically arranged fibers, the annulus fibrosus, that enclose a gelatinous, mucopolysaccharide nucleus pulposus. Forces exerted on the disk are evenly distributed within the containment of the disk. The functions of the intervertebral disk are twofold: constant intradiskal pressure maintains separation of the two adjacent vertebrae, and mobility of the nucleus pulposus facilitates vertebral motion. For example, during flexion the nucleus pulposus moves posteriorly and during extension it moves anteriorly.

The loss of blood supply to the disk normally occurs between the ages of 20 and 30 years. In adults, the disk receives its nutrition by diffusion of solutes through the vertebral end-plates and by the imbibing properties of the nucleus pulposus. The annulus fibrosus attaches to the edges of hyaline cartilage of adjacent vertebral end-plates by the insertion of annular fibers. The disk is ensheathed by periosteum, which has two thickenings, the anterior and posterior longitudinal ligaments.

The annulus fibrosus is innervated by twigs of the recurrent sinovertebral nerve and by skeletal branches of the primary central rami. It contains both free (nocioceptive) nerve endings and complex surface receptors, thought by Bogduk to be used for proprioception.

Intervertebral disk degeneration is often initiated simply by wear and tear. Repeated microtrauma, especially when induced by rotational forces, further predisposes the disk to damage. Typically, circumferential tears appear in the outer portion of the annulus. The weakened annulus, no longer able to contain the nucleus pulposus under pressure, may bulge. After severe or repeated stress, circumferential tears may coalesce, forming a radial tear through which nuclear material can herniate. The loss of disk height with herniation disrupts normal joint function, initiating a cycle of progressive degeneration and joint instability.

POSTERIOR FACET JOINTS

Posterior facet joints are typical synovial joints formed by the inferior and superior facets. The articular capsule is richly innervated by twigs from the recurrent sinovertebral nerve and branches of the primary dorsal ramus of the mixed spinal nerve, each supplying at least two facet joints.

Kirkaldy-Willis often describes degenerative changes in the three-joint complex as occurring in three phases. Key to this model is the recognition that the posterior facet joints and intervertebral disk are intimately related. Instability of one, whether due to degenerative processes or trauma, will always affect the other. During the first phase, repeated microtrauma leads to synovitis and hypomobility of the posterior facet joints. Progression of this process produces instability and capsular laxity, with possible subluxation of the posterior joints. Stage three is heralded by an attempt at stability of the involved joints, accomplished by fibrosis and the formation of osteophytes. Osteophyte formation on the superior facets produces lateral stenosis, whereas osteophyte formation on the inferior facets limits the central canal.

Similar changes occur at the disk. These include annular tears with possible herniation, advanced disk degeneration, and osteophyte formation. The final result is spondylosis at one or more levels.

SPINAL NERVES

There are 31 pairs of spinal nerves; five are in the lumbar area. Each pair exits the spine through the intervertebral canal just below the vertebral body it is named for. Hence, a herniated L4-L5 disk compresses the L5 nerve root. The lumbar spinal nerve roots arise from a series of filaments that blend together to form distinct ventral and dorsal roots. These travel through the subarachnoid space until they exit at the intervertebral canal.

As the nerve roots traverse the subarachnoid space they acquire meningeal coverings—the pia mater, arachnoid, and finally dura mater. Just lateral to the dorsal root ganglion, the dural investments of the two nerve roots combine to form a common sheath around the mixed spinal nerve, and the dura mater becomes continuous with the epineurium. Proximal to the dorsal root ganglion, each of the mixed spinal nerves divides into a primary ventral ramus and a primary dorsal ramus. The primary ventral rami proceed to the lumbar or sacral plexus. They also send skeletal branches to the posterolateral and lateral aspects of the intervertebral disk, anterior longitudinal ligament, and periosteum.

The smaller primary dorsal rami have medial, intermediate, and lateral branches. The medial branch passes under the mammiloaccessory ligament on its way to the lumbar intrinsic muscles. Deep to the multifidus muscle a branch arises to supply sensory innervation to the interspinous ligament and posterior facet joints both above and below each branch. The intermediate branches supply the lumbar fibers of the longissimus muscles. The first through fourth lumbar primary dorsal rami innervate the iliocostalis muscles by their lateral branches. The first through third lateral branches continue past the iliac crest to provide sensation to the skin of the lateral buttock as far as the greater trochanter.

The recurrent sinovertebral nerve is formed by twigs from the anterior primary rami (somatic input) and the gray ramus communicantes (autonomic innervation). It reenters the intervertebral canal to innervate the posterior longitudinal ligament, posterior and posterolateral disk, anterior meninges, the nerve root sleeve as far as the intervertebral foramen, the ligamentum flavum, and the posterior facet joints.

Four large mixed nerves innervate the entire lower extremity. The second through fourth lumbar primary ventral rami, after exiting the intervertebral foramen, travel within the body of the psoas muscle and form the lumbar plexus with its two divisions. The obturator nerve (anterior division) innervates the hip adductors and the gracilis muscle; the femoral nerve (posterior division) innervates the hip flexors and knee extensors.

The lumbosacral plexus is formed by the primary ventral rami of the fourth and fifth lumbar nerves and the first through third sacral nerves. It also forms two large mixed nerves that are initially bound by a common sheath. The sciatic nerve exits the pelvis through the greater sciatic foramen. It travels beneath the piriformis muscle into the posterior thigh. Just proximal to the popliteal fossa, the common peroneal (posterior division) and tibial (anterior division) components of the sciatic nerve separate. The tibial nerve innervates the foot, ankle, and knee flexors; the common peroneal nerve supplies the toe and ankle extensors as well as ankle evertors by way of its superficial and deep branches.

Any of these nerves may become inflamed. The resulting peripheral neuritis is a potential source of confusion with the lower extremity pain, numbness, or paresthesias associated with a lumbar radiculopathy. Sciatic neuritis will be discussed in greater detail in the section on the piriformis syndrome.

Physical Examination

The diagnosis of lumbar radiculopathy is based on a thorough history and physical examination. Sciatica is not difficult to diagnose. However, accurate delineation of the etiology of the symptoms is not only challenging but is essential for an effective treatment plan. The physical examination outlined below is performed in conjunction with a routine physical examination, with special emphasis on the musculoskeletal and nervous systems.

GAIT

Observe the patient during the swing and stance phases of gait, looking for ease of motion. Note antalgia, ataxia, "simian gait," and signs of neurologic deficit such as foot drop. Have the patient walk on his toes and heels and squat to assess the S1, L5, and L4 nerve roots respectively.

STANDING

Observe static symmetry. Examine the lordotic and kyphotic curves. Is scoliosis present? Evaluate the gross range of motion in flexion, extension, side bending, and rotation. Perform a standing flexion test. Note any guarding or overdramatization of pain.

SEATED

Examiner in Front of the Patient

Test the deep tendon reflexes at L4 (patellar tendon) and S1 (Achilles tendon). Asymmetry may indicate neural compromise. With the patient seated, perform the 90-degree straight leg raising test. This is less obvious to the patient and should be compared with results on a supine straight leg raising test.

Generally assess the muscle strength of all lower extremity muscle groups. Note any asymmetry. The myotomes as described by Magee are L2—hip flexion, L3—knee extension, L4—ankle dorsiflexion and inversion, L5—great toe extension, S1—plantar flexion, ankle eversion, and hip extension, and S2—knee flexion.

Check sensation in response to both dull and sharp stimuli. Check joint position sense; it can be altered peripherally in diabetes mellitus or centrally with posterior column damage (i.e., subacute combined degeneration). Note any muscle atrophy or fasciculations.

Examiner in Back of the Patient

Note skin temperature, drag, and consistency of the paravertebral muscles (ropy v. boggy). Test gross range of motion and lumbar intersegmental vertebral motion. Perform the seated flexion test.

SUPINE

The straight leg raising test with and without dorsiflexion helps to delineate sciatic nerve irritation (positive with dorsiflexion) from hamstring muscle contracture. Note the performance of the nondysfunctional leg on the straight leg raising test. The Thomas test for psoas muscle contracture and the FABERE test for hip joint pathology are performed. Palpate the greater trochanteric area for trochanteric bursitis. Palpate for tender points at the tensor fascia latae and iliotibial bands, and perform the Ober test. Check for anterior tender points (Jones test). Roll your fingers over the skin of the iliac crests. Point tenderness may indicate Maigne's syndrome. The Hoover test may be used when malingering is suspected.

PRONE

Palpate for paravertebral muscle consistency (ropy vs. boggy) and for changes in tissue texture. Evaluate for sacral motion restriction. Note accentuation or flattening of the normal lumbar lordosis, and perform a spring test. Palpate for tender points at the intervertebral disk spaces, the transverse and spinous processes, the lumbosacral junction, the lumbar and sacral tender areas (Jones tender points), and over the piriformis, gluteal, and quadratus lumborum muscles. Perianal or saddle paresthesia may indicate a cauda equina syndrome.

OTHER TESTS

A rectal examination may be performed to evaluate sphincter tone, prostate enlargement, occult blood, masses, and piriformis tenderness. Check for testicular masses.

Adjunctive tests should include blood and urine chemistries; supine or standing (postural) anteroposterior, lateral, and indicated oblique radiography of the lumbar spine and pelvis; and computed tomography (CT), magnetic resonance imaging (MRI), or myelography. Chest radiography, skeletal scintigraphy, angiography, and diskography are performed as needed, as are tests of the erythrocyte sedimentation rate, C-reactive protein assays, rheumatoid factor assays, serum protein electrophoresis, serum immunoelectrophoresis, acid phosphatase or prostate-specific antigen assays, lumbar puncture, and HLA typing.

Herniated Nucleus Pulposus

Intervertebral disk herniation can occur in three directions: posterolaterally, purely laterally, and centrally. Posterolateral disk herniation is most common. It often presents as sharp pain of sudden or gradual onset. Increased intraabdominal pressure accompanying a cough, sneeze, lifting, or a Valsalva maneuver will accentuate symptoms. The L5–S1 and L4–L5 disks account for 95% of disk herniation in the lumbar region. The lower lumbar segments bear more weight and act as a fulcrum for forward and backward bending; therefore, they are subjected to greater mechanical stress.

Because of this distribution, radicular symptoms typically present as sciatica or low back pain that radiates to the hip, buttock, posterior thigh, and sometimes the leg and foot. Persistent radiculopathy without back pain may occur once the

nuclear material has passed the posterior longitudinal ligament. Atypical pain patterns, such as anterior thigh and groin pain, may be associated with disk herniation at a higher level or with a massive midline herniation.

PHYSICAL FINDINGS

The patient may stand with the affected leg slightly flexed and may walk with an antalgic gait, which reduces tension on the sciatic nerve and its connective tissue wrappings. Protrusion of the disk lateral to the nerve root causes side bending away from the involved side. Disk protrusion medial to the nerve root causes side bending toward the lesion. Protective paravertebral muscle spasm with flattening of the normal lumbar lordosis and decreased range of motion is common. A compensatory scoliosis and pelvic side shift with forward flexion are usually present.

The straight leg raising test is most specific for disk herniation affecting the L4, L5, S1, and S2 nerve roots. The straight leg raising test produces tension along the sciatic nerve, the lumbosacral nerve roots, and dura mater. Unilateral straight leg raising between 0 and 35 degrees places some tension on the sciatic nerve; between 35 and 70 degrees it maximally involves the sciatic nerve, its nerve roots, and the dura. Pain associated with unilateral straight leg raising beyond 70 degrees is most likely joint pain.

A positive straight leg raising test is one that produces pain radiating along the distribution of the sciatic nerve. However, a positive test result is not coequivalent with disk herniation, just as a negative test result does not exclude the possibility of disk herniation. One study by Hudgins found a 64% correlation of results on the straight leg raising test with herniation demonstrated by CT. On the other hand, 97% of patients with positive results on a straight leg raising test of an apparently normal leg had herniated disks demonstrated on CT. Kosteljanetz et al reported that 43 (88%) of 49 patients with positive results on the straight leg raising test and 19 (95%) of 20 patients with a positive test of the apparently normal leg had disk herniation confirmed surgically.

Neurologic deficit is an important physical finding that helps differentiate radicular from referred pain. Motor weakness, sensory deficit, or reflex changes depend on the level of the involved nerve roots and the extent of the herniation.

The clinical diagnosis can be confirmed with CT, myelography, or MRI. Asymptomatic disk defects have been shown by CT and myelography to occur in up to 25% of the general population. Thus, none of these imaging studies is diagnostic, and clinical correlation is mandatory. CT and MRI have been shown by Mikheal et al to be of equal value in demonstrating herniated intervertebral disks. MRI offered more detail on the degree of disk degeneration and was more accurate in demonstrating small, nonherniated disk protrusions. CT, however, demonstrated purely lateral disk herniation previously missed with MRI. Foristall et al found MRI with surface coil to be more accurate than contrast-enhanced CT in 25 patients diagnosed at surgery as having herniated disks.

Myelography has not been completely replaced by CT or MRI and remains an important diagnostic modality. Since the substitution of water-based for oil-based dye, the incidence of arachnoiditis secondary to myelography has decreased.

Most patients with disk herniation can be treated conservatively. Conservative treatment includes bed rest (less than one week), moist heat or ice, nonsteroidal anti-inflammatory agents, and dose pack corticosteroids or muscle relaxants in the acute phase, followed by osteopathic manipulation and an exercise program. Prolonged bed rest, traction, corsets, most centrally acting muscle relaxants, and ultrasound treatment are of debated therapeutic efficacy.

The results of manipulative treatment, osteopathic or nonosteopathic, are mixed. Siehl and Bradford treated over 700 patients between 1950 and 1960 with manipulation under anesthesia. Of these, 185 were diagnosed as having a herniated disk, 171 with myelography. Most of the patients were followed for at least two years. Twenty-six percent of the 186 responded with good results (i.e., they were able to resume normal activities relatively symptom free), while 44% of the patients had fair results (they resumed a relatively normal activity level but with some residual symptoms). The remaining 30% responded poorly. These patients showed little to no improvement, reported exacerbation, or had early recurrence of symptoms.

Similarly, Chrisman et al treated 39 patients with rotatory manipulation under anesthesis, one treatment each. The diagnosis of herniated disk was made in 27 patients both clinically and with myelography. The remaining 12 patients had normal myelograms and were diagnosed from clinical findings alone. Approximately one third of the patients with an abnormal myelogram responded favorably. Ten of the 12 with a normal myelogram also had good to excellent results. In general, those with normal myelograms consistently did better.

Myelography was performed both before and after rotatory manipulation. No reduction of herniation was noted. However, in several operations rotatory manipulation was performed and was noted to cause the two adjacent lamina, on either side of the herniated disk, to move apart at least 5 mm. The authors proposed that stretching of the lower fibers of the ligamentum flavum and the superolateral position of the posterior joint capsule, rather than an actual reduction in herniation, was a possible mechanism for symptom relief. They also discussed the possibility of adhesions over the spinal nerve roots as a cause for radicular symptoms that are freed by rotatory manipulation.

Steiner has stressed the distinction between a reducible versus a nonreducible herniated disk, or a protruding versus a degenerated or sequestered disk. As long as the annulus has retained its inherent elasticity and the disk herniation is not fragmented or massive, it should be reducible with manipulation. However, only clinical or subjective improvement has been reported; the disk lesion has not demonstrably resolved on CT or myelography.

Surgery is indicated when there is progressive neurologic deficit or moderate to severe neurologic deficit (e.g., bowel or bladder dysfunction, foot drop, paralysis), or persistent, intolerable radicular symptoms despite an adequate trial of manipulation.

Weber reported that surgery offers more of a short-term than long-term solution. On four- to ten-year follow-ups of patients in a randomized study who had been treated surgically, the same functional capacity and complaints existed as in patients treated nonoperatively. By contrast, Herron reported that careful patient selection, accurate preoperative diagnosis, and the absence of psychosocial impairment greatly increased the likelihood of surgical success. The risk of a poor surgical outcome is associated with lack of clinical correlation, abnormal pain drawing, a pending Workmen's Compensation case, and a psychological profile indicating hysteria, hypochondriasis, or somatization.

Osteopathic manipulation is directed toward eliminating or reducing muscle spasm and restoring normal joint motion. These goals can be achieved through a combination of specifically applied soft tissue techniques. Once muscle spasm has been sufficiently relieved, high velocity, low amplitude thrusting techniques are often necessary to normalize joint motion. Trigger points can be treated with a vapocoolant spray and injection of a local anesthetic.

CENTRAL DISK HERNIATION

When large enough, central disk herniation produces a compressive lesion of the cauda equina at one or more levels. The cauda equina syndrome is characterized by bilateral or unilateral sciatica, "saddle" anesthesia, and lower extremity weakness that may progress to paraplegia with bowel and bladder incontinence. Physical examination may reveal unilateral or bilateral weakness and decreased sensation in the lower extremities, decreased anal sphincter tone, urinary retention, saddle paresthesia, a positive straight leg raising test on the dysfunctional or nondysfunctional side, and bilaterally depressed deep tendon reflexes. Definitive diagnosis requires CT or MRI.

Reported cases of cauda equina syndrome secondary to central disk herniation range from 1% to 16% of all herniated lumbar disks. There is no indication for conservative treatment. Prompt and accurate diagnosis is essential to ensure quick surgical decompression. Irreparable damage to bladder function is likely unless surgical decompression is performed within 12 hours of the initial loss of bladder control.

Spinal Stenosis

LATERAL SPINAL STENOSIS

Lateral spinal stenosis can involve any one of the three segments of the lateral spinal canal: the entrance zone (spinal canal), the midzone (nerve root canal), or the exit zone (intervertebral foramen). As with a herniated disk, lateral stenosis most commonly occurs at the L4–L5 or L5–S1 levels. The patient usually complains of unilateral or bilateral sciatica without concurrent low back pain. The symptoms are exacerbated by extension and rotation of the lumbar spine and are often in-

termittent. Neurologic deficit, if present, is usually mild. However, progressive degeneration can result in fixed stenosis with constant resting pain and dysesthesia.

Lateral radiographs may show decreased intervertebral disk height and/or enlarged superior articular processes or spondylolisthesis. Oblique X-ray is best to demonstrate spondylolysis. CT or MRI will usually demonstrate stenosis of any one of the three portions of the lateral spinal canal.

Conservative treatment includes an exercise program with the avoidance of rotational exercises, instruction in back care, and an abdominal support. Manipulative treatment was shown by Kirkaldy-Willis and Cassidy to offer significant relief of symptoms in 50% of patients diagnosed with lateral spinal stenosis. If the condition is severe enough, laminectomy is indicated.

CENTRAL SPINAL STENOSIS

Central spinal stenosis is also called pseudoclaudication or neurogenic claudication. The symptoms are similar to those of intermittent claudication due to occlusive aortoiliac disease. However, there are differentiating features between the two. The pain of neurogenic claudication is usually described as a burning or numbness in the low back and buttock which is exacerbated by walking up an incline and by extending of the lumbar spine. Relief is reported after 20 to 30 minutes of rest and by sitting with the hips and trunk flexed. The patient may walk in a "simian" posture with his trunk flexed at the hips.

Vascular intermittent claudication, on the other hand, typically manifests as an aching or cramplike pain in the hips, thighs, and buttocks with radiation into the calves. The pain is usually initiated by walking and is relieved within a few minutes of resting. Spinal motion (e.g., extension) does not exacerbate symptoms.

Physical examination in a patient with vascular disease may demonstrate femoral bruits, decreased peripheral pulses, and cool, pale lower extremities, with one leg usually worse than the other. Neurologic deficit is absent. In contrast, neurogenic claudication is often significant for unilateral or bilateral radicular symptoms. Deep tendon reflexes may be depressed at more than one spinal level. If the deep tendon reflexes are initially normal, an abnormality may be revealed when tested immediately after exercise. A neurogenic bladder also frequently accompanies neurogenic claudication. Although subtle, a history of frequency, urgency, or incomplete bladder emptying is an indication. Perianal anesthesia and hypotonicity of the anal sphincter may also be present.

Some authors have suggested that degenerative changes of the spine are accompanied by hypertension of the vertebral venous plexuses. The pain experienced in central stenosis may be the result of edema with subsequent compression of the small nerves innervating vertebrae, the annulus fibrosus, and ligaments, as well as compression of the vertebral arterial supply, producing ischemia of the cauda equida.

Conservative therapy includes an exercise program emphasizing lumbar flexion, and abdominal support. Kirkaldy-Willis and Cassidy found that high velocity, low amplitude thrusting techniques offered significant symptom relief in five of 11 patients with central spinal stenosis. Soft tissue and articular techniques and occasionally thrusting techniques are used to treat palpable findings such as muscle spasm, decreased joint mobility, and tender points. Flexion should be encouraged and extension avoided, as either may exacerbate symptoms. Surgery is generally indicated in cases of pain refractory to conservative measures, marked exercise intolerance, significant muscle weakness, numbness or paresthesia, and bladder or bowel dysfunction.

The resolution of symptoms in some patients treated by high velocity, low amplitude thrusting techniques for documented spinal stenosis raises two important questions. The manipulation itself does not reduce bony stenosis. Therefore, what is the actual source of symptoms in these patients, and are the symptoms relieved? Only speculative answers are available. Are radicular symptoms due to abnormal fascial and dural strains or to adhesions that compress the arterial, venous, and nerve supply to the vertebrae, spinal cord, disks, and posterior joints? Do radicular symptoms represent an abnormal sympathetic reflex mediated by the sinovertebral nerves? In normalizing the articular relationship of the dysfunctional vertebral segment and those adjacent to it, are fascial or dorsal strains that compress the vascular and nerve supply being reduced, thereby relieving venous congestion, edema, ischemia, and nerve compression? Are ligaments, muscles, and the posterior facet joint capsule being stretched? Are adhesions being broken?

The posterior facet joints, sacroiliac joints and muscles are all potential sources of primary low back pain with radiation to the lower extremities. By means not entirely understood, each can produce pseudoradicular pain. The pseudoradicular syndromes differ from true radicular syndromes in that they lack the tension signs and neurologic deficit common to the true radiculopathies. Furthermore, referred pain is characterized as deep, boring, and diffuse, whereas radicular pain is described as sharp and well defined.

Sacroiliac Joint Syndrome

Sacroiliac joint syndrome is due to somatic dysfunction of this joint and must be differentiated from lumbar radiculopathy. Sacral motion is restricted, and changes in tissue texture occur over the sacroiliac joint. The patient's pain may be reproduced during the examination. Associated spasm of one or more muscles attaching to the sacrum is usually present. These muscles include the piriformis, gluteus maximus, coccygeal, iliac, and erector spinae via the thoracolumbar fascia. Muscle spasm and trigger points, if bilateral, are usually worse on the side of the dysfunction.

Symptoms include pain at the sacroiliac area with possible radiation to the lower extremity. Neurologic deficit does not accompany this syndrome. The condition is diagnosed from clinical findings and a favorable response to osteopathic manipulation. Radiography is useful to rule out other pathologic conditions and early ankylosing spondylitis.

Manipulative treatment includes any of the soft tissue techniques: myofascial, muscle energy, counterstrain for tender points, myofascial release, facilitated positional release, and, when indicated, thrusting techniques.

The use of a vapocoolant spray and injection of a local anesthetic into the affected joint may be therapeutic as well as diagnostic. The cause of sacroiliac joint pain is not clear. It has been speculated to originate from the joint itself or to be secondary to prolonged contraction of one of the muscles that attach to it.

Posterior Facet Joint Syndrome

Posterior facet joint syndrome is also not a true radiculopathy; however, its presentation is similar to that of other causes of radiating pain.

Posterior facet joint syndrome and sacroiliac syndrome are the most common causes of low back pain referred to the lower extremities. Proposed causes include synovitis and the pinching of folds of synovial tissue (pseudomenisci) within the facet joints, degenerative changes of the facet joint, and spinal segmental instability.

Less clearly understood is the cause of radiating pain associated with posterior facet joint pathology. Innervation of the facet joints by the recurrent sinovertebral nerve and its branches overlaps considerably. This was demonstrated by McCall et al, who found the distribution of pain following pericapsular and intraarticular injection of the L1–L2 and L4–L5 posterior facet joints with normal saline to have a significant amount of overlap. Clinically, specific pain patterns corresponding to a specific lumbar level have generally not been shown.

Maignes syndrome is one Parisian doctor's claim to fame for describing a lesion at the T12–L1 posterior facet joints. In addition to local pain and tenderness in the region of the facet joints, there is irritation of the superior cluneal nerves, producing tenderness over the iliac crest of the involved side.

The typical history associated with posterior facet joint syndrome is unilateral or bilateral low back pain (usually at the L4–S1 levels), often radiating to the buttock, trochanteric region, and posterior thigh or groin and occasionally extending as far as the calf or ankle. Complaints of muscle weakness or sensory loss do not typically accompany this syndrome. The physical examination generally reveals motion restriction of one or more vertebral segments, local paravertebral muscle spasm, focal paraspinal tenderness, limited spinal range of motion, and exacerbation of pain with lateral side bending or extension and rotation on the symptomatic side. Straight leg raising is often limited, probably because of accompanying hamstring muscle spasm. Findings on neurologic examination are normal or minimally abnormal. Oblique and lateral radiographs may reveal abnormal posterior facets.

Posterior facet joint syndrome is diagnosed initially from the history and physical examination findings. Without radiography, the diagnosis is often presumptive and is based on the patient's response to manipulative treatment or facet joint injection with a corticosteroid and a local anesthetic agent under fluoroscopy. This type of injec-

tion may relieve symptoms in 20% to 50% of suspected cases of posterior facet joint syndrome.

Osteopathic manipulation is effective in the treatment of the facet syndrome. It is directed toward specific palpatory findings. Kirkaldy-Willis and Cassidy conducted a prospective study of high velocity, low amplitude thrusting techniques in 283 patients with chronic low back and radicular pain. Results were reported for specific diagnoses—sacroiliac joint and/or posterior facet joint syndrome, lateral stenosis (fixed or dynamic), and central stenosis. Some 79% of 56 patients with posterior facet joint syndrome, 92% of 69 patients with sacroiliac joint syndrome, and 88% of 48 patients with both joint syndromes reported significant improvement in symptoms and ability to resume daily activities. Daily treatment for two weeks was most efficacious. Patients who did not respond to this regimen were unlikely to respond to manipulative treatment. No patient's condition was worsened by the thrusting therapy.

Piriformis Syndrome

Piriformis syndrome is a peripheral neuritis of the sciatic nerve caused by an abnormal condition of the piriformis muscle. The piriformis muscle is an external rotator and abductor of the thigh, located deep to the gluteal muscles. It originates on the anterolateral border of the sacrum, at the sacroiliac joint capsule, and on the anterior portion of the sacrotuberous ligament, and inserts into the superomedial aspect of the greater trochanter of the femur.

After passing through the greater sciatic foramen, the sciatic nerve courses under the piriformis muscle on its way to the posterior thigh. Factors thought to cause sciatic nerve irritation or inflammation include piriformis muscle spasm or contracture, local trauma to the buttocks, repeated mechanical stressors (e.g., running), sacral base unleveling or pelvic instability, excessive local pressure, especially in thin or cachectic patients ("hip pocket neuritis"), anatomic variation, and local perineural inflammation secondary to the endogenous release of vasoactive substances from an inflamed piriformis muscle.

In approximately 10% of the general population the common peroneal and tibial components of the sciatic nerve remain separate. One, usually the common peroneal, passes directly through the piriformis muscle. In another 10%, the piriformis muscle arises from two tendinous origins, with the sciatic nerve passing between them.

The piriformis syndrome produces symptoms easily confused with those of a herniated lumbar disk or facet joint pathology. The patient often complains of hip and buttock pain radiating down the posterior thigh, possibly to the calf or foot. Low back pain is usually not a major component. The piriformis syndrome generally differs from disk herniation by the absence of neurologic deficit. Rarely, severe piriformis compression produces a sciatic nerve palsy and all of the accompanying neurologic sequelae.

On physical examination muscle strength, sensation, and deep tendon reflexes are normal (unless the syndrome is extreme). Most notable is exquisite tenderness with or without trigger points anywhere along the piriformis muscle. When palpated, these trigger points may reproduce the radicular pain. Gluteal tender points may also be present.

Contracture of the piriformis muscle can be grossly assessed with the patient prone. Flex the knees to 90 degrees and, while holding the ankles, internally rotate both hip joints until resistance is met. Compare the relative freedom of motions on each side. Sacral motion is often restricted.

Osteopathic manipulative medicine is especially effective in the treatment of this syndrome. Manipulation is directed toward palpatory findings, not subjective complaints. A combination of soft tissue techniques such as muscle energy treatment, active and passive myofascial techniques to the lumbar and lumbosacral region, counterstrain treatment for tender points, and myofascial release of the sacrum and pelvis, as well as thrusting techniques, when indicated, are especially effective. Trigger points can be treated with a vapocoolant spray and local injection of an anesthetic.

SPONDYLOLISTHESIS AND SPONDYLOLYSIS
Barbara Polstein

The term *spondylolisthesis* is derived from the Greek words *spondyl*, meaning spine, and *olisthesis*, meaning to fall or to slip. Spondylolisthesis refers to forward slippage of one vertebral body over the vertebral body immediately below it. Retrolisthesis, or backward displacement, is much less common but can occur. *Spondylolysis* refers to fracture and separation of the pars interarticularis of the vertebral arch.

Spondylolisthesis occurs in 20% to 70% of patients with spondylolysis. Spondylolisthesis is usually found in the lumbar spine and occasionally in the cervical spine. If found in the thoracic region, it is always secondary to trauma. Approximately 75% of all cases occur with L5 slipping on S1, 20% with L4 slipping on L5, and 5% at higher levels (Figs. 29-5 and 29-6).

Classification
Wiltze, Newman, and McNab have classified spondylolisthesis into five categories, according to etiology. These are described below.

DYSPLASTIC SPONDYLOLISTHESIS
Dysplastic spondylolisthesis is a congenital abnormality of the first sacral or fifth lumbar neural arch. Unable to withstand normal forces exerted on the lumbar spine, this defect permits slippage of the L5–S1 facet joint articulation during childhood or adolescence. Approximately 25% to 35% of symptomatic children have dysplastic spondylolisthesis. Standing lateral radiographs show subluxation with forward slipping of the entire neural arch of L5, including the spinous process. Progression of slippage may occur with attenuation of the pedicles. If the posterior elements and lamina are present, spondylolisthesis does not usually exceed 25%. If it does, cauda equina syndrome or frank paralysis can result.

ISTHMIC SPONDYLOLISTHESIS
Isthmic spondylolisthesis is a primary defect of the pars interarticularis (located within the lamina). There are three types:

1. Elongation of the pars interarticularis
2. Fatigue fracture of the pars interarticularis

A

Figure 29-5. (**A**) Spondylolysis and spondylolisthesis of L5 on S1. (Adapted from Rothman R, Simeon AF. 1982. The Spine, 2d ed., Vol. 1. Philadelphia: Saunders, pp. 263–284.) (**B**) Radiograph of same condition.

B

3. Acute fracture of the pars interarticularis secondary to trauma

Isthmic spondylolisthesis is the most common type of spondylolisthesis in the general population less than 50 years of age. It is thought to be an inherited defect of the cartilaginous model of the vertebral arch. The familial incidence of spondylolysis with or without spondylolisthesis ranges from 27% to 69%. This is in contrast to a 4.4% to 6.0% occurrence in the general population. Some authors report a male/female ratio of 2:1 or 3:1; others have found no sex difference. The most common age of onset of spondylolysis is between five and seven years. Onset is generally painless. The condition seldom is seen in children less than five years old. This observation supports the belief that spondylolysis and spondylolisthesis are not anomalies present at birth.

Fredrickson et al found that approximately 90% to 95% of 500 cases of spondylolysis with or without spondylolisthesis involved L5 on S1. Approximately 75% of the cases were bilateral. No patient with unilateral spondylolysis had concurrent spondylolisthesis.

Analysis of various mechanical loads on the lumbar spine by Dickerson and others has shown that the L5 vertebra, particularly the pars interarticularis, is subject to the greatest mechanical stress. It is easy to imagine how a defect in the L5 vertebra might predispose it to elongation or to spondylolytic cracks in the pars interarticularis. Farfan et al identified three mechanisms thought to result in disruption of the neural arch: unbalanced shear force, forced rotation, and flexion overload.

Progression of spondylolisthesis is most rapid at 10 to 15 years of age, during adolescent growth. Like spondylolysis, it is also generally painless. From 16% to 31% of children with spondylolysis or spondylolisthesis have a significant history of trauma to the low back. Progression of slippage after 20 years of age is rare.

Fredrickson and others have shown that 7% of patients with pars interarticularis defects have concurrent lumbarization or sacralization of the

Figure 29-6. Cross-sectional view of bilateral spondylolysis at the pars interarticularis. (Adapted, with permission, from Rosse, Kay. 1980. The Musculosketeal System in Health and Disease. New York: Harper and Row, p. 132.)

spine. Spina bifida occulta is also 13 times more prevalent in patients with spondylolysis or spondylolisthesis.

DEGENERATIVE SPONDYLOLISTHESIS
This condition is most common in persons aged 50 years and older. Forward displacement of the vertebra is caused by degenerative changes in the posterior facet joints. Commonly, L4 slips on L5. There is a reported female/male ratio of 4:1. Degenerative spondylolisthesis at the L4–L5 level is four times more common in patients with sacralization of the fifth lumbar vertebra. This is because sacralization of L5 subjects the L4 vertebra to greater mechanical forces.

It is believed that degenerative spondylolisthesis is the result of spondylosis. Degeneration with erosion of the posterior facet joints and degenerative changes in the disk eventually allow the inferior facets and body of the L4 vertebra to slip forward on the L5 vertebra. Degenerative spondylolisthesis usually does not exceed 30%

unless there is a history of previous back surgery, in which case disruption of the lamina or pseudo-arthrosis formation exacerbates instability.

TRAUMATIC SPONDYLOLISTHESIS
Traumatic spondylolisthesis involves acute fracture anywhere in the neural arch other than the pars interarticularis, e.g., the pedicle or the inferior or superior articular facets.

PATHOLOGIC FRACTURE
Pathologic fracture may occur with localized or generalized bone disease anywhere in the neural arch. General causes include metastatic bone disease, Paget's disease, and spinal tuberculosis. A localized cause is fracture of the vertebra one level above a previous spinal fusion.

Findings and Examination
Most cases of spondylolysis and spondylolisthesis in children and adolescents are painless. About a quarter of all cases have low back pain with or without radiation to the lower extremity. Very few seek medical attention before the age of 20. In the majority of cases, symptoms associated with spondylolisthesis begin during the second or third decade of life.

The most common symptom is persistent low back ache with or without radiation to the buttocks, posterior thigh, and occasionally to the leg and foot. These symptoms are aggravated by standing for long periods of time or by increased activity, and are relieved by rest.

The sole complaint of radicular pain or neurologic deficit is less common. Neurologic deficit (motor weakness, sensory loss, and deep tendon reflex depression or loss) in isthmic spondylolisthesis has been attributed by Gill and colleagues to an aberrant fibrocartilaginous mass at the lysed or elongated pars interarticularis. In degenerative spondylolisthesis, the pedicles of the forwardly displaced vertebra compress the nerve root at the same level in a guillotine-like manner. A third cause of nerve root compression is intervertebral disk herniation. Spondylolisthesis produces instability, which in turn causes greater stress, with subsequent degenerative changes in the disk and facet joints. Typically, herniation of the L4 disk occurs with spondylolisthesis of L5 on S1.

Hamstring muscle spasm of varying degree is frequently seen with spondylolysis or spondylolisthesis, occurring in 80% of symptomatic chil-

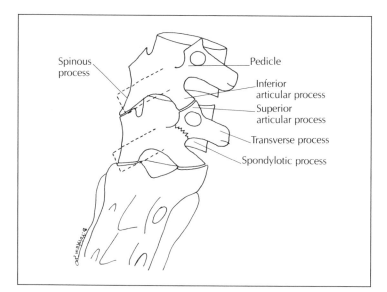

Figure 29-7. Spondylolysis of the L5 pars interarticularis, oblique view. Note the appearance of a collar around the neck of a Scotty dog. (Adapted from McGee, 1987, p. 212.)

dren. The hamstring muscles are secondary hip extensors and the major knee flexors. Contracture produces limited forward flexion at the hips, diminished knee extension, and backward tilting of the pelvis. If severe enough, the result is a characteristic stiff-legged, short-strided gait with the hips rotating forward with each step. This gait has been referred to by Wiltze as the pelvic waddle. Some children with hamstring involvement run instead of walk, or walk on their toes with their knees flexed. These children may also sleep with their knees and hips markedly flexed.

The mechanism of hamstring muscle involvement is not clearly understood. Some believe it is due to nerve root irritation. Others suspect it is a mechanical attempt by the body to stabilize the lumbosacral articulation. The postural and gait changes associated with hamstring muscle spasm spontaneously resolve following spinal fusion without the need for nerve root decompression. The straight leg raising test is often positive with minimal degrees of flexion, reflecting the severity of hamstring muscle spasm.

Diagnosis

The diagnosis of spondylolysis and spondylolisthesis is made with standing radiography of the lumbar spine, which best demonstrates the degree of spondylolisthesis. Bilateral oblique views al-

low for the diagnosis of spondylolysis. A spondylolytic defect of the pars interarticularis appears as a collar around the neck of the scotty dog (Fig. 29-7).

Lowe et al compared recumbent and standing lateral roentgenograms in 50 patients with spondylolisthesis. Approximately 26% of the patients showed dynamic changes with a 2-mm or greater increase in forward displacement on standing. A comparison of supine and standing radiographs will help evaluate the degree of instability of the defect. Patients with a greater degree of slippage on weight-bearing also tended to have more severe symptoms.

One system of grading spondylolisthesis is on a scale of I to IV. This grading system estimates the degree of forward slip of one vertebra over another on standing lateral radiographs of the lumbar spine. The sacrum or vertebral body below the slipped segment is divided into four equal parts. In grade I spondylolisthesis, vertebral displacement is between 0% and 25% of the anteroposterior (AP) diameter of the vertebra below; in grade II, between 25% and 50%; in grade III, between 50% and 75%; and in grade IV, greater than 75% (Fig. 29-8).

A more accurate measurement, expresses spondylolisthesis as a percentage (Fig. 29-9). *A* is that portion of the AP diameter of the lower segment over which the upper segment has slipped; *A'* is

Figure 29-8. Spondylolisthesis, grades I to IV.

Figure 29-9. The degree of forward slippage is expressed as the percentage $\dfrac{A}{A'} \times 100$.

the total AP diameter of the lower segment. This method of measurement is preferred for accurate follow-up of the progression of the spondylolisthesis. It is only possible if roentgenograms are taken the same way each time. Other methods of measuring progression are shown in Figure 29-10.

Patients with grade I or early grade II spondylolisthesis often have relatively normal physical examinations. Limited forward flexion and hamstring muscle tightness might be the only abnormal physical findings. It is usually not until late grade II or grade III slippage occurs that postural deformity becomes apparent. Typically there are marked exaggeration of the lumbar lordosis, backward tilting of the pelvis, and forward thrusting of the lower abdomen. A transverse abdominal crease at the level of the umbilicus is often present.

In isthmic spondylolisthesis, a stepoff or depression directly above the spinous process of the slipped segment (L5) may be palpated. In the degenerative type, the posterior elements are displaced with the rest of the vertebra. Therefore, this stepoff will be palpable just below the spinous process of the slipped segment. In more advanced cases, nerve root irritation causes protective muscle spasm in the lower back, producing a compensatory scoliosis. If not treated, this functional scoliosis can convert into a structural scoliosis.

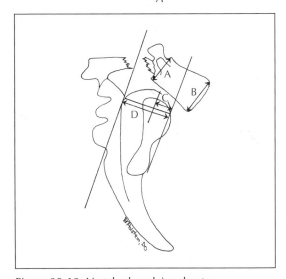

Figure 29-10. Vertebral wedging due to spondylolisthesis is calculated as the percentage $\dfrac{A}{B} \times 100$. The percent rounding of the sacral base is calculated as $\dfrac{C}{D} \times 100$. Both measurements have been used as a method of following the progression of slippage of L5 on S1. (Figs 29-9 and 29-10 adapted from Wiltze LL, Winter RB. 1983. Terminology and measurement of spondylolisthes. J. Bone Joint Surg. 65:6.)

Treatment

The majority of symptomatic patients respond to conservative treatment without the need for surgical stabilization. Conservative therapy for spondylolisthesis includes:

1. A daily exercise program, including the Williams flexion exercises and quarter situps.
2. Weight loss in overweight patients, to help relieve postural stress on the spondylolytic defect.
3. Osteopathic treatment: Manipulative treatment will probably not reduce the lesion. However, it can help to identify the other sources of referred pain that commonly accompany spondylolisthesis or spondylolysis. These include the posterior facet joints (typically one level above the defect), the sacroiliac joints, and myofascial trigger points.

The posterior facet joint and SI joint syndromes are diagnosed clinically, primarily from the presence of motion restriction and lack of neurologic deficit. Myofascial syndromes are recognized from the presence of trigger points. All identified somatic dysfunctions should be treated. Alleviation or significant reduction of the patient's symptoms after one or two treatments confirms the diagnosis.

Surgery is indicated for the following:

1. Symptomatic grade I or II spondylolisthesis unrelieved by an adequate trial of conservative therapy.
2. Progression of forward displacement.
3. Grade III spondylolisthesis.
4. Postural deformity or significant gait abnormality due to hamstring spasm not relieved by physical therapy.

It is important to follow any progression of spondylolisthesis. This is accomplished by serial radiographs with measurement of the percentage of forward slip, as described earlier. Instability of L5 on S1 is responsible for wear and tear of these vertebrae. Gradual erosion of both the anterior and posterior portions of the sacral base produces a rounded or dome shape. The body of L5 becomes wedge shaped, with the posterior portion narrower than the anterior portion. Both of these changes reflect the degree of slip.

Forward slippage can occur laterally as well as in a purely anterior direction. The *slip angle*, or the angular relationship between L5 and S1, is measured at the intersection of one line drawn along the posterior aspect of S1 and another along the anterior aspect of the body of L5.

Progression is also noted from accentuation of the lumbar lordosis and an increase in the lumbosacral angle. These changes can be followed by measuring the percent of rounding of the sacrum, wedging of the fifth lumbar vertebra, angle of lumbar lordosis, and the lumbosacral angle.

COCCYGODYNIA
Paula D. Scariati

In 1859, Sir J. V. Simpson coined the term *coccygodynia,* using it to describe persistent pain in the coccyx. He noted that when injury to the coccyx or coccygeal joint occurred, or when the surrounding tissue was inflamed, contraction of the muscles attached to the coccyx would elicit the characteristic pain of coccygodynia. Further observations since that time have confirmed the presence of spasm of the levator ani and coccygeus muscles in a significant percentage of cases of coccygodynia.

Anatomy

THE BONY PELVIS

The word *coccyx* comes from the Greek word *kokkue*, meaning cuckoo, as the coccyx resembles a cuckoo's beak. The coccyx is a result of fusion of four evolutionarily separate vertebrae. It is not unusual to visualize the coccyx as three to five distinct vertebrae in a child, but by adulthood, these bones are united into a single bone. In later life, the coccyx may even fuse with the sacrum. The coccyx is a triangular osseous formation that is concave anteriorly, following the curve of the sacrum.

The bones of the pelvis vary from male to female. The female pelvis is more delicate than the male pelvis. The sacrum is shorter, wider, and less curved. The greater sciatic notch has a greater diameter; the ischial tuberosities are wider apart and everted; and the inferior aperture is larger, and hence the coccyx is more variable in position. The position of the sacrum and coccyx in the female tends to be backward and thus more prone to trauma. The male pelvis has a narrower sciatic notch and the inclination of the sacrum and coccyx is forward into the pelvic cavity tucked between the ischia. This shields the coccyx from external trauma to a great extent in males.

THE MUSCLES

The pelvic diaphragm is a thin sheet of muscle consisting of the coccygeus muscle posteriorly and the more extensive levator ani muscle anterolaterally. Its halves form the sloping floor of the pelvis through which the urethra, vagina, and anal canal pass. The diaphragm closes the inferior pelvic outlet somewhat as a funnel would were it placed in the pelvic cavity.

Levator Ani

This broad, thin muscle unites with its contralateral partner to form the largest portion of the pelvic diaphragm.

Origin: pelvic surface of the body of the pubis to the ischial spine.
Insertion: central perineal tendon, wall of the anal canal, anococcygeal ligament, and coccyx.
Innervation: fibers from the third and fourth sacral nerves which enter its pelvic surface, and the inferior rectal nerve (a branch of the pudendal nerve which originates from S2–S4 nerve roots), which enters its perineal surface.

Functions: The muscular pelvic diaphragm supports the pelvic viscera and resists the inferior thrust accompanying increases in intraabdominal pressure (e.g., such as occurs during coughing, defecation and normal thoracolumbar respiration). Parts of the levator ani also support the prostate (males) and the posterior wall of the vagina (females), holds the anorectal junction anteriorly, and supports the fetal head during parturition while the cervix of the uterus is dilating.

Coccygeus

This triangular sheet of muscle lies against and blends with the posterior portion of the levator ani. It forms the smaller, posterior portion of the pelvic diaphragm.

Origin: pelvic surfaces of the ischial spine and the sacrospinal ligament.
Insertion: lateral margins of the fifth sacral vertebra and the coccyx.
Innervation: branches from the ventral rami of the fourth and fifth sacral nerves.
Function: supports the coccyx. In women, it pulls the coccyx forward after it has been pressed posteriorly during childbirth.

Physiology

In *Visceral Manipulation*, Jean-Pierre Barral and Pierre Mercier define the sacrococcygeal articulation as a diarthrosis with an articular motion of up to 30 degrees. This joint is surrounded by anterior, posterior, and lateral sacrococcygeal ligaments which allow good mobility while ensuring appropriate tension on the coccyx and associated structures. The motion of this joint is best exemplified during childbirth, where its posterior flexion allows some vital centimeters to be gained. On a daily basis, the sacrococcygeal joint and pelvic diaphragm play a role in copulation, defecation, and micturition. They also contribute to lumbosacral biomechanics, and thus coccygeal dysfunction can manifest as lumbosacral restriction.

Motion at the sacrococcygeal articulation can be restricted to various degrees following retraction or spasm of the soft tissue structures that attach to or help to maintain the joint. Coccygeal displacement can impede pelvic physiology. For example, when the coccyx moves closer to the pubic symphysis (e.g., anterior flexion), the pelvic diaphragm becomes lax and loses tone. The levator ani and coccygeal muscles lose power, and thus the structures that pierce the diaphragm are affected. It is not uncommon for patients to complain of incontinence of stool and urine, impotence (males), and painful intercourse (females).

Etiology

The causes of coccygodynia are many. They include infections such as tuberculosis and osteomyelitis, fractures, dislocations, ligamentous tears, postnatal injuries and other types of trauma.

Signs and Symptoms

The presenting signs and symptoms of coccygodynia are consistent regardless of the etiology.

ACUTE COCCYGODYNIA
A. Symptoms
　1. Pain with sitting
　2. Pain with bowel movements
　3. Proctalgia fugax
　4. Tenesmus (rarer)
　5. Painful intercourse
　6. Occasionally, pain when lying supine, if the sacrococcygeal joint is very convex (the prone position may afford some relief from pain)
B. Signs
　1. Point tenderness at the tip of the coccyx, sacrococcygeal joint, and along the coccygeal ligaments
　2. Muscle pain in the levator ani and coccygeus muscles
　3. Decreased range of motion in the sacrococcygeal joint
　4. Hypermobile distal coccygeal segments secondary to ligamentous tear or fracture
　5. Side bending–rotation lesions of the sacrococcygeal joint
　6. Sharp pain on distraction and compression of the coccyx
　7. Pain with passive flexion or extension of the coccyx

CHRONIC COCCYGODYNIA
A. Some or all of the signs and symptoms of acute coccygodynia

B. Gastrointestinal
　1. Constipation
　2. Hemorrhoids secondary to decreased venous drainage
　3. Proctalgia fugax
　4. Incontinence
C. Genitourinary
　1. Urethral syndromes—nonspecific urinary tract infections secondary to stasis or poor drainage
　2. Urethritis secondary to spasm of the periurethral muscles
　3. Decreased venous and lymphatic drainage
　4. Incontinence
　5. Impotence
　6. Cystitis
　7. Prostatitis
D. Gynecology
　1. Painful intercourse
　2. Pelvic anhedonia—loss of orgasm secondary to nervous system shock (loss of genital vasomotor response and decrease in uterovaginal mobility)
　3. Ligamentous strain causing congestion
　4. Uterine retroversion
E. Musculoskeletal
　1. Stretched iliolumbar ligaments. If the coccyx is restricted, the sacrotuberous ligament cannot stretch as the ischia spread during the act of sitting. Instead, the iliolumbar ligaments are forced to accommodate.
　2. Spasm of associated adjacent muscles (e.g., the piriform muscle, which has its origin on the anterior surface of the sacrum)
F. Psychology
　Depression—Generalized devitalization secondary to a decrease in the mobility of the entire body or a decrease in the craniosacral respiratory impulse

Evaluation

Evaluation begins as the patient walks in the door. Does he walk stiffly and sit cautiously? A complete history is important. The physician must inquire as to any signs and symptoms relative to the genitourinary and gastrointestinal systems, as well as sexual dysfunctions.

Next the mobility of the coccyx is tested. An external route is employed first. A rectal examination is done only if necessary. The patient sits with his legs hanging slightly apart so that the sacrococcygeal attachments are taut. With his index finger, the physician follows the patient's gluteal crease to a point 1 cm posterior to the anus. At the tip of the coccyx, located at this point, a posterosuperior force is exerted. Sharp pain is an indication of dysfunction and a reason to perform a rectal examination.

To facilitate rectal examination, the patient is placed in the lateral decubitis position with his legs slightly separated. Donning a lubricated glove, the physician enters the rectum with his index finger, leaving the finger in the rectal ampulla with the pad posteriorly against the coccyx and sacrum. The mobility of the sacrococcygeal articulation is checked by placing a thumb, externally, parallel to the index finger. The coccyx is moved anteriorly and then side to side. Anterior restrictions are the most common, but lateral displacements also occur.

Range of motion testing of the coccyx evaluates the integrity of the sacrococcygeal joint and the associated ligaments and muscles. Normally there are asymmetries and minimal tenderness.

Osteopathic Manipulative Techniques

Conservative, noninvasive treatment of coccygodynia seems to produce the best results. Some authors have proposed coccygotomies and injections as first-line therapy. This seems premature and irrational when one considers the combined cure/improvement rate of manipulation in various studies is anywhere from 50% to 100%.

MOBILIZATION OF THE
SACROCOCCYGEAL JOINT
1. Patient position: lying on the table in the lateral decubitus position.
2. Physician position: standing beside the table, facing the back of the patient.
3. **Technique:**
   a. The physician places the palm of his cephalad hand on the patient's sacrum (used for counterpressure).
   b. The physician inserts the index finger of his other hand gently into the patient's rectum.
   c. Thereafter different techniques are used.
      i. For anterior displacement, the tip of the coccyx is pushed posteriorly and up.
      ii. For posterior displacement, the tip of the coccyx is pushed anteriorly.
      iii. For lateral displacement, the coccyx is mobilized from side to side.
      iv. For pure fixation, the coccyx is moved in an anterior-posterior motion.
   d. With each repetition, the force exerted is increased to help facilitate the fullest motion possible at the sacrococcygeal joint.
   e. All the techniques are done gently. The goal is to free stiffened tissue, release joint restriction, and restore full mobility.

RELEASE OF THE PELVIC DIAPHRAGM AND
ASSOCIATED MUSCLES
1. Patient position: lying on the table in the lateral decubitus position.
2. Physician position: standing beside the table, facing the back of the patient.
3. **Technique:**
   a. The physician inserts the full length of his index finger into the patient's rectum. (The physician should position the palm of his other hand on the patient's sacrum as a stabilizing force.)
   b. The physician exerts a lateroposterior pressure with a concomitant horizontal stroking motion to the fibers of the levator ani and coccygeus muscles.
   c. The piriformis is immediately beyond the sacrospinous ligament and is touched by fingertip in such a manner that lateral motion of the finger will stroke lengthwise those portions of the muscles in the pelvis.
   d. It is wise to begin this technique as lightly as possible, as the muscles involved are tender. Pressure may be increased in the course of several treatments.

MYOFASCIAL RELEASE OF THE
PELVIC DIAPHRAGM
This technique may be done from an external approach. The principles were described earlier.

Dysfunctions of the coccyx and the sacrococcygeal joint can cause increased tension on the dural tube, which in turn can affect attachments of the tube (dura) in the spine and cranium. Upledger and Vredevoogd found a cause-and-effect relationship between sacrococcygeal somatic dysfunction and pain of the head and back.

TOTAL TREATMENT PROGRAM
1. Osteopathic manipulative treatment every other day for seven to ten days.

2. Improved posture, because sitting erect pulls the buttocks together and causes natural cushioning.
3. Laxatives for constipation.
4. Hot sitz baths daily for seven to ten days.
5. Tricyclics for depression.

Conclusion

Coccygodynia is a painful symptom complex that can affect major organ systems. It is the job of osteopathic physicians to look at the entire picture and realize the far-reaching interactions. Only by restoring proper structure is the body allowed its fullest potential to heal.

DYSMENORRHEA

Mary E. Hitchcock

Painful menstruation in the absence of pelvic organ pathology is known as idiopathic or primary dysmenorrhea. The pain is relative and depends largely upon the susceptibility of the individual. Because dysmenorrhea is a subjective symptom, the degree of pain must be gauged from the behavior of the patient during the attack. To be termed dysmenorrhea, there must be a change in mode of living for days or hours, necessitating relief. It is essential to rule out, by careful gynecologic examination, polyps, cervical strictures, hydrosalpinx, and other organic changes that may be responsible for dysmenorrhea.

Primary dysmenorrhea has been estimated to occur in 3% to 47% of menstruating females. This wide range could be due to the different standards employed by different investigators.

Premenstrual tension includes a variety of symptoms in the days preceding menstruation. It manifests in breast tenderness, abdominal bloating, weight gain, and some swelling of the lower extremities. Fluid retention results from secretion of estrogen during the first three weeks of the cycle, with a relative deficiency of progesterone at this time, and from sodium ion retention due to an increase in steroid hormone activity in the later part of the cycle.

The osteopathic physician has a unique position in the diagnosis and treatment of menstrual disorders. There may be musculoskeletal changes suggestive of dysfunction of pelvic viscera. According to Burns, "Sensory impulses from injured or diseased viscera are recognized to cause reflex contraction of skeletal muscles. Any stimulation of the somatic sensory nerves may affect the skeletal muscles, the visceral muscles, the blood vessels, and the glands which receive innervation from the same cord level either directly or via the sympathetic ganglia."

In those segments of the cord supplying innervation to somatic structures that have shown altered mobility and palpable changes in texture, a lower reflex threshold exists that is called facilitation. These areas require minimum stimulation to sustain neuronal activity. The muscles innervated by these facilitated motoneuron pools are in contraction when their counterparts in other segments are at rest, and they continue to contract long after the physiologic demand has passed (Korr, 1974).

The response to treatment and progress can be noted on palpation of the somatic tissues whose innervation is the same as those of the female pelvic viscera. This flows from the sympathetic nerves at the level of the thoracic segments ten, eleven, twelve, and first and second lumbar segments, carrying most of the sensory fibers for the uterus. The parasympathetic supply is through the pelvic nerve from the level of S2 and S3. Synapses with neurons of the spinothalamic tract send impulses to higher centers of pain in the brain.

One aspect of the monthly cycle is the release of an ovum. Another is preparation of the endometrium of the uterus for implantation, if the ovum becomes fertilized. These processes are dependent on gonadotropic hormones, which are released from the pituitary gland starting at about age eight. The monthly sexual cycle begins between the ages of 11 and 14 years. The gonadotropins are controlled by follicle stimulating hormone (FSH), leuteinizing hormone (LH), and luteotropic inhibiting factor (LTH) of the pituitary. These regulate estrogen and progesterone activity, controlling the menstrual cycle.

Causes of Dysmenorrhea

The predisposing causes are varied and include the following:

1. An imbalance in the estrogen-progesterone ratio.
2. With endometrial changes, after regression of the corpus luteum, there may be endometrial fragments behaving as foreign bodies with resultant colicky contractions.
3. If hyperplasia exists, fibrous tissue may decrease contractions, causing venous stasis with nerve irritation. Infantile uterus with partial obliteration of the cervical canal may be the cause.
4. Positional changes of the uterus, especially anteflexion.
5. Fear and anxiety regarding menstruation.
6. Faulty posture, sedentary habits, or poor muscle tone, leading to weakness of uterine support.
7. Autonomic imbalance, resulting from musculoskeletal abnormalities, can increase irritability of the uterus, causing pain. The peak of each contraction coincides with the greatest degree of discomfort.

Diagnosis

There is usually a history of progressive menstrual pain with onset at or near menarche, with no pelvic abnormality. Pain usually starts shortly before the appearance of flow and peaks within 24 hours. Occasionally, premenstrual pain subsides with inauguration of the flow. Pain is colicky and intermittent and may be concentrated in the lower abdomen, back, or umbilical region or radiate down the legs. There is a vagus–pelvic nerve connection that may express itself in nausea.

Structural examination may disclose an abnormality in the area of the tenth thoracic vertebra down through the second lumbar vertebra. Stress in this area may be palpated in myofascial tissues.

Manipulative Treatment

The osteopathic approach emphasizes two fundamental principles: The dependence of health on structural integrity, and the ability of the body to heal itself.

To explain the trophic influence of nerves on the organs and tissues supplied by them, Korr reported, "Our research clearly implicates certain proteins which are synthesized in the peripheral nerve cells . . . and are transported down the length of the axon into the tissue cells. Protein synthesis may be altered by mechanical stress affecting tissues and organs with which they are neurologically related. The osteopathic philosophy contends that the body has all the elements for adaptation and compensation."

The whole patient must be appraised in examining the musculoskeletal system. Changes cannot occur in one organ or tissue without affecting others through communication of the visceral and somatic systems. Osteopathic treatment is directed toward normalization of musculoskeletal function and restoration of normal physiology through reflex mechanisms.

Dysmenorrhea can be favorably affected by manipulative treatment directed to the levels of T10 through L2 and the sacral areas. Hormonal imbalance may be influenced favorably by correction of the thoracic abnormalities as well. Postganglionic sympathetic fibers rise in the superior cervical ganglia, following the internal carotid vessels to the adenohypophysis. The adrenal gland function can be altered by abnormal vasomotor efferents in the lower thoracic spine, disturbing the balance of this gland with the hypothalamus and pituitary glands.

The round ligaments pass forward and outward through the internal abdominal ring and along the inguinal canal. Steady pressure on tissues overlying the pubic symphysis area may give marked relief.

Leg length differences cause muscle spasm of lumbar paravertebral tissues. By placing a lift under the heel of the short leg, the weight-bearing point is shifted, relieving the muscle spasm.

Normalizing treatment in the thoracic and lumbar areas affects the sympathetic outflow involving the uterus. Treatment should be directed toward release of spasm and to spinal articular mobility, including the articulations of the pelvis.

The lymphatic pump improves blood and lymph circulation, moving the endometrial debris through these elements, when that is one of the causes of dysmenorrhea.

McCole uses rapid percussion at the thoracolumbar junction to relieve menstrual cramps. Bimanual correction of uterine displacement should

Figure 29-11. Sacral pressure for the relief of dysmenorrhea.

Figure 29-12. Deep inhibiting pressure on tissues overlying the pubic symphysis.

Figure 29-13. Self-treatment by sacral pressure using a book.

Figure 29-14. Increasing sacral pressure by flexing legs on trunk.

be carried out when indicated. Inhibitory pressure over lower thoracic, lumbar, and sacral vertebral structures may be used to quiet uterine contractions at the height of painful menstruation. With the patient prone, the physician maintains deep steady pressure on the sacrum until the contractions are released (Fig. 29-11). Pressure on the syphysis pubis with patient supine may relieve lower abdominal and lumbar discomfort (Fig. 29-12). To maintain sacral pressure, the supine patient may place a book under her sacrum (Figs. 29-13 and 29-14).

Accepted treatment for dysmenorrhea includes mental and physical rest, exercise, and appropriate management of thyroid imbalance if present. Estrogen and progesterone are used, as are certain surgical procedures at times. An oral contraceptive regimen has had some success, but because of its influence on other organ systems of the body it has certain inherent dangers. Antispasmodics, muscle relaxants, mood elevating drugs, diuretics, and analgesics are frequently used. There has been a fair degree of success in the use of the nonsteroidal anti-inflammatory drugs in the treatment of dysmenorrhea. Various conventional medical measures have been hopefully advanced and reluctantly discarded.

Manipulative techniques, exercise, and attention to disparity of leg length may offer relief of dysmenorrhea without the dangers of some surgical and medical measures used in orthodox medicine. The osteopathic concept that a healthy body has the ability through reflex mechanisms that are causing pain, to restore normal function has particular application to the treatment of dysmenorrhea.

THE OBSTETRIC PATIENT
Mary E. Hitchcock

Osteopathic care throughout pregnancy provides the woman with the special benefit of adjusting the functions of her body to the demands of a progressing pregnancy. Seemingly minor problems, especially those in the back, may be the beginning of a lifetime of musculoskeletal difficulties.

The pelvis is the foundation upon which the entire spinal column is balanced. Forward tilting of the pelvis occurs in pregnancy, with a resulting increased lumbar lordosis as a counterbalance. This may lead to acute or chronic backache. Lordosis is commonly more marked in women than men, and obesity and a growing fetus compound the curve (Fig. 29-11). Alterations in posture affect ligamentous and disk structures of the spinal column, necessitating excessive muscle strain to maintain proper balance. As the uterus enlarges, the abdominal musculature becomes distended, losing tonicity.

Anatomy

The body is designed to resist gravity through a main center of gravity and two subsidiary centers (Fig. 29-12). The main center is at the lumbosacral area, the others are at the dorsolumbar and cervicodorsal crossover points. These three points are responsible for anteroposterior balance with the center of gravity and for this reason are subject to greater stress than other spinal areas.

Stretching and pulling of the abdominal muscles and their fascia results in depression of the anterior thorax. This is compensated for by an increase in anteroposterior and transverse dimensions of the chest. The position of the heart changes, and respiratory and circulatory functions are changed. These alterations may lead to constipation, edema of the lower extremities, and backache.

At the thoracolumbar junction, the dorsal vertebrae bear almost as much weight as the vertebrae of the lumbar area, yet they are smaller and weaker. In addition, the transverse processes of the thoracic area are smaller than those below. The longer lumbar transverse processes, together with the iliac crests and the ribs above them, pro-

Figure 29-15. Pregnancy increases the curvature of the spine, especially the lumbar lordosis.

vide powerful leverage to muscles that move the thoracolumbar region. Because this area is located approximately at the middle of the spine, greater leverage can be brought to bear against it than anywhere else in the spine.

The lumbosacral joint, the main center of gravity, is another region of sharp transition that is subjected to increased strain because it lies between the mobile lumbar spine and the rigid sacrum. The key muscle for erect posture is the iliopsoas. It is capable of exerting tremendous

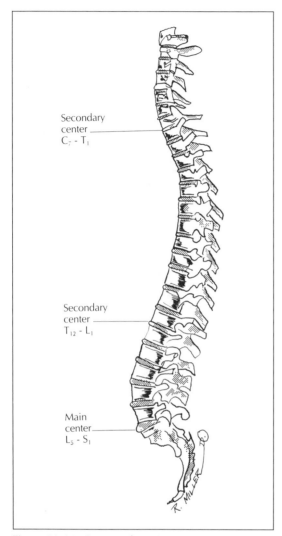

Secondary
center
C_7 - T_1

Secondary
center
T_{12} - L_1

Main
center
L_5 - S_1

Figure 29-16. Centers of gravity.

force. The iliopsoas is worthy of special mention in the approach to back pain in pregnancy. Its point of origin on the lumbar vertebra is close to the axis of flexion and extension of the lumbar spine. It is called on to compensate for imbalance between anterior abdominal muscles and posterior spinal muscles in stabilizing the lumbar portion of the spine. The psoas is important in maintaining the fetus in the upper abdomen; equally important is relaxation of this muscle at term, permitting engagement of the fetus in the true pelvis.

Thus, corrective manipulation of spinal struc-

tures that control and maintain the pelvic tilt is important in the management of pregnancy. Although lumbar and sacral backaches are the most common musculoskeletal complaints of pregnancy, the thoracic spine and the cervical spine are also frequent areas of involvement. Rib cage pain, upper and mid-thoracic fatigue, and discomfort result from the stooped posture and slouching shoulders caused by the enlarging breasts and the compensatory increased thoracic kyphosis.

Cervical spine symptoms are less frequent, but chronic neck fatigue involving the trapezius and upper back muscles occurs with the compensatory cervical lordosis necessary for maintaining the head in the erect position.

Coccygodynia may be encountered as a result of altered posture, or because in the seated position the added weight placed on the coccyx strains the sacrococcygeal joint. This may be due to too little natural cushioning or because the lower coccygeal segment is prominent or straight.

During delivery the hip, pelvic, and abdominal musculature undergoes maximum physical strain, with resulting stress on the back, pelvic, and sacroiliac ligaments. The lithotomy position places additional strain on pelvic ligaments. Coupled with an increase in intraabdominal pressure, stresses are placed on structures of the lumbosacral area.

Using manipulative treatment, the osteopathic physician has the opportunity to normalize the spinal complex and thus influence homeostasis, which may have been altered through abnormal vasomotor reflexes resulting from autonomic imbalance and impaired respiration. Lymphatic flow is aided by affecting lymphatic channels through intermittent force on the chest wall, using the thoracoabdominal lymph pump, or by the action of body musculature, produced through force against the plantar surfaces of the feet, using the Dalrymple technique.

Sympathetic innervation to the female pelvic structures is derived from nerves at the spinal levels of T10–T12 and L1–L2. Parasympathetic innervation arises from S2–S4 over the pelvic nerve (Fig. 29-17).

Traditionally, treatment has been limited to soft tissue relaxation with correction of isolated somatic dysfunctions. Emphasis should be placed on relief of gravitational strain, improving respiration, and facilitation of drainage of blood and lymph.

Figure 29-17. Sympathetic and parasympathetic innervation of the female pelvis.

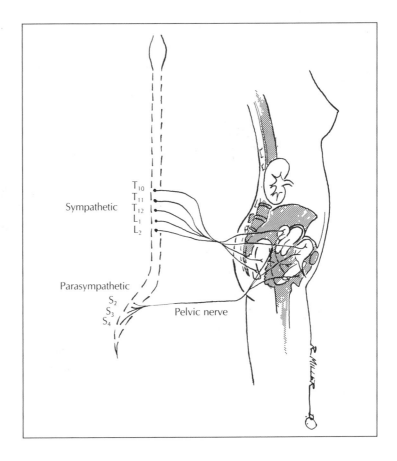

Sympathetic

T₁₀
T₁₁
T₁₂
L₁
L₂

Parasympathetic

S₂
S₃
S₄

Pelvic nerve

Treatment

Sacral rocking may be used to release sacral restrictions, both before delivery and during early delivery (Fig. 29-18). Lumbar counterpressure can be used during contractions, up to 7 or 8 cm of cervical dilation (Fig. 29-19).

After delivery, the woman's legs are removed from the stirrups and her hips are put through adduction, internal rotation, and extension, in that order (Figs. 29-20 and 29-21). This prevents sacroiliac dysfunction, which may result from the increased elasticity of pelvic ligaments under strain.

Manipulation is also used postpartum as early as four or five hours after a caesarean section, and then three times a day, to alleviate hyperextension of the lumbar spine.

EXCEPTIONS TO MANIPULATION

There are few exceptions to the use of manipulation during pregnancy, but these exceptions are extremely important.

1. Do not treat during premature labor. Stimulation of spinal nerves may be sufficient to continue a labor that might have been stopped by complete rest.

2. Do not treat in the presence of abruptio placentae. This occurs after the 20th week of gestation and most commonly in the last 10 weeks of pregnancy. Any detachment earlier in pregnancy is regarded as abortion. When symptoms of shock or changes in fetal activity and heart sounds occur, placenta previa should be suspected.

3. Do not treat if membranes rupture without labor. Without amniotic fluid protection, the fetus is vulnerable to outside trauma.

4. Ectopic pregnancy requires surgery. The treatment is preparation for surgery as early as possible.

Figure 29-18. Sacral rocking on obstetric patient.

Figure 29-19. Lumbar counterpressure.

Figure 29-20. Adduction and internal rotation of the hips.

Figure 29-21. Adduction, internal rotation, and extension of the hips.

Osteopathic manipulative treatment is complementary to classes in preparation for natural childbirth if these methods are desired. It is concerned with strengthening the musculoskeletal system by preventing back problems, strengthening weakened abdominal muscles, improving diminished respiratory function and stasis of the venous circulation, and edema of the lower extremities, all of which may occur in pregnancy, whatever the birth method.

Too often, little thought is given to the mother after delivery. Cumulative strain on low back structures may manifest in the postpartum period. There is a sudden return toward the normal curve of the spine, but muscle tone and ligamentous strains are slower to readjust to the stooping, bending, and lifting necessary in caring for the child. This can result in low back dysfunction.

Exercises

A well-designed postpartum regimen should be instituted before discharge, with three to six months of gradual exercise designed to hasten return of muscle power and prevent ligament and disk disability. Along with manipulation, exercise can do much to mitigate postpartum musculoskeletal problems. Exercises are designed primarily to improve circulation and restoring muscle tone and are used in conjunction with postural reeducation. Simple bed exercises may begin shortly after delivery.

A few hours after delivery, the patient is instructed to pull her shoulders together, attempting to approximate the scapulae. This produces motion of the chest cage and can be done with the patient sitting in bed (Fig. 29-22). The next day the woman lies in bed with her knees bent and

Figure 29-22. Approximation of the scapulae.

Figure 29-23. Tilting the pelvis posteriorly by flattening the lumbar lordosis.

raises the buttocks an inch or so, pressing the lumbar area against the bed and thus tilting the pelvis (Fig. 29-23). In about one week she may stand with legs apart and twist her trunk from right to left and back about 10 times (Fig. 29-24). In the same position, she may bend the trunk sideways, then forward, repeating 10 times (Figs. 29-25 and 29-26).

Two weeks after delivery, the woman continues exercises while lying on the floor. Her legs should be straight and her arms out to the side. She reaches with one knee to the opposite arm, returns, and does the same with the other arm and knee (Fig. 29-27). All exercises should be repeated 10 times.

A useful exercise is psoas stretching. When the iliopsoas is severely contracted, an initial stretching exercise is suggested. The unaffected leg is placed at a height of two to two and one-half feet from the floor, on a chair or stool. The affected leg is stretched about three feet behind in neutral rotation attitude. With continual exercise, the foot is gradually rotated internally. The woman applies pressure over the affected buttock, exercising full body weight at the level of the compromised hip (Fig. 29-28). When the contraction allows, this may be done without using a chair or stool.

A second, passive exercise is to lie supine on a rolled-up towel that has been placed at the dor-

Figure 29-24. Trunk twists.

Figure 29-25. Bending the trunk sideways.

Figure 29-26. Forward bending of the trunk.

Figure 29-27. Trunk twists while lying on the floor.

Figure 29-28. Iliopsoas stretch.

solumbar junction. This should relieve the flexion stress accumulated during the day, because most activity involves flexion of the spine.

Leg raising with the legs not more than 6 inches from the floor will strengthen abdominal muscles (Fig. 29-29). If the legs are raised higher it involves the psoas in flexion, which is not desirable in some low back problems.

An attempt should be made to produce motion in spinal segmental areas where there is limitation of motion, within the physiologic parameters of that segment, and thus help restore normal feedback to the central nervous system.

Figure 29-29. Strengthening the abdominal muscles.

Summary

With few exceptions, manipulative treatment during pregnancy differs little from that given to patients with similar musculoskeletal problems. In early pregnancy the woman will experience no difficulty in being positioned for treatment of any kind, but with an increase in the size of the fetus, techniques requiring the prone position must be altered. The patient may be treated in either the lateral recumbent position or by using seated muscle energy techniques.

THE PULMONARY PATIENT

Eileen L. DiGiovanna

Treating the pulmonary patient, particularly one with chronic disease, is a challenge to the physician. Utilization of osteopathic manipulation adds a dimension to the care of patients with respiratory problems.

Pulmonary conditions may be divided into the acute, infectious type and the chronic, progressive type. Acute pulmonary diseases include the various pneumonias and infectious bronchitis. These are of rather sudden onset and are bacterial or viral in etiology. Chronic pulmonary diseases are frequently gradual in onset and slowly progressive. Although persons with these conditions are susceptible to secondary infections, the primary cause is seldom of an infectious nature. Included are asthma and chronic obstructive pulmonary diseases (COPDs) such as chronic bronchitis and emphysema.

Other pulmonary conditions, such as lung cancer, pulmonary embolus, and tuberculosis, are less likely to respond with manipulation, although it may prove a valuable adjunctive treatment.

Somatic Diagnosis of Pulmonary Diseases

Osteopathic somatic dysfunction diagnosis may be a valuable tool in identifying the presence of pulmonary pathology. Numerous studies have been done over the years to find the best somatic predictors of respiratory disease. Myron Beal reviewed many previous studies as well as reporting one of his own. The most consistent findings were at T2–T7, with significant representation at C2–C3. Beal found somatic dysfunction of two or more adjacent vertebrae in this region, deep muscle splinting, and resistance to compressive springing of the involved area. These areas represent viscerosomatic reflexes from the lung to the soma.

When evaluating the pulmonary patient, it is also important to evaluate all components involved in respiration, including rib motion, ability of the spine to straighten during inspiration, diaphragmatic motion, and accessory muscles of respiration such as the scalenes, sternocleidomastoids, and abdominal muscles.

The physician should keep in mind that there is more involved in respiration than just thoracic cage motion. For tissues to be healthy, they require the following:

1. Good arterial supply
2. Motor and sensory impulses
3. Trophins
4. Adequate biochemical environment
5. Venous and lymphatic return

Each of these needs to be evaluated and addressed.

Entities

BRONCHITIS AND PNEUMONIA

Although the causes and manifestations may differ, the goals of therapy are relatively the same in any of these conditions:

1. To improve lymphatic and venous flow
2. To improve arterial circulation to carry immune system products to the lungs
3. To ease removal of accumulated bronchial secretions and phlegm
4. To decrease the workload of breathing

Osteopathic manipulation should address these goals to assist the body's fight against infection.

Various forms of lymphatic pump or thoracic pump will aid in improving venous and lymphatic flow as well as favorably affecting arterial circulation. Rib raising techniques may be used to free bronchial secretions so they may be more easily expectorated. The workload of breathing may be decreased by improving the compliance of the thorax — that is, by freeing the ribs, vertebrae, clavicles, and sternum to restore the intrinsic elastic forces in the thorax.

BRONCHIAL ASTHMA

Asthma represents a group of symptoms of various causes. The lungs of asthmatics are highly sensitized and react to such varied stimuli as allergens, irritants, emotion, and exercise. Whatever the trigger, the allergic attack is manifested through spasm of the bronchioles, edema of the mucous membrane, and increased production of thick, tenacious mucus. These three incidences create difficulty in emptying air out of the alveoli, with resultant dyspnea and a wheezing sound on expiration.

In managing an acute attack of asthma, it is essential to address the patient's immediate needs first. Medications such as epinephrine should be given. Then, as breathing quiets, rib raising is useful in easing the patient's respiratory efforts and in loosening mucous plugs.

Between acute attacks, it is important to treat all components of the respiratory system. In particular, all viscerosomatic reflex areas should be treated to prevent possible abnormal sympathetic feedback to the lungs. Possible increased vagal involvement may be treated by freeing the occipitoatlantal area.

Because of the emotional involvement in asthma

as an etiologic factor and the fear elicited by the dyspnea, the very act of placing the hands on the patient will have beneficial effects and serve to calm him as you treat. This alone can be a significant therapeutic factor.

CHRONIC OBSTRUCTIVE PULMONARY DISEASE

As a result of cigarette smoking and pollution, COPD has become a major cause of pulmonary illness in the world today. It is of insidious onset and is devastating to its victims. Dyspnea may become quite significant. As dyspnea increases, physical activity is curtailed. Chronic bronchitis produces large amounts of thick mucus, emphysema produces lesser amounts.

Musculoskeletal changes occur during the course of the disease. The chest assumes a barrel shape in which the AP diameter equals the transverse diameter. The accessory muscles of respiration gradually hypertrophy. Hypertrophied scalene muscles may cause neurovascular compression at the scalene triangle. Rib motion is markedly restricted and eventually contributes to the dyspnea. The thoracic spine becomes kyphotic and immobile. Motion of the diaphragm is restricted.

Osteopathic manipulation contributes to the overall well-being of the patient, even though the basic pathophysiology may not be reversible. The thoracic spine is treated to restore mobility and to address the viscerosomatic reflex changes in the upper thoracic spine. Rib motion may be improved with muscle energy techniques. It may be well to avoid thrusting techniques, as many COPD patients require corticosteroids, which may lead to osteoporosis. Rib raising techniques are helpful. Fascial release of the diaphragm should be done. Thoracic pumping will improve lymphatic flow and the expectoration of tenacious mucus.

The cervical area should be treated, with attention given to the accessory respiratory muscles. The clavicles should be freed and any sternal restrictions treated.

Upper extremity motion restriction may be found in chronic lung disease. Sternal release and Spencer techniques may be used to improve this.

After osteopathic manipulation, COPD patients frequently report a subjective increase in their sense of well-being. They experience less effort breathing and improved physical functioning.

Because of the relationship of the musculoskeletal system to the respiratory system, the osteopathic physician must evaluate all components of each system when diagnosing and treating the pulmonary patient.

THE CARDIAC PATIENT
Dennis Cardone

The comprehensive approach of osteopathic medicine is particularly applicable to the cardiac patient. For many years osteopathic physicians have observed an interrelationship between visceral and somatic disturbances. This interrelationship can be applied to heart disease. A palpable somatic dysfunction might suggest the presence or impending development of heart disease. Furthermore, correlating the somatic component with a specific cardiac abnormality might be valuable in assessing the efficacy of treatment by taking the rate of disappearance of the somatic component as a reflection of improved cardiac physiology.

Anatomy and Physiology

The nerve supply to the heart comprises both sympathetic and parasympathetic fibers. Preganglionic sympathetic efferents arise from the upper five thoracic segments of the spinal cord. Parasympathetic innervation is via branches of the right and left vagus nerve.

Visceral afferents from the heart terminate in the upper five thoracic segments of the spinal cord. These are the same cord segments that give rise to preganglionic sympathetic efferents and segmentally related somatic spinal nerves.

A reflex pathway is established between somatic tissue and the involved viscus. Theoretically, a somatic dysfunction may produce and maintain a visceral dysfunction, and a visceral dysfunction may produce and maintain a somatic dysfunction.

Evaluation

Studies have shown a causal relationship between heart disease and specific somatic dysfunctions. An increased incidence of distinctive, segmental patterns of somatic dysfunction has been demonstrated in patients with heart disease. The spinal segments most frequently involved are T1–T5 on the left. The somatic changes involve the skin, subcutaneous tissue, and muscle. The palpable changes can include increased firmness, increased skin drag, warmth, ropiness, bogginess, edema, muscle hypertonicity, and decreased mobility.

The evaluation of the patient with a cardiac disorder includes a complete structural analysis, since specific levels of the spine are affected by distant segments. Special attention should be directed to the upper thoracic region.

The osteopathic physician must recognize and manage abnormal influences on the sympathetic and parasympathetic nervous systems, and remove the visceral portion of the reflex arc from the abnormal stimuli of the somatic spinal complex (osteopathic lesion). Manipulative treatment is aimed at correcting somatic dysfunctions.

Palpation of the precordium should be part of every physical examination. It should include palpation of the apex beat. Abnormal apex beats, determined by location, amplitude, duration, and components of the beat, are associated with specific disease states. Ectopic impulses, right ventricular impulses, palpable heart sounds, exaggerated precordial movements, thrills, and inward retractions of the precordium also alert the physician to cardiac abnormalities and aid in the diagnosis of heart disease.

The fingers are relatively insensitive to movements of the precordium. These movements are of large amplitude and low frequency (less than 5 Hz). Sensitivity is directly related to frequency. As the frequency increases, different neurons activated by changes in velocity enhance palpatory perception. In the normal apex beat, only the high frequency, early systolic portion is palpable. Precordial palpation, even with its limited sensitivity, is still a valuable part of the physical examination.

Structural changes can provide valuable clues to a variety of heart disease. Some of these structural changes are described below.

Coarctation of the aorta: greater muscular development of the upper extremities than the lower extremities.

Ventricular septal defect—Children: bilateral prominence of the anterior part of the chest with bulging of the upper two thirds of the sternum and an indrawing of the lower third.

Ventricular septal defect—Adults: unilateral bulge at the fourth and fifth intercostal spaces at the lower left sternal border.

Atrial septal defect: bulging in the area of the second and third intercostal spaces at the left sternal border.

Constrictive pericarditis or isolated tricuspid valve regurgitation: indrawing of the precordium during systole.

Structural changes: seen in diseases, other than heart disease, that are associated with secondary cardiac involvement.

The physician must be aware that not all painful somatic symptoms of the anterior chest wall are related to heart disease. In addition to the heart, chest pain may originate in the lungs or other organs of the chest, the upper abdominal viscera, or the musculoskeletal system, particularly the neck, thorax, and shoulders. Psychogenic disorders may also be associated with chest pain.

The correct diagnosis of chest pain can often be made following a detailed history and palpation of the anterior chest wall. Characteristics that help differentiate chest pain include duration, quality, intensity, location, precipitating factors, relieving factors, and the size of the area of discomfort. The severity of symptoms often does not coincide with the gravity of its cause. Musculoskeletal disorders are responsible for more cases of chest pain than are any other disease entities. Most of these disorders respond to osteopathic manipulative treatment.

Osteopathic manipulative treatment should be included in the possible prevention of and treatment of heart disease. It should be used in combination with pharmacotherapy or other therapeutic modalities when they are indicated.

References

WHIPLASH

Becker RE. 1958. Whiplash injuries. In: Yearbook of Selected Osteopathic Papers. Carmel, Calif: Academy of Applied Osteopathy, pp 65–68.

———. 1961. Whiplash injury. In: Yearbook of Selected Osteopathic Papers. Carmel, Calif: Academy of Applied Osteopathy, pp 90–98.

Cailliet R. 1981. Neck and Arm Pain. Philadelphia: F.A. Davis Co.

Harakal JH. 1975. An osteopathically integrated approach to the whiplash complex. J Am Osteopath Assoc 74:59–73.

Heilig D. 1963. Whiplash, mechanics of injury: Management of cervical and dorsal involvement. J Am Osteopath Assoc 63:52–59.

Lalli JJ. 1972. Cervical vertebral syndromes. J Am Osteopath Assoc 72:43–50.

Macnab MB. 1971. The whiplash syndrome. Orthop Clin North Am 2:389–403.

McKeever DC. 1960. The so-called whiplash injury. Orthopedics 2:14.

Mealy K, Brennan H, Fenelon GCC. 1986. Early mobilization of whiplash injuries. Br Med J 292:656–657.

HEADACHE

Friedman AP. 1979. Tice's Practice of Medicine. Vol X. Hagerstown, Pa: Harper & Row Publishers.

Guyton AC. 1981. Textbook of Medical Physiology. Philadelphia: W.B. Saunders Co.

Isselbacker KJ, et al. 1980. Harrison's Principles of Internal Medicine, 9th ed. New York: McGraw-Hill Book Co.

Jones LH. 1981. Strain and Counterstrain. Colorado Springs: American Academy of Osteopathy.

Magoun HI. 1951. Osteopathy in the Cranial Field. Kirksville, Mo: Journal Printing Co.

———. 1978. Practical Osteopathic Procedures. Kirksville, Mo: Journal Printing Co.

Upledger JE, Vredevoogd JD. 1983. Craniosacral Therapy. Seattle: Eastland Press.

Warwick R. 1973. Gray's Anatomy, 35th British ed. Philadelphia: W.B. Saunders Co.

Wyngaarden JB, ed. et al. 1982. Cecil Textbook of Medicine. Philadelphia: W.B. Saunders Co.

SCOLIOSIS

Arbuckle BE. 1970. Scoliosis capitis. Am Osteopath Assoc 70:131–137.

Ascani E, et al. 1986. Natural history of untreated idiopathic scoliosis after skeletal maturity. Spine 11:784–789.

Brookes HL, Bunnel WD, Mitchell FL. 1981. You can help patients with scoliosis. Patient Care 11:111–127.

Bunnel WD. 1986. The natural history of idiopathic scoliosis before skeletal maturity. Spine 11:773–776.

Fryette HH. 1978. Principles of Osteopathic Technique. Kirksville, Mo: Journal Printing Co.

Kahanovitz N, et al. 1986. Lateral electrical surface stimulation (TENS) compliance in adolescent female scoliosis patients. Spine 11:753–755.

Kein HA. 1972. Scoliosis. Ciba Found Symp 24:2–32.

Magoun HI. 1978. Practical Osteopathic Procedures. Kirksville, Mo: Journal Printing Co.

McCollough NC III. 1986. Nonoperative treatment of idiopathic scoliosis using surface electric stimulation. Spine 11:802–803.

Meranda JT. 1988. Evaluation and management of childhood scoliosis. Female Patient 13:49–60.

Ogilvie JW. 1984. Conservative management of childhood scoliosis. J Musculoskel Med 1:67–77.

Picault C, et al. 1986. Natural history of scolioses in girls and boys. Spine 11:777–778.

Roaf R. 1987. Posture. New York: Academic Press.

Schiowitz S, et al. 1983. Biomechanics of vertebral motion. In: An Osteopathic Approach to Diagnosis and Treatment. Old Westbury, N.Y.: New York College of Osteopathic Medicine.

Stiachano WF. 1953. Scoliosis. In: Yearbook of the American Academy of Osteopathy. Vol 52. pp 377–378.

Sullivan JA, et al. 1986. Further evaluation of the scolition treatment of idiopathic adolescent scoliosis. Spine 8:903–906.

Weinstein SL. 1986. Idiopathic scoliosis: Natural history. Spine 11:780–783.

THORACIC OUTLET SYNDROME

Cailliet R. 1977. Neck and Arm Pain, 2nd ed. Philadelphia: F.A. Davis.

Sheon RP, Moskowitz RW, Goldberg VM. 1982. Soft Tissue Rheumatic Pain: Recognition, Management, Prevention.

Turek SL. 1984. Orthopaedics: Principles and Their Application, 4th ed. Philadelphia: Lippincott.

Tyson RR, Kaplan AF. 1975. Modern concepts of diagnosis and treatment of thoracic outlet syndrome. Orthop Clin North Am 6(2).

LUMBAR RADICULOPATHIES

Arnoldi X, et al. 1976. Lumbar spinal stenosis and nerve root entrapment. Clin Orthop 115:4.

Bernard T, Kirkaldy-Willis WH. 1987. Recognizing specific characteristics of nonspecific back pain. Clin Orthop 217:266.

Cathie AG. 1974. American Academy of Osteopathy 1974 Year Book. Special manipulative procedures for the normalization of the L-S and S-1 areas. AAO Year Book 1974, pp 131–139.

Cathie A. 1950. Anatomical relationships of the sciatic nerve. Academy of Applied Osteopathy Year Book, pp 70–72.

————. Academy of Applied Osteopathy Yearbook 1952, Academy of Applied Osteopathy.

Chrisman D, et al. 1964. A study of the results following rotary manipulation in the lumbar intervertebral disc syndrome. J Bone Joint Surg [Am] 46:557–524.

Davis H. 1950. Technic for the removal of still lesions usually found in the S-1 area and associated low back conditions. Academy of Applied Osteopathy Year Book. Academy of Applied Osteopathy, pp 73–75.

Dooley JF, et al. 1988. Nerve root infiltration in the diagnosis of radicular pain. Spine 13:79–83.

Doran DML, Newell DJ. 1975. Manipulation in the treatment of low back pain: A multicenter study. Br Med J 2:161.

Dvorak J, Gauchat M-H, Valach L. 1988. The outcome of surgery for lumbar disc herniation: I. A 4–17 year follow-up with emphasis on somatic aspects. Spine 13:1418.

Eaton J. 1952. Differential diagnosis of low back syndrome. Academy of Applied Osteopathy Year Book. 1952. Academy of Applied Osteopathy, pp 79–85.

Frymoyer J. 1988. Back pain and sciatica: Medical progress. N Engl J Med 318:291.

Hadler N, et al. 1987. A benefit of spinal manipulation as adjunctive therapy for acute low back pain: A stratified controlled trial. Spine 12:703.

Haldeman S. 1983. Spinal manipulative therapy: Status report, Clin Orthop 179:62.

Helbig T, Lee C. 1988. Lumbar facet syndrome. Spine 13:61–64.

Hockburger R. 1986. The lowdown on low back pain. Emerg Med. 18:123.

Hoeler FK, Tobis JS, Buerger AA. 1981. Spinal manipulation for low back pain. JAMA 245:1835.

Jackson R, Jacobs R, Montesano P. 1988. Facet joint injection: A prospective, statistical study. Spine 13:966.

Johnson J, et al. 1988. Extraspinal pathology and incidental disc herniation in patients with sciatica. Spine 13:393.

Kirkaldy-Willis WH. 1981. Musculoskeletal disorders: A three-article symposium. Postgrad Med 70:166.

————. 1978. Five common back disorders. How to diagnose and treat them. Geriatrics. 33:32–41.

————, Hill RJ. 1987. A more precise diagnosis for low back pain. Spine 4:102.

————, McIvor G. 1976. Editorial: Lumbar spinal stenosis. Clin Orthop 115:2.

————, ed. 1988. Managing Low Back Pain, 2nd ed. Edinburgh: Churchill Livingstone.

Kosteljanetz M, et al. 1988. The clinical significance of straight leg raising (Lasegue's sign) in the diagnosis of prolapsed lumbar discs. Spine 13:393.

Kostiuk JP, et al. 1986. Cauda equina syndrome and lumbar disc herniation. J Bone Joint Surg [Am] 68:386.

Kuo PP-F, Loh Z-C. 1987. Treatment of lumbar intervertebral disc protrusions by manipulation. Clin Orthop 215:47.

Lee CK, Rauschning W, Glenn W. 1988. Lateral lumbar spinal canal stenosis: Classification, pathology, anatomy, and surgical decompression. Spine 13:313.

Levine RL, Schutta HS. 1987. Lumbo-sacral root syndromes. In Camins MB, O'Leary PF, eds. The Lumbar Spine. New York: Raven Press, pp 163–170.

Mensor MC. 1955. Non-operative treatment, including manipulation, for lumbar intervertebral disc syndrome. J Bone Joint Surg 1955;37-A:925.

Mooney V. 1983. Syndromes of low back disease. Orthop Clin North Am 14:505–515.

————, Robertson J. 1976. The facet syndrome. Clin Orthop 11:149.

Nakano K. 1987. Sciatic nerve entrapment: The piriformis syndrome. J Musculoskel Med 33.

Paris S. 1983. Spinal manipulative therapy. Clin Orthop 179:55.

Porter RW, Miller CG. 1988. Neurologic claudication and root claudication treated with calcitonin: A double blind trial. Spine 13:1061.

Selby DK. 1983. When to operate and what to operate on. Orthop Clin North Am 14:577.

Siehl D. 1967. Manipulation of the spine under general anesthesia. American Academy of Osteopathy Yearbook 1967. M. Barnes (ed.). Carmel: American Academy of Osteopathy. 147–151.

Simons P, Traudl J. 1983. Myofascial origins of low back pain: Parts 1–3. Postgrad Med 73:66.

Soliday H. 1978. Review of low back pain and treatment in general practice. Osteopath Med 2.

Spitzer W, LeBlanc F, Dupuis M. 1987. Scientific approach to the assessment and management of activity related spinal disorders: A monograph for clinicians. Spine (suppl), vol 12.

Steiner C. 1977. Ambulatory treatment of disc syndrome. J Am Osteopath Assoc 77:290–299.

————. 1987. Piriformis syndrome: Pathogenesis, diagnosis, and treatment. J Am Osteopath Assoc 87:318–323.

Weinstein X, et al. 1986. Lumbar disc herniation. J Bone Joint Surg [Am] 68:43.

Yong-Hing K, Kirkaldy-Willis WH. 1983. Pathophysiology of degenerative disease of the lumbar spine. Orthop Clin North Am 14:491.

SPONDYLOLISTHESIS AND SPONDYLOLYSIS

Dietrich M, Kurowski P. 1985. The importance of mechanical factor in the etiology of spondylolysis. Spine 10:532.

Farfan HF, Osteria V, Lamy C. 1976. The mechanical etiology of spondylolysis and spondylolisthesis. Clin Orthop Rel Res 117:40.

Fredrickson B, Mettolick W, Lusicky J. 1984. The natural history of spondylolysis and spondylolisthesis. J Bone Joint Surg [Am] 66(5):699.

Kirkaldy-Willis WH, ed. 1988. Managing Low Back Pain, 2nd ed. Edinburgh: Churchill Livingstone.

Lowe R, et al. 1976. Standing roentgenograms in spondylolisthesis. Clin Orthop Rel Res 117:80.

McGee D. 1987. Orthopedic Physical Assessment. Philadelphia: W.B. Saunders Co.

Mierau D, et al. 1987. A comparison of the effectiveness of spinal manipulative therapy for low back pain patients with and without spondylolisthesis. J Manip Phys Ther 10(2):49.

Rothman R, Simeone AF. 1982. The Spine, 2nd ed. Vol. 1. Philadelphia: W.B. Saunders Co, pp 263–284.

Soren A, Waugh T. 1985. Spondylolisthesis and related disorders: A correlative study of 105 patients. Clin Orthop Rel Res 193:171.

Turners R, Bianco A. 1971. Spondylolysis and spondylolisthesis in children and teen-agers. J Bone Joint Surg [Am] 53:1298.

Wiltze L, Newman P, McNab I. 1976. Classification of spondylolysis and spondylolisthesis. Clin Orthop Rel Res 117:23.

———, Winter R. 1983. Terminology and measurement of spondylolisthesis. J Bone Joint Surg [Am] 65(6):768.

COCCYGODYNIA

Barral JP, Mercier P. 1988. Visceral Manipulation. Seattle: Eastland Press.

Borgia CA. 1964. Coccydynia: Its diagnosis and treatment. Milit Med 335–338.

Dubrovsky B, et al. 1985. Spinal control of pelvic floor muscles. Exp Neurol 88:277–287.

Duncan GA. Painful coccyx. Arch Surg 1088–1104.

Edwards M. Trauma of the coccyx and coccygodynia. Am J Surg 42:591–594.

Karpinski MRK, Piggott H. 1985. Greater trochanteric pain syndrome. J Bone Joint Surg [Br] 67.

Llourie J, et al. 1985. Avascular necrosis of the coccyx: A cause of coccygodynia. Br J Clin Pract 247–248.

Nicosia JF, Abcarian H. 1985. Levator syndrome: A treatment that works. Dis Colon Rectum 28:406–408.

Postacchin F, Massobrio M, Marco. 1983. Idiopathic coccygodynia. J Bone Joint Surg [Am].

Sinaki M, et al. 1977. Tension myalgia of the pelvic floor. Mayo Clin Proc 52:717–722.

Stern FH. 1967. Coccygodynia among the geriatric population. J Am Geriatr Soc 15:100–102.

Thiele GH. 1937. Coccygodynia and pain in the superior gluteal region. JAMA 1271–1275.

Upledger JE, Vredevoogd JD. 1983. Craniosacral therapy. Seattle: Eastland.

Wilensky T. The levator ani, coccygeus and piriformis muscles. Am J Surg 59:44–49.

DYSMENORRHEA

Burns L. 1911. Studies in the Osteopathic Sciences. Vol. 2. The Nerve Centers. Cincinnati: Monfort & Co.

———, et al. 1917. A contribution to the study of the pathology of the vertebral lesion. Chicago: A.F. Still Research Institute, Bulletin 4.

Campbell EDM, Dickinson CJ, Slater JDH, eds. 1968. Clinical Physiology, ed 3. Philadelphia: F.A. Davis Co.

Guyton AC. 1966. Textbook of Medical Physiology, ed. 3. Philadelphia: W.B. Saunders Co.

Hoag JM. 1969. Concepts of osteopathic medicine. In Hoag JM, Cole WV, Bradford SG, eds. Osteopathic Medicine. New York: McGraw Hill Book Co.

Israel S. 1967. Diagnosis and Treatment of Menstrual Disorders and Sterility, ed. 5. New York: Harper & Row.

Korr IM. 1974. Research and practice a century later. Andrew Taylor Still Memorial Lecture. J Am Osteopath Assoc 73:362–369.

McCole GM. 1972. A Handbook of Osteopathic Guidelines for Student and Physician. American Academy of Osteopathy Yearbook 1972. Colorado Springs, Co: American Academy of Osteopathy. pp 27–154.

THE OBSTETRIC PATIENT

Delinger F. 1975. Osteopathic principles and practice. Philadelphia College of Osteopathic Medicine 00:000–000.

Kappler RE. 1973. Role of psoas mechanism in low-back complaints. J Am Osteopath Assoc 72:794–801.

Michele A-A. 1962. Iliopsoas: Development of Anomalies in Man. St. Louis: Charles C Thomas, Publisher.

Siehl D. 1972. Conservative treatment of the risk syndrome. J Am Osteopath Assoc 71:589–593.

THE PULMONARY PATIENT

Beal M, Morlock J. 1984. Somatic dysfunction associated with pulmonary disease. J Am Osteopath Assoc 84:179–183.

Greenman P. 1977. Manipulative therapy for the thoracic cage. Osteopath Ann 3:140–149.

Howell RK, Allen TW, Kappler RE. 1975. The influence of osteopathic manipulative therapy in the management of patients with chronic obstructive lung disease. J Am Osteopath Assoc 74:757–760.

Kline JA. 1959. An examination of the management of bronchial asthma. American Academy of Osteopathy Yearbook 1959. M. Barnes (Ed.). Carmel: American Academy of Osteopathy, pp 127–132.

Magoun HI. 1978. Practical Osteopathic Procedures. Kirksville, Mo: Journal Printing Co.

Stiles E. 1981. Manipulative management of chronic lung disease. Osteopath Ann 9:300–304.

Zink J. 1977. Respiratory and circulatory care: The conceptual model. Osteopath Ann 3:108–112.

THE CARDIAC PATIENT

Beal MC. 1983. Palpatory testing for somatic dysfunction in patients with cardiovascular disease. J Am Osteopath Assoc 82(11):73–82.

Hurst JW. 1986. The Heart, 6th ed. New York: McGraw-Hill Book Co.

Nicholas A. 1987. A somatic component to myocardial infarction. J Am Osteopath Assoc 87:62–68.

Miller WD. 1975. Functional aspects of coronary circulation.

Walton WJ. 1972. Textbook of Osteopathic Diagnosis and Technique Procedures, 2nd ed. St. Louis: Mattheues Book Co.

30

Alternative Modes of Treatment

TRIGGER POINT THERAPY
Joseph A. DiGiovanna

Trigger point therapy gained prominence as an important modality in treating myofascial pain in the 1960s. Although it had been a recognized type of therapy for many years, it was brought to the forefront by Janet Travell, who treated John F. Kennedy, the President of the United States. For years, Travell worked to document the existence of the myofascial trigger point. Although trigger points could be palpated and treated successfully, no scientific data were available. Eventually David Simons, Clinical Professor of Physical Medicine and Rehabilitation at the University of California, supplied much of the needed neurophysiologic information, and trigger point therapy became an accepted therapeutic modality. Travell and Simons cooperated, in writing a book on the diagnosis, treatment, and aftercare of patients with trigger points. *Myofascial Pain and Dysfunction: The Trigger Point Manual* was published in 1983.

What Is a Trigger Point?
A trigger point is best described as an area of hypersensitivity in a muscle from which impulses travel to the central nervous system, giving rise to referred pain. The area from which the pain arises is the *trigger point*. The area at which pain is noticed is the *reference point*. The reference point and the trigger point may be in the same area; however, in most instances the reference point is distant.

A trigger point may be latent or clinically active. A latent trigger point may exist for a long time without producing symptoms. It may become clinically active—symptomatic—if disturbed by any one of many factors, which will be described later. A clinically active trigger point has the capacity to refer pain.

In the examination of a clinically active trigger point, one or several of the following may be noted:

1. On palpation, a hard, usually rounded (although it may form various shapes) mass is felt. This area is sensitive or painful to the patient.
2. The clinician may feel a tremor or fasiculation under the palpating finger.
3. When pressure is applied to the trigger point, the patient may complain of pain not only under the palpating finger but at a distant area (reference area). Pain felt only at the reference area is an indication that a specific pathway exists. Therefore, before trigger point therapy is

started on any patient, the clinician should review the various pathways. If a patient complains of pain at a distant or reference area, the clinician will then be able to locate the trigger point.

Causes of Trigger Points

Causes of trigger points include the following:

1. Acute injury to tissue from a fall, an automobile accident, a strain, and so forth.
2. Excessive repetitive movements.
3. Another primary point, causing a secondary trigger point.
4. Nervous tension or stress.
5. A previously latent, asymptomatic trigger point that is activated by any of the above.
6. A preexisting Jones tender point. There is some question as to whether the Jones tender point is an early untreated trigger point. I feel that an untreated, longstanding tender point may undergo certain chronic changes, at which time it may be classified as a trigger point requiring intensive treatment. Studies done by Miehlke and reported by Travell and Simons indicate that the myofascial trigger point process begins as a neuromuscular dysfunction, but can evolve into a histologically demonstrable dystrophic phase. Miehlke's study related the clinical symptoms to the biopsy findings. It supported the fact that the initial dysfunctional phase, after a period of time, develops into the dystrophic phase.

Trigger points are not dependent on muscular activity to exist, as demonstrated by autopsy studies of trigger point tissue. Trigger points are true pathologic entities. Some of the changes noted in such tissues at autopsy were fatty infiltration, an increased number of nuclei, fibrosis, and serous exudates and mucopolysaccharide deposits.

Treatment

Several methods of therapy are presently being used by physicians. The specific method depends on several factors, including the duration of the trigger point, its location, the expertise of the physician, and the cooperation of the patient.

Travell used the spray and stretch technique

initially, first with ethyl chloride and subsequently with fluorimethane, which causes less freezing to the skin and is not flammable. Later she used injection therapy. At present, Travell often uses a combination of techniques. Hans Kraus, initially an advocate of injection therapy, often uses both modalities. Other types of modalities are transcutaneous electrical nerve stimulation, ultrasound, and electrical muscle stimulation. The use of fluorimethane and injection therapy is discussed in more detail.

FLUORIMETHANE

Fluorimethane is a vapocoolant spray that is applied in the following manner:

1. First the nozzle function is checked. When depressed, the nozzle should produce a direct stream that travels approximately three feet.
2. The skin is sprayed from the trigger point to the reference point, at a 45-degree angle, at a rate of 4 inches per second, in one direction only.
3. Three or four sweeps are made while the area being treated is simultaneously stretched gently. This process should be repeated three to four times. An effective method is to use passive stretching after the first series of sweeps, isometric resistant contractions after the second series of sweeps, and isokinetic resistant contractions after the third series of sweeps.
4. The treatment should not be rushed.
5. Myofascial treatment, muscle energy techniques, counterstrain treatment, high velocity techniques, fascial release, or facilitated positional release may be used as indicated.
6. The patient should be sent home with instructions for a series of gentle, progressive stretching exercises.
7. Follow-up treatment should be within a week or less.
8. The patient should be warned of a possible exacerbation of pain in the first 24 to 48 hours. If pain occurs, ice should be applied intermittently to the trigger point for the first 24 hours, followed by wet warm compresses for the next 24 hours. Analgesics may be given.

INJECTION THERAPY

Trigger points may be treated by direct injection of lidocaine. The size and length of the needle are determined by the site being injected. For a large muscle mass, such as in the hip, a 1½-inch, 22- or 23-gauge needle may be used. If the upper border of the trapezius or an intercostal muscle is to be injected, a ⅝-inch, 25-gauge needle is usually used. Care must be taken to avoid injecting into the lung.

Technique

Approximately 1½ to 3 ml of 1% lidocaine is injected into the trigger point and the four quadrants surrounding it in equal amounts. Always aspirate before injecting. Most patients will respond to the lidocaine; however, a short-acting steroid may be added. I usually use lidocaine alone for the first or second treatment. If the response is poor, a steroid may be added.

The patient should be warned of possible increased pain the following day, although in most cases there is improvement. If there is increased pain, ice should be applied intermittently for 24 hours, followed by moist heat for 24 hours. If the trigger point does not completely resolve, it may be reinjected in approximately one week.

The combination of fluorimethane spray and lidocaine injection may be used, although either may be used alone.

MECHANISM OF ACTION

Although the exact mechanism of action of trigger point therapy is not known, several theories have been proposed. At present, the theory of greatest acceptance hypothesizes interruption of the reflex arc by the action of the modality utilized. Afferent sensory nerve fibers travel from the muscle to the spinal cord. The fibers are classified as A fibers and C fibers. Stimulation of the A fibers, the large myelinated fibers, decreases pain. (These fibers respond to phasic stimulation.) Stimulation of the C fibers, the small unmyelinated fibers, results in increased pain, such as occurs when one burns his fingers. Efferent fibers return to the muscle from the cord. Interruption of the cycle either toward or away from the cord, i.e., either the afferent or the efferent fibers, breaks the pain cycle, and the pain is relieved. If the cause of the pain is not addressed, the pain cycle will most likely return, or a new pain cycle will be established.

A second theory suggests that trigger point treatment releases endorphins, which decrease the pain. Clinical experience indicates that one or more mechanisms of action are operative, because symptoms and pain are relieved when trigger points are appropriately treated.

ACUPUNCTURE*
Raymond Goldstein

Acupuncture originated in China about 4,000 to 5,000 years ago. The definitive treatise on Chinese Medicine is the *Nei Ching*, whose authorship is attributed to the Yellow Emperor and his physicians. It is written in the form of questions and answers and embraces, besides medicine and therapy, hygiene, pathology, physiology, politics, and economics.

The oldest records of acupuncture are found on bone etchings from about 1600 B.C. The first book of acupuncture, which contains a wealth of detail,

*This material is from a lecture outline by Raymond Goldstein, osteopathic physician and licensed acupuncturist, who studied Oriental medicine in the United States, Hong Kong, Japan, Korea, and Taiwan.

is the *Hungdi Neiging Suwen*, written about 200 B.C.

Acupuncture is not the exclusive possession of the Chinese. The Papyrus Ebers, an Egyptian medical treatise from 1550 B.C., refers to a book on the subject of vessels which could be the 12 meridians. The Bantu of South Africa scratched the surface of the body to cure certain diseases. In the treatment of sciatica, some Arabs cauterized a specific part of the ear with a hot metal probe (auriculotherapy, or ear acupuncture). A cannabalistic tribe in isolated areas of Brazil shot tiny arrows with a blow pipe at specific parts of the body. However, the Chinese are the only ones that have developed a fairly complete systematic method.

Two opposing philosophies of life were prevalent in China at the time of Confucius: a feudalistic philosophy, which resisted structural changes, and Taoism, a system of mysticism, magic, democratic ideas, and science mediating on the order of naturalism, a wholistic viewpoint.

Oriental medicine defines good health as a state of energy balance within the human body. The primary components of all physiologic activities, characterized quantitatively and qualitatively, are manifested in the polar forms of Yin and Yang (negative and positive). The undifferentiated basic state of energy with its great potential is Tao—the concept of the total, whole unit.

According to the *Nei Ching*, the universe is an oscillation of the forces of Yin and Yang and their changes. The universe is a macrocosm to Earth; the earth is a macrocosm to us, we are microcosms in a macrocosm. We are microcosms with 365 acupuncture points. Portions of the body also are microcosms. The ear lobe, the face, the scalp, each hand, and each foot are reflections of the body as a whole. Each unit has acupuncture points through which the whole body may be treated. For example, a fetus turned upside down is placed in concept over the ear lobe and its organ placement in the ear helps the prober find specific organs for needling. This is called auriculotherapy.

There is no absolute Yin or Yang. There is relativity and inseparability; there is a small portion of each within the other. Every Yang has a little Yin in it and every Yin has a little Yang in it.

Extrapolating from this energy thought, the Chinese conceived of Yin as negative, female, cold, dark, and passive, that which is deep or hidden, on the right side of the body, water, inhibiting, parasympathetic; and Yang as heat, active, male, on the surface of the body, fire, on the left side of the body, sympathetic, stimulating. The earth and moon are associated with Yin, the sun and sky with Yang.

The interaction of Yin and Yang energy circulating through the body activates specific organs and tissues. Any imbalance in the relative amounts of Yin and Yang was considered the root of all pathology.

The skin, the external side of the body, and the back were considered Yang; the internal side of the body and the ventral side was considered Yin.

The Chinese ideogram for energy is called CH'i and is a combination of two ideograms, the first for gas or oxygen, the second for rice or food. The combination of oxygen and food formed energy—no different from Western thought. Acceleration or deceleration in the flow of energy caused disease. When energy slows down it is damned up; and conversely, a speeding up of energy flow causes a later depletion. Imbalances in the rate of energy flow are corrected with accurate and precise needling.

The dynamic force of energy is constantly circulating through the body in 14 specific pathways called meridians. These meridians are not dissectable as a nerve fiber, yet they exist in the same anatomic relationship in all people regardless of size or shape. Along each meridian are specifically located acupuncture points at exact locations. The use of these points is exact and precise.

The meridians are vertically arranged and intercommunicate as a vast network, gathering the body into one functioning unit. They are distributed front and back, on the right and left sides, and internally and externally. Since the medial side of the body is considered Yin, there are three meridians on the medial side of the forearm designated as Yin meridians. The three lateral meridians are Yang meridians. The three Yin meridians of the hand travel from the chest to the hand and Yang meridians (three) travel from the hand to the head.

In the lower extremity there are again three Yin and three Yang meridians on the medial and lateral aspects. There are six meridians on each extremity, two exactly in the midline, front and back. The midline meridians have no connection with any of the organs. The one in the back is called the conception vessel. The rest of the meridians are coupled. They are as follows: lung with large intestine, heart with small intestine, stomach with spleen, bladder with kidney, heart constrictor with triple warmer, gallbladder with liver.

Solid organs are coupled with hollow organs. The solid organs are considered Yin and are centrally located in the body. Their functions are protective and are concerned with maintenance of body function and circulation. Examples of solid organs are the heart, liver, spleen, lung, kidney, and heart constrictor. The hollow organs are dorsally located. Their main function is to receive and digest food and to excrete wastes. The hollow organs comprise the stomach, gallbladder, small intestine, large intestine, bladder, and triple warmer.

It was believed that energy originated in the lung with the infant's first breath. This started its flow along a Yin meridian to the hands bilaterally, and then through its coupled meridian from the hand to the head along a Yang meridian, then along a Yin meridian from the head to the foot bilaterally again, then from the foot back to the lung along a Yang meridian. The completed 12-meridian pathway occurred within a period of 12 hours and therefore was a diurnal flow. The energy traversed an entire meridian before entering the next meridian, in this manner coursing through the entire 12 meridians.

On each meridian there are a number of points at which site needling is done. However, each meridian has connecting points to other meridians so that energy can jump out of circuit. There are specific alarm points on each meridian indicating that a specific organ is involved with disease. Reflex points indicate whether the energy is balanced on the meridian. Of course, there are forbidden points.

According to Chinese philosophical thought, the universe created itself but remained in a state of chaos. The abstract motivator *Tao* altered this macrocosmic chaos to one of balance and harmony by dividing it into positive and negative elements, Yin and Yang. This is the first principle of acupuncture. The human microcosm reflects the macrocosm.

CHAPMAN'S REFLEXES
Eileen L. DiGiovanna

Frank Chapman graduated from the American School of Osteopathy in 1897. In his practice he became aware of areas in the soft tissues of the body that were palpably different from the surrounding tissue. As various investigators have proposed reflex linkage of somatic structures with visceral structures, so Chapman believed his gangliaform contractures were neurolymphatic reflexes. Each reflex area seemed to be consistently related to a specific viscera. Particularly significant to Chapman was the interrelatedness with the endocrine system.

The reflex area can be palpated in the deep fascia at specific points on the anterior and posterior parts of the body. The areas feel tense and are about the size of a small bean. The patient describes tenderness as pressure is applied to the area.

Many osteopathic physicians find Chapman's reflexes of particular use in the differential diagnosis of visceral disease. By knowing the patterns of distribution of reflex areas they are able to relate the reflex area to a specific viscera. For example, reflex areas, along the lateral thigh are related to colon problems. The gallbladder produces a reflex in the forearm just below the elbow. Chapman and his successor, Charles Owens, believed these reflex areas lay in lymphoid tissues. A student, H.R. Small, who worked with Owens, reported, "In the intercostal space between the anterior and posterior fascia is located some lymphoid tissue. It is within this tissue that a Chapman's Reflex will be found."

Fred Mitchell describes the method of treatment in his foreword to Owen's book, *An Endocrine Interpretation of Chapman's Reflexes*. The pad of the finger is placed over the area to be treated, and "firm gentle contact is maintained and a rotary motion imparted to the finger through the arm and hand so as to express the fluid content of the locus into the surrounding tissues (i.e., dissipate the swelling)." Each reflex area involved with a particular viscus must be treated.

Today many physicians believe there is a relationship among trigger points, acupuncture points, Jones tender points, and Chapman's reflexes. Precisely what the relationship may be is unknown. George Northup states in an editorial, "One cannot escape the feeling that all of these seemingly diverse observations are but views of the same iceberg, the tip of which we are beginning to see without understanding either its magnitude or its depth of importance."

References

Gunn CC, Milbrandt WE. 1977. Tenderness at motor points: An aid in the diagnosis of pain in the shoulder referred from the cervical spine. J Am Osteopath Assoc 77:196–212.

Johnson DM. 1979. Time, gravity, and the motion barrier. Osteopath Ann 7(1):31–44.

Kraus H. 1970. Clinical Treatment of Back and Neck Pain. New York: McGraw-Hill Book Co.

Northup GW. 1977. Same subject—different views, (editorial). J Am Osteopath Assoc 77:288–289.

Northup TL. 1941. Role of the reflexes in manipulative therapy. J Am Osteopath Assoc 40:521–524.

Owens C. 1980. An Endocrine Interpretation of Chapman's Reflexes. American Academy of Osteopathy.

Reeves JL, Jaeger B, Poletti CE. 1984. Trigger points in headache. Aches Pains 5:22–25.

Travell JG, Simons DG. 1983. Myofascial Pain and Dysfunction: The Trigger Point Manual. Baltimore: Williams & Wilkins Co.

Index

ISBN 0-397-51001-2